Organ Transplantation: Current Clinical and Immunological Concepts

Organ Transplantation: Current Clinical and Immunological Concepts

Edited by

Leslie Brent and Robert A. Sells

Baillière Tindall

London Philadelphia Toronto Sydney Tokyo

This book is printed on acid free paper. ∞

Baillière Tindall 24–28 Oval Road
W. B. Saunders London NW1 7DX

The Curtis Center
Independence Square West
Philadelphia, PA 19106-3399

55 Horner Avenue
Toronto, Ontario M8Z 4X6, Canada

Pty Limited, 30–52 Smidmore St
Marrickville, NSW 2204, Australia

Harcourt Brace Jovanovich Japan Inc.
Ichibancho Central Building, 22–1 Ichibancho
Chiyoda-ku, Tokyo 102, Japan

First published 1989

British Library Cataloguing in Publication Data is available

ISBN 0-7020-1393-5

Filmset by Bath Typesetting Limited, Bath
and printed in Great Britain by Galliard (Printers) Ltd, Great Yarmouth, Norfolk

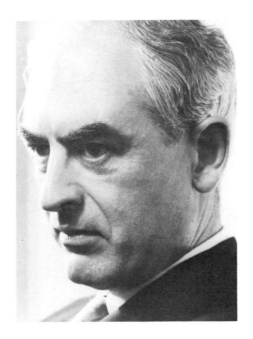

DEDICATION

We dedicate this volume to the memory of Peter Brian Medawar, whose manifold scientific contributions have led the way in establishing the science of transplantation immunology and cellular immunology.

L.B.
R.A.S.

Contents

Appendices

Contributors

W. J. Armitage Department of Ophthalmology, Bristol Eye Hospital, Lower Maudlin Street, Bristol BS1 2LX, UK.

B. A. Bradley United Kingdom Transplant Service, Southmead, Bristol, UK.

L. Brent BSc, PhD, FIBiol, Hon MRCP, Professor of Immunology, Department of Immunology, St Mary's Hospital Medical School, London W2 1PG, UK.

D. J. Cook PhD, Department of Surgery, PO Box 629, MCV Station, Medical College of Virginia, Richmond, VA 23298, USA.

A. B. Cosimi MD, FACS, Harvard Medical School; Transplant Unit of the General Surgical Service, Massachusetts General Hospital, Boston, MA 02114, USA.

T. de Witte Department of Haematology, University Hospital, Nijmegen, The Netherlands.

D. L. Easty MD, FRCS, Professor of Ophthalmology, Department of Ophthalmology, Bristol Eye Hospital, Lower Maudlin Street, Bristol BS1 2LX, UK.

J. W. Fabre MB, BS, B Med Sc, PhD, Director of Research, Blond McIndoe Centre, Queen Victoria Hospital, East Grinstead, Sussex RH19 3DZ, UK.

W. E. Fibbe Department of Paediatrics, University Medical Centre, PO Box 9600, 2300 RC Leiden, The Netherlands.

R. G. Gill Barbara Davis Center for Childhood Diabetes, 4200 East 9th Avenue, Box B140, Denver, CO 80262, USA.

J. M. Goldman Professor, Haematology Department, Royal Postgraduate Medical School; Honorary Consultant Physician, Hammersmith Hospital, Du Cane Road, London W12 0HS, UK.

E. C. Gordon-Smith MA, FRCPath, FRCP, Department of Haematology, St George's Hospital Medical School, Cranmer Terrace, Tooting, London SW17 0RE, UK.

S. M. Gore PhD, MRC Biostatics Unit, Hills Road, Cambridge CB2 2GH, UK.

B. D. Kahan PhD, MD, Professor of Surgery, The University of Texas, Medical School of Houston, Houston, TX 77030, USA.

J. W. Kupiec-Weglinski MD, PhD, Associate Professor of Surgery, Harvard Medical School, Department of Surgery, Brigham and Women's Hospital, 75 Francis Street, Boston, MA 02115, USA.

K. J. Lafferty PhD, Professor of Microbiology/Immunology, Barbara Davis Center for Childhood Diabetes, 4200 East 9th Avenue, Box B140, Denver, CO 80262, USA.

R. D. G. Leslie MD, FRCP, Consultant Physician, Charing Cross and Westminster Medical School, London SW1P 2AR, UK.

R. Y. Moore MD, PhD, Professor and Chairman, Department of Neurology HSC, State University of New York at Stony Brook, Stony Brook, NY 11794, USA.

P. J. Morris PhD, FRCS, FRACS, FACS (Hon.), Nuffield Professor of Surgery, Nuffield Department of Surgery, John Radcliffe Hospital, Oxford OX3 9DU, UK.

S. J. Moss Department of Ophthalmology, Bristol Eye Hospital, Lower Maudlin Street, Bristol BS1 2LX, UK.

K. C. Moudry-Munns RNC, CCRN, BSN, University of Minnesota Hospital and Clinic, 420 Delaware Street SE, Box 280, Minneapolis, MN 55455, USA.

G. Opelz MD, Professor of Immunology, Department of Transplantation Immunology, Institute of Immunology, University of Heidelberg, Im Neuenheimer Feld 305, D-6900 Heidelberg, FRG.

C. A. Rogers United Kingdom Transplant Service, Southmead, Bristol, UK.

K. Rolles MA, MS, FRCS, Consultant Surgeon, Royal Free Hospital and School of Medicine, Pond Street, London NW3, UK.

R. H. Rubin MD, Associate Professor of Medicine, Harvard Medical School; Chief of Infectious Disease for Transplantation, Massachusetts General Hospital, Boston, MA 02114, USA.

R. A. Sells FRCS, Director, Renal Transplant Unit, Royal Liverpool Hospital, Prescot Street, Liverpool L7 8XP, UK.

E. Simpson MA, Vet MB, Research Scientist with MRC, Section Head, Transplantation Biology Section, Clinical Research Centre, Watford Road, Harrow, Middlesex HA1 3UJ, UK.

R. Storb MD, Professor of Medicine, UW, Fred Hutchinson Cancer Research Center, 1124 Columbia Street, Seattle, WA 98104, USA.

T. B. Strom MD, Department of Medicine, Beth Israel Hospital and Harvard Medical School, Boston, MA 02215, USA.

K. M. Sullivan MD, Fred Hutchinson Cancer Research Center, 1124 Columbia Street, Seattle, WA 98104, USA.

D. E. R. Sutherland MD, PhD, Professor of Surgery, University of Minnesota Hospital and Clinics, 420 Delaware Street SE, Box 280, Minneapolis, MN 55455, USA.

P. I. Terasaki PhD, Professor of Surgery, UCLA School of Medicine, UCLA Tissue Typing Laboratory, 950 Veteran Avenue, Los Angeles, CA 90024, USA.

N. L. Tilney MD, Professor of Surgery, Harvard Medical School, Brigham and Women's Hospital, 75 Francis Street, Boston, MA 02115, USA.

A. Ting PhD, Nuffield Department of Surgery, John Radcliffe Hospital, Oxford OX3 9DU, UK.

J. M. J. J. Vossen Department of Paediatrics, University Medical Centre, PO Box 9600, 2300 RC Leiden, The Netherlands.

J. Wallwork BSc, MBChB, FRCS(E), MA, Consultant Cardiothoracic Surgeon, Papworth Hospital, Papworth Everard, Cambridge CB3 8RE, UK.

D. Weatherall MD, FRCP, FRS, Nuffield Professor of Clinical Medicine, University of Oxford; Nuffield Department of Clinical Medicine, John Radcliffe Hospital, Oxford OX3 9DU, UK.

A. J. Wing FRCP, Consultant Physician, St Thomas' Hospital, London SE1 7EH, UK.

F. E. Zwaan MD, PhD, Head, Bone Marrow Transplant Unit for Adults, University Medical Centre, PO Box 9600, 2300 RC Leiden, The Netherlands.

Preface

In considering the contents of this book we decided against a comprehensive approach to a topic that is not only vast but still developing. Although no doubt useful as reference texts, comprehensive tomes are usually well out of date by the time they are read. We have, instead, chosen those areas in the field of organ transplantation that are of the greatest importance, either because much has already been achieved or because they are vital growing points. Because organ transplantation is intimately, indeed inseparably, linked with the basic immunological, immunogenetic and pathological mechanisms that form the critical barrier to transplantation, we have included appropriate chapters dealing with these mechanisms. Only when these mechanisms are fully understood will it be possible to enter the promised land in which potentially harmful immunosuppressive drugs can at last be spurned.

This book is thus somewhat selective. We have been fortunate to gain the co-operation of a number of distinguished workers to whom we wish to express our appreciation for having written their chapters quickly and for accepting our rigorous editing with good grace. As a result this book is pretty well up to date and the reader will find numerous 1988 references in the bibliographies. It should also be eminently readable.

The book has several novel features. First, most illustrations have been redrawn by an artist and the volume derives a sense of unity and continuity from this. We are grateful to Mr J. Bridger-Chalker for his expert help. Second, Chapter 8 deals with several issues that are either controversial or relatively new. Third, the three appendices should be of considerable interest in that they provide clinical data in digestible form and, in the case of Appendix III, brief accounts (with full references) of the early history of the most important events in clinical transplantation and transplantation immunology.

We believe that this book will be of interest not only to those actively involved in clinical transplantation or in transplantation immunology, but to all – students as well as those well established in their fields – who wish to know about the state of the art and what the future holds. We hope that it will encourage physicians, surgeons and scientists to enter an area that is of great benefit to mankind and that offers formidable intellectual challenges and opportunities.

Endeavours in the field of organ transplantation have not only contributed to the solution of medical and surgical dilemmas, but have been a potent influence in the development of modern immunology. Although sometimes disputed (see, for example, the Panel Discussion, Sir Peter Medawar Memorial Symposium, *Immunology Letters* (1989), *21*, pp. 81–89) there can be little doubt that immunology has had – and will continue to have in even greater measure – an impact on organ transplantation; the reverse is equally true. This book therefore encapsulates this symbiotic relationship.

We thank our publishers for having succeeded in publishing this volume in a commendably short time, and our secretaries Ms M. Kelson and Ms A. Clarke for their invaluable help.

Leslie Brent
London

Robert A Sells
Liverpool

1 Major and Minor Histocompatibility Antigens

ALAN TING
ELIZABETH SIMPSON

The HLA system is the human major histocompatibility complex (MHC), and analogous complexes are found in all mammalian species. It is termed the MHC because it is the genetic system which encodes the expression of the most important cell surface antigens recognized as foreign on an allograft and towards which the host's rejection response is directed. Apart from their role in tissue and organ transplantation the HLA antigens are involved in numerous other vital functions such as cell co-operation in the initiation of the immune response, the destruction of virus-infected cells and in disease susceptibility. We will discuss the role of HLA antigens in transplantation and the part these molecules play in the recognition of minor histocompatibility and other antigens.

MAJOR HISTOCOMPATIBILITY ANTIGENS

Genetics and Structures of HLA Antigens

The genes which encode HLA antigens are located on the short arm of chromosome 6. Six loci can now be identified (Figure 1), their relative positions on the chromosome starting from the centromere being DP, DQ, DR, B, C and A. The antigens encoded by the A, B and C loci are referred to as class I antigens and those encoded by the DR, DQ and DP as class II antigens. Both class I and class II antigens are members of the Ig superfamily of molecules, which are transmembrane glycoproteins arranged as a series of domains at the exterior surface of the cell (see Figures 1 and 2 and the section on T cell responses to minor H antigens). Between the DR and B there are loci which code for the complement components Bf, C2, C4, and for the 21-hydroxylase enzyme. Well over a hundred HLA antigens can be detected, and this large number of alleles (listed in Table 1) makes the HLA system one of the most polymorphic systems found in man.

HLA antigens are inherited as co-dominant alleles. Recombination between the loci does occur and the frequency is about 1% between A and B, 0.8% between B and DR, and about 10% between DQ and DP. The abnormally high frequency of DQ–DP recombinants is thought to be due to a recombination 'hot spot', for the loci are known to be in close proximity in this area. Because the six loci are relatively closely linked they are usually inherited *en bloc* by the offspring from each parent. The HLA antigens encoded by the genes of one chromosome are termed an HLA haplotype and each individual therefore has two HLA haplotypes. If the paternal haplotypes are designated E and F and the maternal haplotypes G and H, then the four different HLA haplotype combinations (genotype) which can be found in the offspring are EG, EH, FG and FH. An understanding of the haplotype inheritance of HLA becomes important when we discuss the evidence showing that HLA is the human MHC.

Table 1.   Recognized HLA antigens. The 'w' prefix indicates that the antigen can be defined but its definition is not as clear as those without the 'w' prefix. The exception is the C locus antigens where the 'w' prefix is added to avoid confusion with the nomenclature of the complement components.

Locus	Antigens
A	1 2 3 9 10 11 w19 23 24 25 26 28 29 30 31 32 w33 w34 w36 w43 w66 w68 w69 w74
B	5 7 8 12 13 14 15 16 17 18 21 w22 27 35 37 38 39 40 w41 w42 44 45 w46 w47 w48 49 w50 51 w52 w53 w54 w55 w56 w57 w58 w59 w60 w61 w62 w63 w64 w65 w67 w70 w71 w72 w73 w75 w76 w4 w6
C	w1 w2 w3 w4 w5 w6 w7 w8 w9 w10 w11
DR	1 2 3 4 5 w6 7 w8 w9 w10 w11 w12 w13 w14 w15 w16 w17 w18 w52 w53
DQ	w1 w2 w3 w4 w5 w6 w7 w8 w9
DP	w1 w2 w3 w4 w5 w6

The class I antigens comprise two polypeptide chains, one with a molecular weight of 45 000 and the other 11 000. The latter is β_2 microglobulin; it is non-polymorphic and it is encoded by a gene on chromosome 15. The heavy chain is polymorphic, gives the 'antigen specificity', and is encoded by genes on chromosome 6. The class II antigens comprise two polypeptide chains; the α chain has a molecular weight of 33 000 and the β chain 28 000. Both molecules are encoded by genes on chromosome 6 (see Figure 1). Polymorphism is caused by amino acid differences in the outer domains of both class I (α_1 and α_2) and class II (α_1 and β_1) molecules (Bjorkman et al, 1987b and Figure 2b).

Detection of HLA Antigens

HLA antigens are conventionally detected by serological techniques using lymphocytes as the target cells. Peripheral blood lymphocytes or separated T lymphocytes are used for class I typing and B lymphocytes for class II typing, because DR and DQ antigens are found on B cells but not on resting T cells. The antibodies to these antigens may be found in the sera of repeatedly transfused patients and in multiparous women. It was the former source that provided Jean Dausset with antibodies for the detection of the first HLA antigen in 1958 (Dausset, 1958). At present most laboratories use the microdroplet lymphocyte cytotoxicity technique pioneered by Terasaki and McClelland (1964). In the last few years attention has focused on the production of monoclonal antibodies to HLA antigens by mouse hybridomas. Some useful HLA reagents have been found but the majority of the antibodies produced react with epitopes shared by a number of HLA

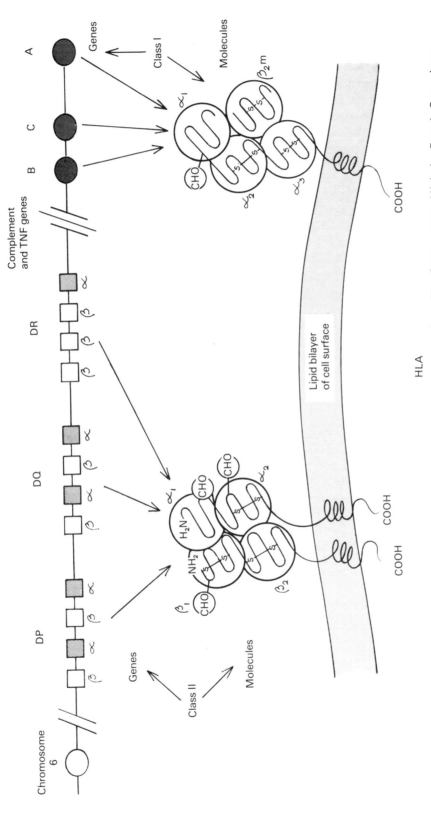

Figure 1. HLA Class I and Class II genes and their transmembrane glycoprotein products. The Class I genes, HLA-A, -B and -C are shown as shaded circles, Class II α chain genes as shaded squares, and Class II β chain genes as open squares. The Class I heavy chain glycoprotein product is shown as a transmembrane molecule with three domains, α_1, α_2 and α_3, associated with a single domain of β_2 microglobulin (β_2m), which is encoded by a gene on chromosome 15. The Class II α and β chains are shown as transmembrane heterodimers each with two domains, α_1 and α_2, β_1 and β_2.

antigens, and so are not useful for HLA typing although they are extremely valuable in biochemical studies. There is also considerable interest in the use of EBV-transformed human B lymphocytes for producing monoclonal antibodies and some useful HLA reagents have been made in this way.

HLA-DP products were first detected by primed lymphocyte testing (PLT; Shaw et al, 1980), and reliable alloantisera are still not available, although some mouse monoclonal antibodies that recognize epitopes common to more than one DP antigen have been produced.

Polymorphisms in HLA class II antigens can be detected at the DNA level using restriction enzymes and DNA probes specific for DR, DQ or DP α or β chain genes (Anderson et al, 1984). A number of enzymes have been used such as Eco R1, HIND III, Taql. The fragments of DNA produced after enzyme digestion are separated by size, using gel electrophoresis, and transferred to nylon or nitrocellulose filters. These filters are hybridized with radiolabelled probes, which adhere to the relevant bands. Using appropriate enzymes and probes, each DR, DQ and DP antigen gives a distinctive band pattern. Although this technique is extremely accurate it cannot be used for the selection of cadaver donors for transplantation as the technique takes at least 5 days to complete.

In the early 1960s it was shown that when the lymphocytes from two unrelated individuals were cultured together both sets would undergo blastogenesis (mixed lymphocyte culture, or MLC; Bach and Hirschhorn, 1964). The determinants responsible for this stimulation were subsequently called HLA-D determinants. They are found on B but not on T lymphocytes and the basis of HLA-D typing is the stimulation of T cells by B cells that are homozygous for a single D determinant, called homozygous typing cells (HTC). In culture, T cells that do not respond to a particular HTC must have the same D determinant as the HTC. Originally it was thought that these determinants (26 have been defined to date) were encoded by a distinct HLA locus but it is now widely accepted that D determinants represent combinations of DR and DQ antigens. The MLC test in vitro represents certain components of the in vivo allograft response.

The tissue distribution of class I and II antigens has been studied extensively, mainly with mouse monoclonal antibodies to monomorphic determinants of HLA (Daar et al, 1984a,b). Class I antigens have a wide distribution being found on almost all tissues; class II antigens on the other hand have a more restricted distribution, being mainly confined to endothelium and dendritic cells in most non-lymphoid tissues.

Evidence that HLA is the Human MHC

Most of the evidence that the HLA system is the human MHC comes from skin graft experiments, kidney transplants from living related donors and bone marrow transplants. Within a family the degree of histocompatibility among the members can be precisely determined, and siblings can share two (HLA identical), one (haploidentical) or no HLA haplotypes. Parents and each offspring share one haplotype and are therefore haploidentical. The most striking proof that HLA is the MHC comes from skin graft experiments in which the immune system of the recipient was not modified either by pretreatment with blood transfusions or by immunosuppression after transplantation. Thus, Ceppellini et al (1969) found that skin from HLA identical sibling donors had a mean survival time of 20 days, whereas haploidentical skin survived for a mean of 13.8 days and skin from siblings with no shared haplotype for only 12.5 days. The latter was similar to that observed with skin from totally unrelated donors (mean of 12.1 days). It was concluded that HLA is the only strong histocompatibility system in man: if this were not the case a quarter of the sibling grafts that were HLA mismatched would have been expected to show prolonged survival, on the assumption that an MHC other than HLA segregated as a single locus independently of HLA.

In living related donor (LRD) kidney transplants an excellent correlation between the number of shared haplotypes and graft outcome has been documented by a number of transplant centres. In patients treated post-transplantation with prednisolone and azathioprine the reported 1-year graft survival rate is 90–95% for HLA-identical siblings, 70–80% for haploidentical siblings and parents, and 60–70% when no haplotypes are shared. The results of haploidentical transplants can be markedly improved by pretreating the recipient with donor-specific blood transfusions, a protocol introduced by Salvatierra et al (1981). Furthermore, the use of cyclosporin has led to an increase in graft survival even in non-transfused patients. It is apparent, therefore, that the influence of HLA on kidney graft survival can be lessened by modifying the host's immune system but this does not mean that the HLA system is not of prime importance.

Until recently bone marrow transplants were almost always carried out between HLA-identical siblings, and identity was usually determined by serological typing and by the MLC test. This strict selection criterion has been used because early transplants with HLA-incompatible siblings either failed or led to severe, usually lethal, graft-versus-host disease (GVHD) (see Chapter 6).

Despite the importance of the HLA system in clinical transplantation it should be noted that even in HLA-identical sibling combinations skin grafts are still invariably rejected, 5–10% of kidney grafts are rejected by the end of the first year even though all patients are immunosuppressed, and bone marrow transplants can be both rejected and cause graft-versus-host disease. These data imply that other histocompatibility antigens must exist in man although, singly, their influence on graft compatibility is not as great as that of the HLA antigens, and they are therefore called minor histocompatibility antigens (see below).

HLA in Cadaveric Renal Transplantation

Based on the results of LRD transplants it is reasonable to expect high cadaver graft survival only in those matched for all HLA loci. This has been seen in some studies (e.g. Cicciarelli et al, 1987), but acceptably high success rates can be achieved with partial matching because there appears to be a gradation in the strength of the antigens encoded by the different loci. The DR antigens are the strongest transplantation antigens followed by B, A and then C. There are few data on DQ matching (although as mentioned above this system does play a role in the MLC reaction) and none on DP. It is fortunate that a high success rate can be achieved with partially-matched grafts because the extreme polymorphism of HLA alleles means that it is rare to find unrelated individuals who are completely HLA identical. Many transplant units match for only the DR antigens, although if a recipient is fortuitously matched for B and/or A antigens that patient will be preferred. Some transplant specialists question the practicability of HLA matching in cadaveric donor programmes and the longer waiting time this imposes, now that high graft survival rates can be achieved with pregraft blood transfusions and/or the use of cyclosporin as standard immunosuppression.

HLA Matching in Cyclosporin-treated Patients

The widespread use of cyclosporin in clinical transplantation has resulted in very high cadaveric graft survival rate, significantly higher than that seen with prednisolone and azathioprine. This has led to a number of transplant units declaring that HLA matching does not add anything to a survival rate that is already very high (e.g. Klintmalm et al, 1985; Taylor RJ et al, 1985). In addition, the sharing of kidneys among transplant units on the basis of HLA matching has dropped markedly in most national and regional organ exhange programmes. This has occurred despite many reports from both multicentre (e.g. Cats et al, 1984; Persijn et al, 1986) and single-centre (Joysey et al, 1985; Madsen et al, 1985) analyses showing that HLA matching, particularly for the DR and B loci antigens, is beneficial even in cyclosporin-treated patients. For example, results from the Collaborative Transplant Study (Opelz, 1987) in which over 10 000 cyclosporin-treated first cadaver transplants were analysed, indicate that those with no B + DR mismatches have a 17% higher 1 year survival rate than those with 4 B + DR mismatches ($p < 0.0001$).

Perhaps graft rejection is no longer the appropriate indicator when measuring the influence of an immunologically measured variable, for overall survival is very high. A more appropriate indicator may be the assessment of the quality of graft function as measured by parameters such as the number of rejection episodes suffered during the first 3 months, the serum creatinine at 3 months or 1 year, or the total amount of immunosuppression received during the first 3 months. In this context it is perhaps interesting to note that the original paper from the Scandinavian group (Lundgren et al, 1986), which cast doubt on the relevance of HLA matching in cyclosporin-treated patients, found a significant correlation between DR matching and the number of rejection episodes but not with eventual graft outcome. On the other hand, Kerman et al (1988) showed no correlation between HLA matching and survival rates, the incidence of rejection episodes, and the serum creatinine at 1, 2 and 3 years post-transplantation. The analyses of HLA matching in cyclosporin-treated patients are recent and there are as yet no data on very long-term results, and these could be more pertinent.

In most analyses of graft survival all graft failures and all patient deaths regardless of the cause are counted as graft loss. Recently Donnelly et al (1987), based on their single-centre analyses, stated that 'Failure to identify and exclude graft loss for non-immunological reasons can give rise to misleading conclusions in analysis of immunoregulatory factors in organ transplantation.' This may be particularly relevant in the cyclosporin era in which few grafts are lost due to immunological rejection and the non-immunological losses may well be greater in number; their inclusion may mask the true role of immunological factors in graft failure. An example of this is seen in an analysis of the Oxford data for the influence of DR matching on graft survival in triple therapy patients (low doses of cyclosporin, prednisolone and azathioprine) when all failures are included and when patients with non-immunological failures are excluded (Table 2). The results show that in this group of 164 recipients of primary cadaver grafts who received triple therapy the overall 1 year graft survival rate is high at 82%. DR matching does not significantly influence graft survival ($p = 0.164$) although the trend is in the 'right direction'. However when the non-immunological failures are excluded the correlation just reaches statistical significance ($p = 0.046$). (The non-immunological failures were mainly renal artery and vein thrombosis and cardiovascular death in patients with functioning grafts.)

Table 2. The influence of HLA-DR matching on first cadaver graft survival in patients immunosuppressed with triple therapy. Analyses were performed with the inclusion (A) and exclusion (B) of failures due to non-immunological causes. The data were analysed by the method of Peto et al (1977).

	No. DR mismatches	No. patients	% Survival (months)			
			3	6	12	24
A	0	44	86	86	86	86
	1	71	87	84	81	75
	2	43	79	79	79	79
B	0	39	97	97	97	97
	1	64	94	94	90	84
	2	39	87	87	87	87

HLA-DRw6 and Immune Responsiveness

Hendriks et al (1983) first reported that DRw6 positive recipients had a significantly poorer chance of graft success than patients without the antigen. This finding aroused considerable interest, for it implied that an HLA antigen may represent an immune-response gene. This 'DRw6 effect' has been confirmed by some units (e.g., Soulillou and Bignon, 1983) but not by others (e.g. Kerman et al, 1985). Hoitsma et al (1984) found that the overall graft survival was no different in DRw6+ and DRw6− patients but that the former had a significantly higher number of rejection episodes than the latter. Hendriks et al (1986) suggested that DRw6+ individuals are high-responders and that DRw6 may represent an immune-response gene. Support for this comes from the work of Darke et al (1983), who found a higher incidence of DRw6 in male responders immunized with Rh-D (50%) than in non-responders (15%), and from the work of Tsakiris et al (1987), who found that non-transfused renal patients who were DRw6+ were more likely to respond to dinitrochlorobenzene than those who were DRw6−. Cook et al (1987) found that DR1 recipients had a significantly higher graft survival rate than DR1 negative recipients and suggested that DR1 is a marker of low immune responsiveness. In contrast, the presence of DR2 and not DR1 has been found to be associated with high graft survival (Kaplan et al, 1983), and in this study DRw6+ patients had the lowest graft survival.

There is ample evidence that HLA class I and II antigens are either immune-response genes or are closely associated with immune-response genes. For example, a number of studies have implicated specific HLA antigens in susceptibility to certain diseases (Tiwari and Terasaki, 1985). Seeking proof of their existence from the results of renal transplantation may not be the ideal situation, because in the majority of cases the patient's immune system has been modified by pretransplant blood transfusions and immunosuppression after transplantation.

Crossmatching for Renal Transplantation

A number of patients awaiting renal transplantation become sensitized to HLA antigens, as indicated by the presence of antibodies cytotoxic for lymphocytes, as a result of blood transfusions, previous pregnancies or a failed graft. In the mid-1960s a number of laboratories found a strong association between a positive crossmatch (the recipient's sera reacting with the donor's lymphocytes) and immediate rejection of the allograft (Terasaki et al, 1964; Williams et al, 1968). As a consequence, performing a crossmatch before transplantation was deemed mandatory and a positive result precluded transplantation. This dogma is not unreasonable considering that HLA antigens are present on endothelial cells lining the blood vessels and could provide a target for pre-existing HLA antibodies. However, the acceptance of this dogma meant that patients with broadly reacting antibodies have had to wait a long time for a crossmatch-negative kidney and in some cases did not receive a transplant at all. Many transplant units still adhere very strictly to this policy although research carried out since the mid-1970s has shown that lymphocytotoxic antibodies are not always harmful to renal allografts, and that under certain conditions successful transplantation can be carried out in the presence of a positive crossmatch. This finding (see below) is a major breakthrough for patients with broadly-reactive antibodies.

Ettenger et al (1976) reported successful transplants with a positive B cell (and negative T cell) crossmatch. It was assumed that the antibodies were against DR antigens although specificity analysis of the antibodies was not carried out. In the same year Cross et al (1976) found a number of patients with lymphocytotoxic autoantibodies that reacted with the donor's cells, too, and their grafts were all successful. Cardella et al (1982) suggested that in patients who develop antibodies but lose them with time the 'old' antibody-positive sera may not be relevant for crossmatching, and that it is the more recently taken sera that give clinically relevant results. These 'peak serum positive, current serum negative' (P+C−) crossmatch transplants are not always successful and a number, particularly second grafts, do suffer early irreversible rejection. Nevertheless, the success rate that has been achieved by Cardella and his colleagues and many other units has certainly led to a re-evaluation of the 'standard' crossmatch protocol of using old and current sera. The immunoglobulin class of the antibody in the peak reactive serum may be an important predictor of graft outcome. IgG antibodies may be associated with graft failure whereas successful outcome has been achieved in the presence of IgM antibodies (Ayoub et al, 1983; Chapman et al, 1986). Reed et al (1987) found that the presence of anti-idiotypic antibodies in the current serum directed at the HLA antibodies in the peak serum was predictive of graft success. In their study the nine patients with such antibodies were all successfully transplanted whereas only one of nine patients without anti-idiotypic antibodies had a successful transplant. There is no doubt that P+C− crossmatch transplants can be successfully performed, but the conditions under which the chances of success are optimal have still to be worked out fully.

Lymphocyte Cytotoxic Autoantibodies

Autoantibodies react with T and B lymphocytes or with B lymphocytes alone: they are not directed at HLA antigens but their specificity is unknown. Development of these antibodies is not associated with pregnancies or transfusions and they may occur 'spontaneously' after viral infections, particularly cytomegalovirus. They are nearly always IgM whereas HLA antibodies are usually IgG, although IgM HLA antibodies may occur in patients on immunosuppression. The incidence of autoantibodies in renal failure patients has been reported to be as high as 42% (Lobo, 1981), but most units find a lower incidence and some none at all. The results of positive crossmatch transplants in Oxford due to these antibodies are shown in Table 3 (cadaver grafts) and Table 4 (LRD grafts). From these and other results it is evident that lymphocytotoxic autoantibodies are not a cause of graft rejection in cadaveric or LRD grafts. This conclusion is valid even if the antibody is present in the patient's serum at the time of transplantation. Further, it is irrelevant whether the antibody reacts with the donor's T and B cells or with B cells only (see Table 4).

Table 3. Survival of first cadaver grafts transplanted in Oxford in the presence of a positive T and B, or B only crossmatch due to autoantibodies. The data were analysed by the method of Peto et al (1977) and the frequencies shown are actuarially derived.

Crossmatch			% Survival (months)			
T	B	No. patients	3	12	36	60
+	+	27	77	65	61	61
−	+	19	84	84	68	57
−	−*	148	77	69	63	57

* Patients who had pregraft cytotoxic antibodies but a negative crossmatch with the donor.

Table 4. Outcome of LRD grafts performed in Oxford in the presence of a positive T and B, or B only crossmatch due to autoantibodies. Two of the 19 grafts were regrafts (one second and one third).

Crossmatch					% Success (months)		
T	B	Peak	Current	No. patients	1	3	6
+	+	+	+	7	100	100	100
+	+	+	−	4*	100	100	100
−	+	+	+	8	100	100	100
−	−			64	97	95	94

* One graft failed at 5 years from chronic rejection.

Table 5. The eight different types of positive crossmatches due to HLA antibodies taking into account the three variables; specificity of the antibody (class I or II), P+C+ or P+C− and, immunoglobulin class (IgG or IgM).

Specificity	Time	Ig class
Class I	P+C+	G
	P+C+	M
	P+C−	G
	P+C−	M
Class II	P+C+	G
	P+C+	M
	P+C−	G
	P+C−	M

A positive crossmatch due to HLA antibodies is more difficult to interpret because a number of variables must be considered before making the decision whether or not to transplant. These variables are: the specificity of the antibody (class I or II), whether the crossmatch is $P+C+$ or $P+C-$, and the immunoglobulin class of the antibody. Table 5 lists the eight different types of positive crossmatches that can occur with these three variables. There is no doubt that in some a transplant can be successfully carried out, while in others early rejection may be expected.

HLA Class I Antibodies

In Oxford we have now performed 24 $P+C-$ crossmatch transplants in which we have shown that the antibody is definitely against HLA class I antigens. Fifteen were IgM antibody and ten (67%) were successful at 3 months; nine were IgG, of which only one (11%) was successful. Based on these data we would certainly be against transplantation if the antibody was of IgG class directed HLA against class I antigens, but would be prepared to go ahead in the presence of a $P+C-$ IgM crossmatch. However, Palmer et al (1987) successfully transplanted three patients after removal of their IgG HLA antibodies by immunoadsorption. These patients were recipients of second grafts and the authors avoided previously mismatched antigens; in addition, kidneys with HLA antigens against which the patients had been known to make anti-HLA antibodies were avoided. Post-transplantation all patients received prophylactic antithymocyte globulin and this may be an important requirement for a successful outcome.

There is no information on $P+C+$ IgM antibodies and most transplant units would not transplant in the presence of a $P+C+$ IgG crossmatch.

HLA Class II Antibodies

The relevance of antibodies against class II antigens is unclear, for a number of reasons. First, many transplant units do not perform a B lymphocyte crossmatch (identifying antibodies against class I and II antigens) and transplant solely on the basis of a T cell result (i.e. identifying only antibodies directed against class I antigens). In these units a number of positive B cell crossmatch transplants would have been performed but whether they were antibodies directed against class II or non-HLA antigens is not known. Second, in most published reports on positive B cell crossmatch transplants the specificity of the antibody has not been determined and in most cases the antibody is probably non-HLA, for these antibodies are more common than class II antibodies in renal patients (d'Apice and Tait, 1980). Class II antigens are found on kidney tissue such as the endothelium of peritubular capillaries (Fuggle et al, 1983) and one may therefore expect class II antibodies to cause rejection. Certainly, early graft failures have been reported (Berg and Möller, 1981; Ahern et al, 1982), but some successful grafts have also been reported (Jeannet et al, 1981). Taylor CJ et al (1987) described a successful transplant in the presence of a positive B-cell crossmatch (an IgG DQw1 antibody) at the time of transplantation. Interestingly, for many months post-transplantation the antibody continued to be present at the same titre as in the pre-transplant serum sample.

The relevance of HLA class II antibodies for renal allografts will remain unclear until further studies have resolved whether the B cell antibody is class II-specific, the immunoglobulin class of the antibodies is defined, and the time interval between the last serum giving a positive crossmatch and transplantation has been fully assessed.

MINOR HISTOCOMPATIBILITY ANTIGENS

The evidence that the HLA complex encodes the major histocompatibility antigens has been presented above. From these data it is, however, clear that other histocompatibility antigens exist, for HLA-matched siblings rejected their sibling's skin grafts (albeit at a slower tempo than between HLA-unmatched siblings), kidney grafts in HLA-matched immunosuppressed recipients are subject to rejection episodes, and bone marrow grafts can suffer rejection or cause GVH disease. (Bone marrow transplantation (BMT) is described in detail in Chapter 6.) Immune reactions between T cells of donor and host, when both share identical HLA haplotypes, define these other histocompatibility (H) antigens, which are referred to as minor H antigens.

T Cell Responses to Minor H Antigens: MHC Restriction

Graft rejection is mediated principally by T cells and not by antibodies, as was originally shown in cell transfer experiments by Mitchison (1954) and by Billingham et al (1954). Although MHC antigens were originally defined by graft rejection, their subsequent analysis in the last 20 years has been made possible because antibodies, too, are made against them. These antibodies permit HLA typing, as described in the first part of this chapter, as well as biochemical, crystallographic and molecular genetic analyses. Unfortunately antibodies are not made to minor H antigens: yet in vivo T-cell responses (graft rejection) to individual minor H antigens has allowed the chromosomal mapping of the genes encoding them in mice, in which breeding experiments establish mouse strains differing from the parental strain at single minor H loci (Bailey, 1975). These loci are scattered throughout the genome, and a minimum of 40 have been identified. The same general picture is likely to be true for man, but because it is not possible to study individual minor H responses in vivo, in vitro T cell responses are the principal means for studies of minor H antigens in man. In both mouse and man it is possible to isolate T cell clones specific for minor antigens from individuals who have been previously exposed in vivo to minor H antigens. In each case the T cells have been found to be MHC restricted, i.e. they recognize the minor H antigen in the context of self MHC molecules, either class I (HLA-A, B or C in man, H-2K, D or L in mouse) or class II (HLA-D in man, H-2IA or IE in mouse).

MHC restricted recognition of minor H antigens strongly suggests that there is a physical association between MHC and minor antigens: it now seems likely that they are peptide fragments of processed cellular molecules, which have become lodged in the antigen-binding groove of the restricting MHC molecule. A representation of this, shown in Figure 2a, is taken from the recently characterized crystal structure of the HLA-A2 molecule, which interestingly appeared to have an unidentified peptide in the antigen-binding groove (Bjorkman et al, 1987a). Figure 2b is a diagrammatic representation of the α_1 and α_2 domains of HLA-A2, showing the groove bound on either side by two α helices, the floor crossed by eight strands of a β pleated sheet. This diagram amplifies the information given in Figure 1 and it is noteworthy that the various polymorphic amino acid substitutions seen in the different alleles of class I molecules lie within the proposed antigen-binding groove, on the inward facing turns of the α helices, or on the strands of the β pleated sheets as they cross the floor of the groove (Bjorkman et al, 1987b). The three dimensional structure of MHC class II molecules can also be modelled on that of class I (Brown et al, 1988), and from this it appears that it is closely similar and could serve to present antigen fragments to T cells in a similar way. This would explain how both class I and class II restricted T cells can recognize minor H antigens. We will return to the implications of T cell recognition of peptides derived from the degradation of self cellular molecules in the antigen-binding groove of MHC molecules in a later section. That antibodies are not made to minor H antigens also becomes more understandable if they are MHC-bound peptides, for we know that whilst the native molecule of influenza nucleoprotein can excite an antibody response, these antibodies fail to block cytotoxic T cell responses to nucleoprotein peptides recognized in the context of class I MHC molecules (Townsend et al, 1986) and assumed to be present in their antigen-binding groove. Antibodies to T cell recognized peptides derived from nucleoprotein are not made during the course of an immune response to virus infection.

Minor H Responses in Clinical Grafting

As there are almost certainly a large number of minor H antigen disparities between any HLA-matched donor–recipient pair, it is difficult to evaluate the contribution of responses to individual antigens to the total host-versus-graft (HVG) or graft-versus-host (GVH) response in vivo. However, experimental work suggests that immunization by grafting or injection of cells between mouse strains matched at the MHC (H-2), but mismatched at multiple minor antigens, results in a very small number of minor H antigens being immunodominant (Wettstein and Bailey, 1982). Their exact identity depends on the particular combination of minor H antigens under study, and on the H-2 type (Wettstein, 1986). This is likely to be true for man, too, and it may simplify the potential problems of typing for minor H antigens.

   T cell clones specific for the male-specific minor H antigen H-Y which is encoded on the human Y chromosome (Simpson et al, 1987), have been isolated from the peripheral blood lymphocytes of a female recipient of a kidney from her HLA-matched brother (Pfeffer et al, 1983). H-Y specific clones have also been isolated from female aplastic anaemia patients receiving bone marrow grafts, which were rejected, from an HLA-matched brother (Goulmy et al, 1977; Goulmy, 1985). T-cell clones to a number of other minor H antigens have been isolated from bone marrow transplant patients receiving HLA-matched grafts, and undergoing either GVH or HVG responses (Zier et al, 1983; Goulmy, 1985, 1988; Elkins et al, 1987). A substantial number of these clones use HLA-A2 as the restriction molecule, and this antigen may therefore be particularly avid for association with various peptides and represent a high-responder type.

   Attempts to evaluate the significance of minor H disparities in vivo have been made by typing donor and recipient pairs of the appropriate HLA type for the minor H antigens identified by T cell clones: the clones thus serve as typing reagents, much in the way that the primed lymphocyte test (PLT) can be used to type for MHC class II antigens (see above). In one series in which 67 pairs of HLA matched siblings in a BMT programme were typed for a single minor H antigen, the clinical results did not correlate with disparities at this locus (Elkins et al, 1987). However, as there are a large number of minor H antigens, this result may not be surprising. In a more extensive series, in which donor–recipient pairs were typed for five different minor H antigens, each identified by a different T-cell clone, there was a significant correlation between severity of GVH reactions and the number of minor H mismatches (Goulmy, 1985). This study has now

is at the moment unclear. What is clear is that allo MHC reactions are extremely heterogeneous with respect to specificity and that this is likely to account for their cumulative abundance.

SUMMARY

Major and minor histocompatibility antigens can cause allograft rejection between genetically incompatible individuals of the same species. Class I and II antigens encoded by the major histocompatibility complex (MHC; HLA in man, H-2 in mouse) excite the strongest reactions involving both T and B cell responses. The T cell responses to them may be very heterogeneous, and represent recognition of MHC molecules to which self peptides are bound. T cell responses to minor histocompatibility (H) antigens are seen both in vivo and in vitro when tissues or organs are exchanged between MHC-matched donor–recipient pairs. Minor H antigens are recognized in association with MHC molecules (MHC restriction) and are likely to be peptides derived from the breakdown of cellular molecules.

For clinical kidney grafting, HLA matching, particularly for class II (HLA-D) antigens, provides the best results in combination with immunosuppression. Discriminant analysis of the specificity of positive crossmatch antibodies allows transplantation of some sensitized patients. For bone marrow transplantation (BMT), exchanges between MHC unmatched pairs present great problems that may involve both GVH and HVG reactions. When BMT is performed using MHC matched pairs, GVH and HVG reactions against minor H antigens can present problems; it may be possible to resolve them if typing for immunodominant minor H antigens were to become generally available.

REFERENCES

Ahern AT, Artruc SB, Della Pelle P et al (1982) Hyperacute rejection of HLA-AB-identical renal allografts associated with B lymphocyte and endothelial reactive antibodies. *Transplantation* 33: 103–106.

Anderson M, Bohmer J, Andersson G et al (1984) Genomic hybridisation with class II transplantation antigen cDNA probes as a complementary technique in tissue typing. *Human Immunology* 11: 57–67.

d'Apice AJF & Tait BD (1980) Most positive B cell crossmatches are not caused by anti-HLA-DR antibodies. *Transplantation* 30: 382–383.

Ayoub GM, Terasaki PI & Tonai RJ (1983) Improvements in detection of sensitization. *Transplantation Proceedings* 15: 1202–1207.

Bach FH & Hirschhorn K (1964) Lymphocyte interactions: A potential histocompatibility test *in vitro*. *Science* 143: 813–814.

Bailey DW (1975) Genetics of histocompatibility in mice I New loci and congenic lines. *Immunogenetics* 2: 249–256.

Berg B & Möller E (1981) Immediate rejection of a HLA-A,B compatible, HLA-DR incompatible kidney with a positive donor–recipient B-cell crossmatch. *Scandinavian Journal of Urology and Nephrology* 54 (Supplement): 36.

Bernhard EJ, Le AT, Yannelli JR et al (1987) The ability of cytotoxic T cells to recognize HLA-A2 1 or HLA-B7 antigens expressed on murine cells correlates with their epitope specificity. *Journal of Immunology* 139: 3614–3621.

Billingham RE, Brent L & Medawar PB (1954) Quantitative studies on tissue transplantation immunity. II. The origin, strength and duration of actively and adoptively acquired immunity. *Proceedings of the Royal Society of London*, Series B. **143**: 58–80.

Bjorkman PJ, Saper MA, Samraoui B et al (1987a) Structure of the human class I histocompatibility antigen, HLA-A2. *Nature* **329**: 506–512.

Bjorkman PJ, Saper MA, Samraoui B et al (1987b) The foreign antigen binding site and T cell recognition regions of class I histocompatibility antigens. *Nature* **329**: 512–518.

Brown JH, Jardetzky T, Saper MA et al (1988) A hypothetical model of the foreign antigen binding site of class II histocompatibility molecules. *Nature* **332**: 845–850.

Cardella CJ, Falk JA, Nicholson MJ, Harding M & Cook GT (1982) Successful renal transplantation in patients with T-cell reactivity to donor. *Lancet* **ii**: 1240–1243.

Cats S, Terasaki P, Perdue S & Mickey MR (1984) Effect of HLA typing and transfusions on cyclosporine-treated renal-allograft recipients. *New England Journal of Medicine* **311**: 675–676.

Ceppellini R, Mattiuz PL, Scudeller G & Visetti M (1969) Experimental allotransplantation in man. I. The role of the HL-A system in different genetic combinations. *Transplantation Proceedings* **1**: 385–389.

Chapman JR, Taylor CJ, Ting A & Morris PJ (1986) Immunoglobulin class and specificity of antibodies causing positive T cell crossmatches: Relationship to renal transplant outcome. *Transplantation* **42**: 608–613.

Cicciarelli J, Terasaki PI & Mickey MR (1987) The effect of zero HLA class I and II mismatching in cyclosporine-treated kidney transplant patients. *Transplantation* **43**: 636–640.

Cook DJ, Cecka M & Terasaki PI (1987) HLA-DR1 recipients have the highest kidney transplant survival. *Transplantation Proceedings* **19**: 675–677.

Cross DE, Greiner R & Whittier FC (1976) Importance of the autocontrol crossmatch in human renal transplantation. *Transplantation* **21**: 307–311.

Daar AS, Fuggle SV, Fabre JW, Ting A & Morris PJ (1984a) The detailed distribution of HLA-ABC antigens in normal human organs. *Transplantation* **38**: 287–292.

Daar AS, Fuggle SV, Fabre JW, Ting A & Morris PJ (1984b) The detailed distribution of MHC class II antigens in normal human organs. *Transplantation* **38**: 293–298.

Darke C, Street J, Sargeant C & Dyer PA (1983) HLA-DR antigens and properdin factor B allotypes in responders and non-responders to the Rhesus-D antigen. *Tissue Antigens* **21**: 333–335.

Dausset J (1958) Iso-leucoanticorps. *Acta Haematologica* **20**: 156–166.

Donnelly P, Henderson R, Fletcher K et al (1987) Specific and non-specific immunoregulatory factors and renal transplantation. *Transplantation* **44**: 523–528.

Elkins WC, Pierson GR & Storb R (1987) Study of a human minor alloantigen in relation to clinical graft versus host diseae. *Bone Marrow Transplantation* **1**: 397–403.

Ettenger RB, Terasaki PI, Opelz G et al (1976) Successful renal allografts across a positive cross-match for donor B-lymphocyte alloantigens. *Lancet* **ii**: 56–58.

Fuggle SV, Errasti P, Daar AS et al (1983) Localisation of MHC (HLA-ABC and DR) antigens in 46 kidneys. Differences in HLA-DR staining of tubules among kidneys. *Transplantation* **35**: 385–390.

Goulmy E (1985) Class I retricted human cytotoxic T lymphocytes directed against minor transplantation antigens and their possible role in organ transplantation. *Progress in Allergy* **36**: 44–72.

Goulmy E (1988) Minor histocompatibility antigens in man and their role in transplantation. In PJ Morris and N Tilney (eds) *Transplant Reviews II*, in press.

Goulmy E, Termijtelen A, Bradley BA & Van Rood JJ (1977) Y-antigen killing by T cells of women is restricted by HLA. *Nature* **226**: 544–545.

Hendriks GFJ, Claas FHJ, Persijn GG et al (1983) HLA-DRw6-positive recipients are high responders in renal transplantation. *Transplantation Proceedings* **15**: 1136–1138.

Hendriks GFJ, Schjreuder GMTh, D'Amaro J & Van Rood JJ (1986) The regulatory role of HLA-DRw6 in renal transplantation. *Tissue Antigens* **27**: 121–130.

Hoitsma AJ, Reekers P, Van Lier HJJ, Van Rens JCM & Koene RAP (1984) HLA-DRw6 and treatment of acute rejection with antithymocyte globulin. *Transplantation* **38**: 25–28.

Jeannet M, Benzonana G & Arni I (1981) Donor-specific B and T lymphocyte antibodies and kidney graft survival. *Transplantation* **31**: 160–163.

Joysey VC, Thiru S & Evans DB (1985) Effect of HLA-DR compatibility on kidney transplants treated with cyclosporin A. *Transplantation Proceedings* **17**: 2187–2192.

Kaplan C, Cartron J, Muller J-V et al (1983) Recipient's HLA-DR phenotype and renal graft outcome. *Transplantation* **36**: 213–214.

Kappler JW, Staerz U, White J & Marrack PC (1988) Self tolerance eliminates T cells specific for Mls-modified products of the major histocompatibility complex. *Nature* **332**: 35–40.

Kerman RH, Van Buren CT, Flechner SM, Lorber MI & Kahan BD (1985) The beneficial effect of cyclosporine on renal transplantation at a single US transplant center. *Transplantation Proceedings* **17**: 2193–2195.

Kerman RH, Van Buren CT, Lewis RM & Kahan BD (1988) Successful transplantation of 100 untransfused cyclosporine-treated primary recipients of cadaveric renal allografts. *Transplantation* **40**: 37–40.

Kisielow P, Bluthmann H, Staerz UD, Steinmetz M & von Boehmer H (1988) Tolerance in T-cell receptor transgenic mice involves deletion of non mature $CD4^+8^+$ thymocytes. *Nature* **333**: 742–746.

Klintmalm G, Brynger H, Flatmark A et al (1985) The blood transfusion, DR matching, and mixed lymphocyte culture effects are not seen in cyclosporine-treated transplant recipients. *Transplantation Proceedings* **17**: 1026–1031.

Langhorne J & Fischer-Lindahl K (1982) Role of non-H-2 antigens in the cytotoxic T cell response to allogeneic H-2. *European Journal of Immunology* **12**: 101–106.

Lobo PI (1981) Nature of autolymphocytotoxins present in renal hemodialysis patients. Their possible role in controlling alloantibody formation. *Transplantation* **32**: 233–237.

Lombardi G, Sidhu S, Lamb JR, Batchelor JR & Lechler R (1989) Co-recognition of endogenous peptide with HLA-DR1 by alloreactive human T cell clones. *Journal of Immunology.* **142**: 753–759.

Lundgren G, Groth CG, Albrechtsen D et al (1986) HLA-matching and pretransplant blood transfusions in cadaveric renal transplantation – A changing picture with cyclosporin. *Lancet* **ii**: 66–69.

MacDonald HR, Schneider R, Lees RK et al (1988) T cell receptor Vβ use predicts reactivity and tolerance to Mls^a-encoded antigens. *Nature* **332**: 40–45.

Madsen M, Graugaard B, Fjeldborg O et al (1985) The impact of HLA-DR antigen matching in cyclosporine-treated recipients of cadaveric renal allografts. A single-center analysis. *Transplantation Proceedings* **17**: 2202–2205.

Marrack P & Kappler J (1988) T cells can distinguish between allogeneic major histocompatibility complex products on different cell types. *Nature* **332**: 840–843.

Matzinger P & Bevan MJ (1977) Why do so many lymphocytes respond to the major histocompatibility antigens? *Cellular Immunology* **29**: 1–5.

Mitchison NA (1954) Passive transfer of transplantation immunity. *Proceedings of the Royal Society of London, Series B* **142**: 72–87.

Opelz G, for the Collaborative Transplant Study (1987) Effect of HLA matching in 10,000 cyclosporine-treated cadaver kidney transplants. *Transplantation Proceedings* **19**: 641–646.

Palmer A, Tabue D, Welsh K et al (1987) Extracorporeal Immunoadsorption of anti-HLA antibodies: Preliminary clinical experience. *Transplantation Proceedings* **19**: 3750–3751.

Persijn GG, Schreuder GMTh, Hendriks GFH et al (1986) Cyclosporin, HLA matching, and transfusions in kidney transplants. *Lancet* **ii**: 915–916.

Peto R, Pike MC, Armitage P et al (1977) Design and analysis of randomized clinical trials requiring prolonged observation of each patient. II. Analysis and examples. *British Journal of Cancer* **35**: 1–39.

Pfeffer PF, Gabrielsen TS, Ahonen J & Thorsby E (1983) Cytotoxic cells recognizing minor histocompatibility antigens in patients rejecting HLA-identical grafts. *Transplantation Proceedings* **15**: 1821–1822.

Reed E, Hardy M, Benvenitsky A et al (1987) Effect of antiidiotypic antibodies to HLA on graft survival in renal allograft recipients. *New England Journal of Medicine* **316**: 1450–1455.

Salvatierra O, Amend W, Vincenti F et al (1981) Pretreatment with donor-specific blood transfusions in related recipients with high MLC. *Transplantation Proceedings* **13**: 142–149.

Shaw S, Pollack MS, Payne SM & Johnson AH (1980) HLA-linked B cell alloantigens of a new segregant series: Population and family studies of the SB antigens. *Human Immunology* **1**: 177–185.

Simonsen M, Skjodt K & Crone M (1985) Compound receptors in the cell membrane: ruminations from the border land of Immunology & Physiology. *Progress in Allergy* **36**: 151–176.

Simpson E (1983) MHC antigens and the genetic control of immune responses. *Transplantation Proceedings* **15**: 186–188.

Simpson E, Chandler P, Goulmy E, Disteche CM, Ferguson-Smith MA & Page DC (1987) Separation of the genetic loci for the H-Y antigen and for testis determination on the human Y chromosome. *Nature* **326**: 876–878.

Soulillou J-P & Bignon J-D (1983) Poor kidney-graft survival in recipients with HLA-DRw6. *New England Journal of Medicine* **308**: 969–970.

Taylor CJ, Chapman JR, Fuggle SV, Ting A & Morris PJ (1987) A positive B cell crossmatch due to IgG anti-HLA-DQ antibody present at the time of transplantation in a successful renal allograft. *Tissue Antigens* **30**: 104–112.

Taylor RJ, Andrews W, Rosenthal JT, Carpenter B & Hakala TR (1985) DR matching in cadaveric renal transplantation with cyclosporine. *Transplantation Proceedings* **17**: 1194–1196.

Terasaki PI & McClelland JD (1964) Microdroplet assay of human serum cytotoxins. *Nature* **204**: 998–1000.

Terasaki PI, Marchioro TL & Starzl TE (1964) Sero-typing of human lymphocyte antigens: Preliminary trials on long-term kidney homograft survivors. In Russell PS & Wynn HJ (eds) *Histocompatibility Testing*, pp 83–96. Washington, DC: National Academy of Sciences-National Research Council.

Tiwari JL & Terasaki PI (1985) *HLA and disease associations*. New York: Springer-Verlag.

Townsend ARM, Rothbard J, Gotch FM et al (1986) The epitopes of influenza nucleoprotein recognized by cytotoxic T lymphocytes can be defined by short synthetic peptides. *Cell* **44**: 959–968.

Tsakiris T, Watson MA, Degiannis D, Briggs JD & Junor BJR (1987) Association between blood transfusion, HLA-DRw6, and response to dinitrochlorobenzene skin test. *Transplantation Proceedings* **19**: 705–707.

Wettstein PJ (1986) Immunodominance in the T-cell response to multiple non H-2 histocompatibility antigens: II Observation of a hierarchy among dominant antigens. *Immunogenetics* **24**: 24–31.

Wettstein PJ & Bailey DW (1982) Immunodominance in the immune response to 'multiple' histocompatibility antigens. *Immunogenetics* **16**: 47–58.

Williams GM, Hume DM, Hudson RP et al (1968) 'Hyperacute' renal-homograft rejection in man. *New England Journal of Medicine* **279**: 611–618.

Zier KS, Elkins WL, Pierson GR & Leo MM (1983) The use of cytotoxic T cell lines to detect the segregation of a human minor alloantigen within families. *Human Immunology* **7**: 117–129.

2 The Immunobiology of Acute Allograft Rejection

N. L. TILNEY
J. W. KUPIEC-WEGLINSKI

Only within the past 50 years have transplant biologists begun to appreciate the full complexities of the phenomenon of acute rejection, that dramatic, multifaceted and powerful series of host immunological responses called into play by, and leading to the destruction of, allografts of genetically foreign tissues. Although some investigators in the first half of the twentieth century described transplantation of kidney grafts in dogs, goats and cats, differences in behaviour between autografts and allografts were not really appreciated until the 1950s when Dempster in London and Simonson in Copenhagen began to provide a biological basis for the rejection response (see Appendix III for history). Indeed, understanding that the host events leading to graft destruction have an immune basis and are moderated primarily by lymphocytes was long in coming; although Murphy in New York in 1926 had described lymphocytes aggregating at the base of skin allografts, Rich at Johns Hopkins, writing a few years later, suggested that they were merely 'phlegmatic spectators watching the turbulent activity of phagocytes'.

The modern era of transplantation biology was opened by Medawar during World War II when he pursued clinical observations with Gibson on skin allografts placed on burnt patients and experimental studies on the behaviour of skin grafts in rabbits (see Appendix III). He described a progressive infiltration of the graft bed by lymphocytes and macrophages which coincided with its destruction about one week after placement in unsensitized recipients. He also found that when skin allografts were transplanted to animals which had previously rejected skin from the same donor, the destruction of these 'second set' grafts was accelerated. In 1955, Scothorne and MacGregor noted that the dramatic changes in lymph nodes draining orthotopic skin allografts included the appearance of large numbers of lymphoid cells in cortical nodules and marked proliferation of plasma cells in medullary cords. At the same time, the assiduous development by Little and Snell of genetically defined inbred strains of mice for the study of immune responses against tumours provided the opportunity to produce reproducible animal models for use in transplantation biology.

Using such inbred strains, Mitchison, and Billingham, Brent and Medawar (see Appendix III) demonstrated that the immune status established in one mouse to a certain tumour or skin graft could be conferred to other members of the host strain by the

ORGAN TRANSPLANTATION: CURRENT CLINICAL AND
IMMUNOLOGICAL CONCEPTS   ISBN 0-7020-1393-5

'transfer' of lymphoid cells from the sensitized individuals. Gowans then showed the small lymphocyte to recirculate and to be the prototypic 'immunologically competent' cell. Since immunity to skin grafts could not be transferred consistently with serum, antibody responses were considered to be of secondary importance in acute rejection. Subsequently, with the progressive elaboration of genetically defined mouse strains, histocompatibility antigens that both stimulate and provide the targets of immune responsiveness have been defined at both cellular and molecular levels. In more recent years, particularly with the rapid advancement in hybridoma technology and increasing availability of monoclonal antibodies (mAbs), investigations have centred upon defining the cellular cascade mediating rejection, as well as the actions, interactions, influences and contributions of cell populations, subpopulations and their various products in this remarkable event.

During the 1940s and 1950s, a few sporadic attempts at kidney transplantations were made in patients; no kidney functioned more than a few days except in a single unmodified individual whose graft sustained him for five months. In 1954, the first successful kidney transplant was performed between identical twins in Boston; this and subsequent twin transplants gave credence to the concept of renal transplantation in humans. In the late 1950s, with gradual appreciation of the significance of the immune responses and with growing evidence that they could be manipulated, a series of transplants was undertaken in Boston and Paris in patients immunosuppressed with total body X-irradiation; however, it was not until 1962, with the initial chemical immuno-suppression experiments, that patient survival and graft function began to improve. Subsequently, the availability of newer and more effective agents alone or in combination, has made successful transplantation of various organs more of a reality.

Several patterns of allograft rejection have been described both experimentally and clinically, each with discrete histopathology, host mechanisms of destruction, temporal patterns and prognosis. Acute rejection, primarily a cellular (T lymphocyte-mediated) phenomenon, occurs after 6–7 days in unsensitized hosts. Hyperacute rejection implies a humoral event manifested by ischaemic graft death secondary to the rapid interaction between cytotoxic antibodies circulating in the presensitized host and antigen expressed on the vascular endothelium of the donor organ. Accelerated rejection probably includes both humoral and cellular components and occurs 1–3 days more quickly than acute rejection in recipients already sensitized against donor antigens. Chronic rejection entails a slow fibrosis of the graft within months or years after placement and may be predominantly humoral. For the purposes of this chapter, the phenomenon of acute rejection will be emphasized, as most is known about its biology.

HOST CELLS MEDIATING ACUTE REJECTION

The histological patterns of acute rejection of all histoincompatible tissues are relatively comparable and show primarily a picture of progressive mononuclear leukocytic infiltration of the graft substance coinciding with its destruction (Figure 1). Within hours of engraftment, a few small lymphocytes infiltrate the area surrounding small vessels; within a few days large numbers of host cells are scattered throughout the foreign tissue. As the inflammatory reaction proceeds, increasing numbers of phagocytic mononuclear cells enter the graft which then undergoes progressive disruption of pericapillary tissues, interstitial inflammation, oedema, diminished blood flow and, ultimately, necrosis. At the same time, numbers of lymphocytes and immunoblasts increase dramatically in host lymphoid compartments of the recipient.

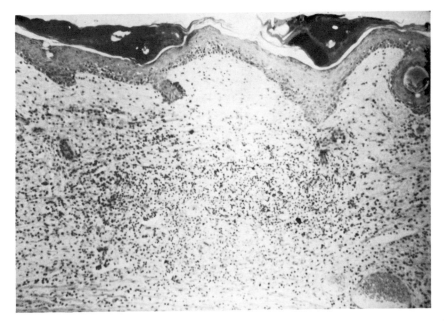

Figure 1. This skin allograft is undergoing acute rejection 5 days after placement, with host mononuclear cells infiltrating the graft bed and dermis from perivascular sources. (Haematoxylin and eosin × 40.)

The identity of the host cells infiltrating acutely rejecting allografts as well as those entering lymphoid organs include T and B lymphocytes, macrophages, and natural killer (NK) cells (Mason and Morris, 1986). That the predominant T cell infiltrate is critical in graft destruction has been emphasized in vitro by its role in direct lymphocyte-mediated cytotoxicity, a cytolytic process which precludes the concurrent need for antibody (Bainbridge and Gowland, 1971; Tilney et al, 1975). The recent availability of specific mAbs has allowed fractionation of the T lymphocyte population into its component subpopulations, the major histocompatibility complex (MHC) class I antigen restricted cytotoxic/suppressor (Tc/s, CD8) and the class II restricted T helper (Th, CD4) phenotypes (Mason, 1988). CD8 and CD4 are current nomenclature for Tc/s and Th lymphocytes, respectively; CD8 is an analogue of OKT8 or LEU-2, LYT-2 and OX8, in the human, mouse and rat, respectively, while CD4 is the analogue of OKT4 or LEU-3, L3T4 and W3/25. However, it should be noted that this terminology, which refers to surface antigens expressed by resting Th and Tc/s cells, wrongly suggests that there is a direct correlation between phenotype and function; it is increasingly apparent that these relationships are not absolute and phenotypes may change dependent upon the state of host responsiveness. Introduction of mAbs against activation markers such as surface receptors has been more helpful in understanding the actual function of various cell subpopulations than identification by phenotype alone, although such probes are still under investigation.

Although Tc/s share a common marker, they may either lyse other cells bearing foreign histocompatibility antigens or suppress both cytotoxic and B lymphocyte functions. Not only may the two functional groups (cytotoxic and suppressor) act simultaneously, but this lymphocyte subpopulation cannot be fractionated using presently available techniques, again emphasizing a lack of correlation between function and phenotype. Whether a single CD8+ population is responsible for these contrasting effects or whether there are separate cytotoxic and suppressor subsets is unknown; it may be that phenotype and function are dependent temporally upon particular conditions of immunological activation or stimulation. In addition to other functions, activated CD4+ cells augment both Tc/s activity and IgG production by B cells through the release of soluble factors, the lymphokines. The most important of these factors in the rejection cascade is interleukin 2 (IL-2, previously known as T cell growth factor), which recognizes and combines with IL-2 receptors (IL-2R) exposed on the surfaces of other activated cell populations and subpopulations, causing their differentiation and proliferation (Wagner et al, 1980).

Cell populations other than T lymphocytes also infiltrate rejecting tissues, although their actual role in the process is less clear. Allostimulated B lymphocytes differentiate into antibody-producing plasma cells and mediate the humoral immune responses by synthesizing and secreting antigen-specific antibodies. NK cells are cytotoxic, non-T, non-B cells which lyse certain tumour cells in culture (Nemlander et al, 1983). They infiltrate organ grafts quickly and show increased activity in vitro following transplantation. However, if they are depleted from the graft and lymphoid compartments of the recipient by specific anti-NK cell antibodies, the inconsequential prolongation of graft survival suggests that these cells are not critical components of the acute rejection response. By contrast, macrophages may act both as accessory cells involved in the initiation of immune responsiveness by antigen presentation and as effector cells causing graft destruction (Figure 2) (Nathan et al, 1980). They play at least four interrelated roles in the host defences: (i) induction of T lymphocyte proliferation, which requires physical association between T cells and antigen-bearing macrophages; (ii) they act as the principal site of control by immune-response genes; (iii) their plasma membrane receptors may help locate antigen–antibody complexes, activate B cells by antigen, or act in antibody-dependent lysis of antibody-coated target cells; (iv) they elaborate biologically active molecules, particularly interleukin 1 (IL-1), that may activate particular lymphocyte populations. In turn, they may become stimulated selectively against the graft through the action of lymphokines released by CD4+ cells.

MECHANISMS OF ALLOGRAFT REJECTION

Like a neurological arc, the immunological host response to foreign grafts has been conceptualized as possessing two limbs, an afferent or sensitizing limb, and an efferent or effector limb (Gowans et al, 1962). Specifically-sensitized effector cells proliferate in host lymphoid compartments following interaction between graft antigen and circulating lymphocytes, then invade the graft via its vasculature and are responsible for, or at least trigger its destruction, probably by marshalling large numbers of non-specific T cells and macrophages.

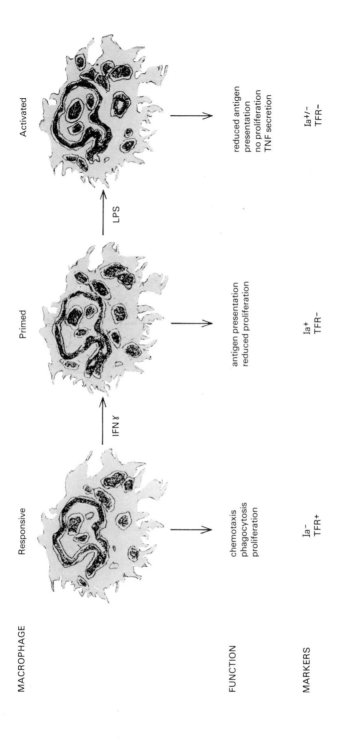

Figure 2. Features of macrophage activation. Ia, MHC class II antigen; IFNγ, γ-interferon; LPS, lipopolysaccharide; TFR, transferrin receptor; TNF, tumour necrosis factor (α). Adapted from Adams and Hamilton, (1987).

MACROPHAGE

Responsive   Primed   Activated

IFN γ   LPS

FUNCTION

chemotaxis
phagocytosis
proliferation

antigen presentation
reduced proliferation

reduced antigen
presentation
no proliferation
TNF secretion

MARKERS

Ia⁻
TFR+

Ia+
TFR−

Ia+/−
TFR−

The Afferent Limb – Antigenic Recognition

Both class I and class II antigens of the MHC are prime targets for immunological attack. They are expressed differentially on graft tissues, may be influenced by factors elaborated by activated host cells and may in turn influence two processes involved simultaneously in triggering graft rejection (Fuggle et al, 1983; Lafferty et al, 1986). First, a response is directed primarily at the relatively ubiquitous class I antigens expressed on parenchymal cells, bone marrow-derived, nucleated 'passenger cells' in the interstitium, and many other tissues as well; these are important in the regulation of lymphocyte activation. Secondly, a response occurs against class II antigens. These are distributed more widely in lymphoid tissues than class I and are expressed on dendritic cells (DC), circulating B lymphocytes, monocytes, and vascular endothelial cells, an especially important target for immune injury as they are exposed continuously to circulating effector cells and their mediators. In general, it apears that allospecific activated CD4+ cells are important but not exclusive in directing effector events involved in graft destruction; their activation requires recognition of class II molecular determinants on the target cell surface.

The expression of MHC antigens can be regulated by various stimuli (Snedire and Schwarz, 1981) (see also Chapter 8). Cell mediators or lymphokines can selectively induce different class II gene products as well as inducing class I differentially over class II. CD8- and CD4-mediated responses are directed predominantly to class I and class II MHC antigens, respectively. Class I may be expressed on almost any cell with the capacity to present antigen to T lymphocytes, while class II expression is found only on bone marrow derived DC in normal rat heart and in Langerhans cells in normal mouse skin; however, these antigens can be induced on vascular endothelium and interstitial monocytes in rejecting grafts (Austyn and Steinman, 1988). In skin, Langerhans cells may activate host T cells which, through mediators, may induce class II MHC antigens on the vascular endothelium. The amount and the location of class I and class II within the transplanted tissue are also important in determining the mechanisms of graft rejection. Similarly, in the rat, class I expression occurs much more rapidly in the transplanted kidney than in the heart and it is 30 times higher than normal by the fifth day after transplantation (Milton et al, 1986). By contrast, class II induction in the kidney develops with kinetics similar to that seen in hearts, with a tenfold increase at the time of rejection.

While T lymphocytes are critical in the afferent limb of immune responsiveness, antigen recognition alone is insufficient to initiate host events. Lafferty et al (1986) have suggested that lymphocyte activation is a two-signal process triggered by the presence of foreign antigens (Figure 3). Transplantation antigen is bound to the surface of T cell receptors (signal 1), which simultaneously receive an inductive (co-stimulating) stimulus (signal 2) from metabolically active, antigen-presenting stimulator cells in the graft. The delivery of both signals causes activation and production of cytotoxic CD8+ cells; indeed, serologically-defined antigens on the surface of allogeneic cells cannot alone cause full differentiation of cytotoxic T cells (Bach et al, 1976). Precursors of this subpopulation, activated by class I antigens, undergo final differentiation after receiving a further signal produced by CD4+ cells which themselves have been activated both by class II antigens and by soluble mediators (IL-1) from activated macrophages. IL-2 elaborated from activated CD4+ is responsible for proliferation of IL-2R-bearing effector cells (Smith, 1984).

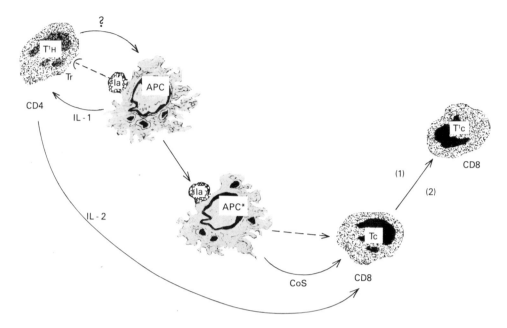

Figure 3.   T lymphocyte activation as a two-signal process. The antigen-primed CD4 cell (T[1]H) interacts with a resting antigen-presenting cell (APC) to induce co-stimulator (CoS) production. The activated APC (APC*) then stimulates the resting CD8 cell (Tc) to become MHC class I-reactive CD8 (T[1]c). This process requires two signals: (1) provided by engagement of T cell receptor (Tr); (2) provided by CoS. (Adapted from Lafferty et al, 1986.)

The Afferent Limb – Dendritic Cells

Antigenic determinants on the various cellular components comprising transplanted tissues and organs can stimulate the host differentially. Isolated leukocytes, vascular endothelium, or epidermal cells can cause vigorous proliferation of histoincompatible leukocytes in vitro and can elicit antibody formation in vivo. Because of their rich content of alloantigen and their capacity to migrate to host lymphoid tissues, the concept has been suggested that 'passenger leukocytes' residing within the graft may be of particular importance to host sensitization (Billingham, 1971). This cell type was defined further when cells with striking dendritic morphology from mouse spleen and afferent lymph in rats were found to stimulate the mixed leukocyte reaction (MLR) strongly and to cause rejection when transferred into syngeneic rats bearing established kidney grafts; transfer of lymphoid cells alone did not affect graft survival (Lechler and Batchelor, 1982). Direct evidence for the identity of DC comes from experiments in which the removal of such cells from mouse pancreatic islets by anti-DC mAb and complement before transplantation renders the islets non-immunogenic (Faustman et al, 1985). Prior administration of DC may also lead to rejection of subsequently grafted tissues. Thus, fetal thymus grafts undergo rejection in mice treated with donor strain DC. However, although cardiac allografts are rejected in an accelerated manner in some strains of mice which have received DC prior to transplantation, transfer of DC could not prevent the beneficial effects of prior blood transfusion (Peugh et al, 1987).

Recent work has further defined this important class of cell; DC (Langerhans cells in the skin), bone marrow-derived, antigen-presenting cells constitutively express class I and class II antigens, and are resident in several tissues. Indeed, survival of skin grafts can be improved when Langerhans cells are reduced either by pretreating the donor with X-radiation, corticosteroids or other leukocytic agents, or when donor-type leukocytes are replaced with host leukocytes following donor pretreatment with lethal X-radiation and reconstitution with host bone marrow (Billingham, 1971). These cells are less sessile than previously thought, as they have recently been shown to migrate from blood to spleen, under control of T lymphocytes, and enter the T cell-dependent areas from the marginal zone (Austyn et al, 1988).

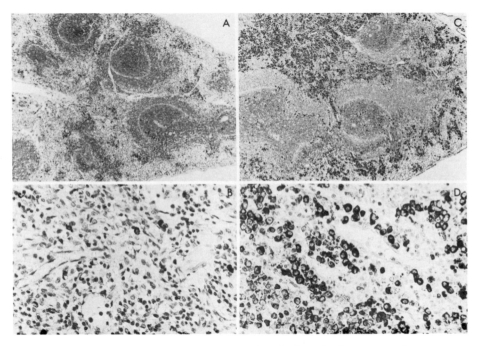

Figure 4.   Splenic morphology of ungrafted and grafted rats is shown using immunoperox-idase, which stains with intracytoplasmic Ig dark. (A) Spleen of normal rat shows white pulp composed of central artery, periarterial sheaths, germinal centres and marginal zone, and the larger red pulp (x40). (B) The periarterial sheath around the central artery contains few immunoperoxidase positive cells (x50). (C) After graft rejection at 7 days, there are large numbers of immunoblasts throughout the red pulp (x40). (D) The marginal zone and red pulp contains clusters of immunoblasts and plasma cells staining positively for Ig, with intervening immunoperoxidase negative small and large lymphocytes. (Adapted from Bald-win et al, 1979.)

Dendritic cells are not the exclusive immunizing component of skin grafts, as transplants of pure epidermal cells are rejected acutely; thus, tissue-specific antigens may be additional components of immunogenicity. Similar antigen systems have been implicated in rejection of organ allografts. An alternative to the route of sensitization of host T cells by 'passenger leukocytes' of the graft is the presentation of graft antigens by the recipient's own antigen-presenting cells, as shown by Sherwood et al (1986) in a series of adoptive transfer recipients.

Routes of Immunization

Differences in host sensitization may account for variations in immunogenicity between skin or organ allografts. Skin grafts are placed on the recipient bed without formal surgical reconstitution of vessels. While lymphatic drainage is re-established quickly, revascularization is not restored for 3–4 days (Scothorne and MacGregor, 1953). During this period, moderate ischaemic changes occur in graft vasculature and epidermis, and granulocytes accumulate at the host–graft interface. Revascularization apparently is not required (or at least is not the sole parameter required) for sensitization by skin, as only a 4-day exposure to a first set skin graft is sufficient to sensitize the host. Hall has suggested that sensitization may occur by the percolation of particulate graft antigen to the regional lymph nodes, a more important factor than migration of passenger leukocytes or recirculating host lymphocytes (Hall, 1967). After cannulating regional lymphatics draining skin allografts and isografts in sheep, he noted that lymph from allografts but not isografts carried much necrotic cellular debris in the absence of a significant increase in viable cells. Indeed, the role of this debris has been thought to be critical in inducing host-responsiveness, as has been demonstrated by transplanting skin to sites of little or no lymphatic drainage which include the anterior chamber of the eye, the brain, the hamster cheek pouch, and vascularized skin pedicles or skin islands with surgically interrupted lymphatics (Barker and Billingham, 1977). Skin grafts placed on such 'immunologically privileged' sites show prolonged survival and produce few immunologically mediated alterations in regional lymph nodes. By contrast, allogeneic skin pedicles, the vessels of which are directly anastomosed to recipient blood vessels but isolated from recipient lymphatics, are rejected promptly.

The direct revascularization of organ allografts produces different conditions for host immunization; Hume found that rejection was not delayed following isolation of the primarily vascularized transplant from recipient lymphatics by encasement in plastic bags (Hume and Egdahl, 1955), while Pedersen and Morris (1970) showed that renal allograft rejection in sheep was not affected by external diversion of efferent lymph from the graft. Immediate revascularization decreases the number of ischaemically injured cells and flushes viable passenger leukocytes directly into the recipient circulation where they are then retained preferentially in host spleen. In addition, prompt revascularization allows a continual exposure of the graft to circulating effector cells. Some of these cells migrate through the organ while cells specifically sensitized to graft antigens may be retained selectively within it, presumably by interaction with endothelial antigens or parenchymal elements (Heslop and Hardy, 1971). Few in number, this sensitized population then triggers infiltration of the graft by large numbers of uncommitted alloaggressive cells which circulate into its substance and remain following interaction with the sensitized cells.

Responses in Lymphoid Tissue

Serial histological studies of peripheral lymphoid tissues of recipients of skin or organ grafts have shown that orthotopic skin grafts elicit vigorous reactions in the regional draining lymph nodes and delayed and milder changes in the spleen (Scothorne and MacGregor, 1953; Billingham et al, 1954); rapid responses in both spleen and lymph nodes occur following organ grafting. The functional relevance of these observations is supported by the observation that rejection of skin grafts can be delayed by lymphadenectomy but not splenectomy; rejection of organ grafts by splenectomy but not lymphadenectomy (Stark et al, 1960; Souther et al, 1974).

Within 12 hours of placement of a skin allograft, obvious changes occur in the regional nodes. Granulocytes accumulate in the medullary sinuses, lymphocytes plug the cortical sinuses, and increasing numbers of lymphocytes traverse the high endothelium of post-capillary venules. Subsequently, lymphocytes proliferate in the thymus-dependent para-cortical areas, primary follicles form, and medullary cords widen with plasma cells. All of these events suggest significant cell traffic between the circulation and the lymph nodes with cells entering in large numbers and leaving in small numbers. Cytotoxic T cell activity, as measured in vitro, occurs in regional draining lymph nodes within 2 days of skin grafting and in the spleen and distant lymph nodes after 6–8 days. IgM antibody titres are first detected in the circulation after 8 days, IgG antibodies after 20 days. While the cytotoxic T cell response declines shortly following rejection, the antibody response persists for several weeks.

Organ allografts trigger a dramatic splenic response (see Figure 4) (Baldwin et al, 1979). Within 2 days after transplantation, large pyroninophilic immunoblasts proliferate in peripheral periarterial lymphoid sheaths and then extend into the red pulp where they proliferate and differentiate into plasma cells which triple the red pulp volume by the time of actual graft rejection. These antibody-producing cells gradually diminish in number following rejection and are replaced by immunoperoxidase negative large and small lymphoid cells. The intensity of splenic involvement is associated with a rapid antibody response, first detected 3–5 days after organ grafting and peaking at 7 days. Cytotoxic T cells in spleen follow a parallel time course (Tilney et al, 1975). Although the actual role of the intense B cell response in acute rejection is not known, it is possible that it contributes to the process.

THE EFFERENT LIMB

The actual events involved in rejection of allografts remain unclear despite serial examinations of histological changes, identification and functional assessment of the cell populations and subpopulations infiltrating the allograft and migrating to host lymphoid tissues, and knowledge of destructive or protective humoral effects. CD8 + and CD4 + lymphocytes, delayed-type hypersensitivity (DTH) reactions, activated macrophages and antibodies have all been implicated in graft destruction (Figure 5) (Häyry et al, 1984).

There has also been much argument concerning the identity of the actual cell types responsible for acute rejection (Tilney et al, 1984; Mason and Morris, 1986; Mason, 1988). Most investigators have found that activated T lymphocytes (found in thymus, thoracic duct, spleen and peripheral blood), but not B lymphocytes (derived from bone marrow), are necessary and sufficient to reproduce the rejection response. The survival of chicken feathers transplanted to athymic T cell-deprived nude mice is especially memorable (Rygaard, 1974). There is still considerable argument, however, as to whether the CD4+ or CD8+ subpopulations of activated T cells bring about rejection. Identification of a predominantly cytotoxic cell infiltrate has been shown by mAb staining in rejecting grafts, suggesting the importance of the CD8+ subset. Some investigators have noted that alloaggressiveness could be reinstituted in otherwise unresponsive hosts by transfer of CD8+ cells, although this fraction produced only attenuated and delayed rejection; others could not duplicate this effect in different models. Other studies have shown that CD4+ cells can be responsible for acute rejection. In several systems, classical acute rejection could be re-established only when the two separate fractions (CD4+ plus CD8+) were recombined in the presence of IL-2 (Mason, 1988).

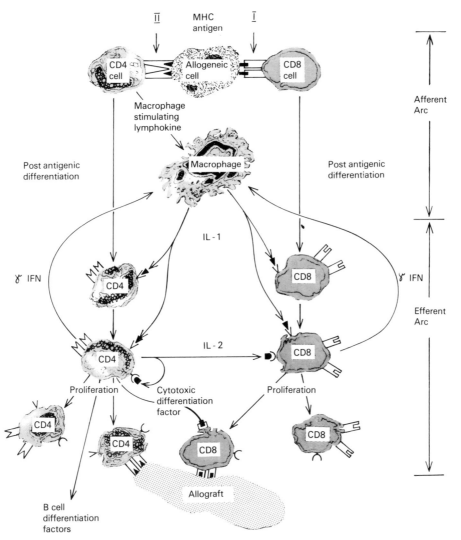

Figure 5. Scheme of allograft rejection response. Antigen-induced interactions between macrophages, CD4+ and CD8+ lymphocytes and their humoral products are critical for the completion of the rejection response.

The relative contribution of particular T cell subpopulations may also depend on the nature of the graft, the degree of host sensitization and the disparity between donor and recipient. Adoptive transfer studies have revealed that the presence of CD4+ cells is critical for rejection of primary organ allografts, but the rejection of a second donor strain allograft may be mediated independently by both CD4+ and CD8+ subsets. In recipients depleted of relevant T cell subsets, CD4+ cells are required to reject class II incompatible grafts, and CD8+ cells are primarily needed for rejection of transplants that differ at class I (Cobbold et al, 1983). It seems increasingly apparent that graft rejection reflects different contributions of not one but multiple effector mechanisms.

Thus, the evidence from multiple studies in many systems places emphasis on the CD4+ T helper cell as the primary, initiating and organizing component of the immune response, and suggests that the Tc/s (CD8+) fraction is later recruited to the graft to complete the process. While Th can mount an independent rejection response (as they do in DTH reactions), they do so more effectively in concert with the CD8+ fraction. Host precursor Tc/s respond to IL-2 elaborated by Th and migrate to the graft progressively throughout the course of rejection. Direct cytotoxicity then assists the coordinated immune system in destroying the allogeneic tissue, after which both T cell subsets may revert to a resting state as memory cells.

CELL MEDIATORS

The critical role of mediators influencing other cell populations and subpopulations in the immunological cascade is becoming increasingly appreciated, particularly with the availability of mAbs directed against the cytokines themselves or receptors for such cytokines. Various effector cell populations may elaborate one or more factors after appropriate stimulation which may in turn act on other cells to activate (or suppress) their activity. Thus, in vitro at least, macrophages which have been activated by graft antigen produce a monokine, interleukin-1, which in turn will stimulate CD4+ cells to give off IL-2.

The next early events of T lymphocyte activation include formation of receptors for insulin, transferrin, IL-1 and IL-2. The development of high affinity surface receptors for IL-2 (IL-2R+) on the majority of CD4+ and CD8+ T cells, some B cells, macrophages and DC is particularly critical (Smith, 1984). Thus, binding of IL-2 to its receptor is followed by internalization of the IL-2/IL-2R complex which transduces the signal for proliferation and clonal expansion of most activated T lymphocytes, driving the entire rejection response forward (Figure 6). It has recently been shown that about 15% of cells infiltrating acutely rejecting rat heart grafts are IL-2R+ (Hancock et al, 1987), and over 20% of lymphocytes express IL-2R in a popliteal lymph node model (Kroczek et al, 1978). That this relatively small population is important in graft rejection has been shown in several species including man (Diamantstein et al, 1987).

Stimulated CD4+ lymphocytes seem primarily responsible for the elaboration of several humoral mediators. It has also been suggested that this subpopulation can itself be subdivided into at least two classes (Th_1 and Th_2) which may elaborate quite distinct lymphokines (Table 1) (Mosmann and Coffman, 1984). One of these, Th_1-derived γ-interferon (IFNγ), has diverse effects on immune responsiveness. It induces class I and class II MHC molecules on selected cell populations, primarily vascular endothelial cells, augments B cell-stimulating lymphocytes, increases antibody production and amplifies macrophage and monocyte activity (Jacob et al, 1987). However, in some experimental models IFNγ antagonizes the action of IL-1 and IL-4. Transfer of cloned IFNγ to an otherwise unresponsive organ graft recipient may produce acute graft loss.

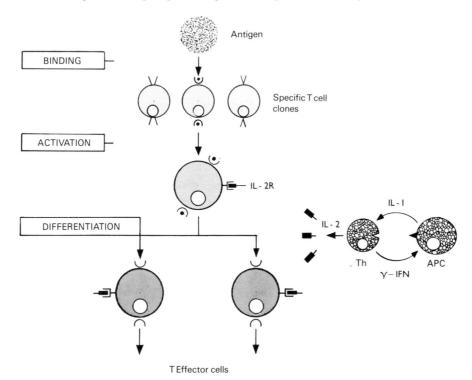

Figure 6.   The central role of IL-2 receptor (IL-2R) in T lymphocyte activation. Acquisition of IL-2R, the target for CD4-derived IL-2, is prerequisite for clonal expansion of T effector cells which are instrumental in the rejection response. APC, antigen presenting cell; γ-IFN, γ-interferon. (Adapted from Tilney et al, 1987.)

Table 1.   Types of murine CD4+ T cells. (Adapted from Mosmann and Coffman, 1984.)

Characteristics	Th$_1$	Th$_2$
Lymphokine production		
IL-2	+	−
IL-3	+	+
IL-4	−	+
IL-5	−	+
IFNγ	+	−
LT	+	−
B cell help	+	++
DTH	+	−

DTH, Delayed-typed hypersensitivity responses; IFNγ, γ-interferon; LT, lymphotoxin (tumour necrosis factor β).

Recent studies have also stressed the role of cytotoxins released by macrophages and leukocytes in states of host cells responsiveness. For instance, these graft-infiltrating cells elaborate tumour necrosis factor (TNF) α (cachectin) and β TNF (lymphocytotoxin), respectively (Lowry and Blais, 1988). As TNFβ synergizes with IFNγ and IL-1, it is possible that these modalities contribute to parenchymal injury during the course of rejection. Finally, TNF released locally by the graft infiltrating cells may, in concert with IFNγ, stimulate MHC allotype expression at the graft site.

IMMUNOREGULATION BY SUPPRESSOR CELLS

The concept of suppression as an active immunoregulatory mechanism originated in studies of tolerance whereby fetal or neonatal animals exposed to specific antigens were unable permanently to react to the same antigen when it was presented in later life. Tolerant states are thymus-dependent; thymocytes from such animals induce specific immunological unresponsiveness following passive transfer into normal hosts while removal of such cells in bulk, such as by thymectomy, has been noted in several models of unresponsiveness to cause abrupt graft rejection (Hendry et al, 1979). It was shown subsequently that many graft recipients, modified non-specifically with various immuno-suppressive modalities, ultimately develop specific unresponsiveness to the graft (Kupiec-Weglinski et al, 1984).

T cells with suppressor characteristics (Ts) are presumably essential in producing and maintaining immunological homeostasis in animals exposed throughout their lives to a panoply of antigenic stimuli. Cells with suppressor activity have been identified in various immunological models and disease states both in vivo and in vitro, and will not be reviewed here. It is also becoming apparent that more than one population of Ts is responsible for inhibition of host responses. Indeed, there may be a complex pathway involving cell-to-cell interactions and their products which may occur sequentially, and may be orchestrated by cells differing in phenotype, MHC restriction and allospecificity. The T suppressor cell pathway, originally identified and described by Dorf and Benacerraf (1984) in a murine DTH model, has been recently adapted by Hutchinson (1986) who showed distinct T cell subsets appearing during the course of prolonged rat renal allograft survival (Figure 7). Three T cell elements have been described: Ts_1 inducer/suppressor cells; Ts_2 transducer cells; Ts_3 auxiliary or effector suppressor cells. In addition to other differences, Ts_1 and Ts_3 have been thought to bear antigen binding receptors that possess idiotype-related determinants, whereas Ts_2 have receptors for anti-idiotype. Some of these Ts subgroups release factors that mediate both specific and non-specific suppression by other cell populations.

Specific Ts have also been noted in many experimental models of unresponsiveness, including neonatally-induced tolerance, and in allograft recipients undergoing total lymphoid irradiation or pretreated with antigen, antibody or both. They have been detected in transplanted animals conditioned with donor blood and antilymphocyte serum or those treated with cyclosporin (Kupiec-Weglinski, 1984). It appears increasingly that the production of Ts by the host acts as a common denominator to maintain long-term unresponsiveness, regardless of the initial methods used to induce this state.

Ts activity even appears during the course of acute allograft rejection. Thus, Hutchinson (1986) found functionally active Ts infiltrating kidney allografts and spleens of unmodified hosts during rejection; Araujo (1985) described similar findings in heart grafted rats. Interestingly, the CD4+ and CD8+ cells were responsible for suppression in the early and late stages of rejection responses in the first model, CD8+ throughout in the second. It has been shown in several models that few phenotypic differences in infiltrating cell populations can be found when acutely-rejecting and long-surviving grafts are compared directly; this suggests that although Ts are present and active, they cannot be identified by available techniques; however, their function can supersede that of effector cells with presumably the same phenotype. Overall it appears that Th initiate the rejection response and exert their influence promptly, while Tc/s are, at least in part, not only responsible for carrying out graft destruction but for halting the systemic processes of immunological stimulation.

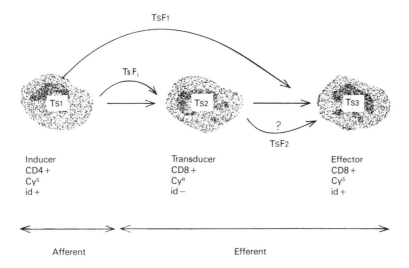

Figure 7. The T suppressor cell (Ts) pathway. Challenge of the recipient with the allograft induces, in addition to the rejection response, CD4+ Ts inducer cells (Ts$_1$). These cyclophosphamide sensitive (Cy^s) id+ cells elaborate an antigen-specific factor (TsF$_1$), which activates CD8+ Ts transducer (Ts$_2$) and Ts effector (Ts$_3$) cells. Ts$_1$ is id− and Cy resistant (Cy^R), whereas Ts$_3$ appears to be id+ and Cy^s. Ts$_1$ acts in the afferent, and Ts$_2$ and Ts$_3$ in the efferent, phase of the immune responses; i.e. Ts$_1$ prolongs test graft survival if transferred before, whereas Ts$_2$ and Ts$_3$ prolong test graft survival if transferred after transplantation. (Adapted from Hutchinson, 1986.)

Thus, there must be a balance between cytotoxicity and suppression in acute host alloresponsiveness, where destruction of allogeneic tissue is ultimately stopped by suppressor mechanisms. The appearance of Ts, regardless of phenotype, in the later stages of rejection apparently represents a host protective mechanism which may be responsible for the resolution of this dramatic event leading to the destruction of transplanted tissues and restoration of the host to immunological homeostasis after the process has become well established. Whether the Ts that emerge during the rejection process represent the same population (though quantitatively different) governing graft acceptance after other types of immunomodulation is unknown, but is a distinct possibility.

CELL MIGRATION PATTERNS DURING ACUTE GRAFT REJECTION

Although the role of T lymphocytes as mediators of acute immune responsiveness has been well established, the mechanisms causing different functional cell populations and subpopulations to accumulate in histoincompatible organ grafts remain unclear. Factors responsible for lymphocyte migration to the allograft may include surface antigen differences between donor and recipient cells, the presence of lymphokines in the graft microenvironment, and the specific predilection of T lymphocyte subsets to a particular graft. Thus, a question that inevitably arises is: are sensitized lymphocytes attracted within allografts because of specific alloantigen recognition or are they retained indiscriminately after entering it from the circulation? When lymphocytes sensitized against disparate donor antigens were radiolabelled differentially in vitro and the mixed suspensions transferred adoptively into rat recipients of two heart or skin allografts of differing genotypes, preferential accumulation of specifically sensitized cells occurred consistently in the appropriate allograft (Tilney et al, 1978); however, the immunospecificity of the cellular accumulation was relatively small. Thus, the cellular interactions induced by the recruited antigen-specific lymphocytes presumably invoke non-specific mechanisms for the retention of other, uncommitted T lymphocytes. These localize indiscriminately, probably as part of a general inflammatory response and, when activated, produce lymphokines chemotactic for other effector lymphocytes and mononuclear cells important in the efferent arc of immunity.

The progressive cellular infiltration of the graft emphasizes the importance of the cell-mediated responses in both recognition and destruction of the antigen. Kinetic studies of rat organ grafts have revealed significant accumulation of adoptively transferred lymphocytes in allografts as early as the first day after transplantation, peaking at day 5, the time when the grafts are undergoing obvious rejection; simultaneous histopathological evaluation has confirmed these migrational patterns (Figure 8). However, it is of interest that despite the dramatic infiltration of host lymphoid cells at day 5, rejecting allografts retransplanted back into a donor strain host recover and go on to survive indefinitely (Kupiec-Weglinski et al, 1985), suggesting that even extensive and well-advanced cellular involvement of the rejecting graft is insufficient to produce its destruction in the absence of sustained host response.

Although 'acute rejection' refers primarily to the destruction of the foreign tissue itself, the process affects profoundly host lymphoid and non-lymphoid tissues. Under physiological conditions normal splenocytes localize more selectively in the spleen than in mesenteric and peripheral lymph nodes; however, during acute rejection of vascularized organ grafts accumulation of radiolabelled cells in the spleen is high in the early stages but declines thereafter, the effect of apparent migration of newly 'armed' cells to the graft site (Kupiec-Weglinski et al, 1982). The spleen is the first effective point of contact between lymphocytes and antigen and is a prominent site for antigen localization and processing. Transferred lymphocytes migrate selectively from the circulation to the splenic microenvironment ('ecotaxis') either through recognition and reaction to antigens or homing to the tissue of origin. In contrast to a subsequently decreased uptake of lymphocytes by the spleen because of active migration to the graft, radioactivity of lymph nodes steadily increases and peaks at the time of actual graft destruction. This lymph node-seeking cell population is enriched for recirculating cells and plays an important role in the recognition phase of rejection, probably as an 'emergency' source of lymphocytes able to move quickly to the site of antigenic challenge.

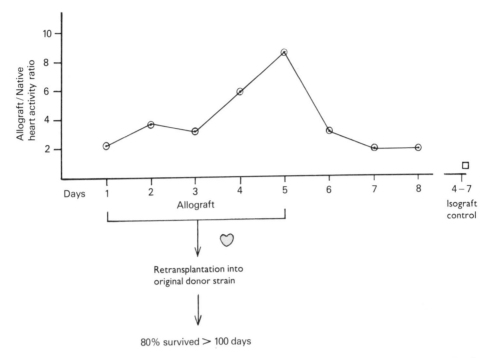

Figure 8. Host–graft relationship – the systemic nature of the rejection response. Radio-actively labelled lymphocytes accumulate progressively in acutely rejecting heart allografts in untreated rats; the peak of infiltration occurs at day 5, i.e. 2–3 days before actual graft loss. However, the majority of these acutely rejecting hearts (day 1–5) will survive indefinitely following retransplantation into normal naive secondary recipients of the original donor strain. Thus, even well-advanced changes at the graft site may be reversed without continu-ous host immunological drive. (Adapted from Kupiec-Weglinski et al, 1985.)

An immunological link between the liver and host lymphoid tissues has also been noted (Kupiec-Weglinski et al, 1982). After splenectomy of recipients acutely rejecting their grafts, adoptively transferred spleen cells that are usually sequestered in the spleen accumulate in higher numbers in the liver; in normal splenectomized rats they are diverted to lymph nodes. Thus, the liver, although not an immunologically active organ, may play a greater role than has been appreciated by serving as a temporary storage area for lymphoid cells rather than a solitary site of their destruction.

SUMMARY

Continuing investigations into acute rejection of allografted tissues has deepened appreciation of the profound complexities of the cascade of host events that lead to dramatic graft destruction, particularly the roles of cell populations and subpopulations, their humoral products and their interactions. Much effort has been expended in recent years in determining the types of cells causing rejection. T lymphocytes are primarily responsible for first set (acute) rejection of MHC incompatible grafts. The relative contribution of particular T cell subsets may depend on the nature of the graft, the degree of host sensitization and the antigenic disparity between donor and recipient; debate continues regarding the individual roles of CD4 (T helper/inducer, Th) and CD8 (T cytotoxic/suppressor, Tc/s) phenotypes in rejection. It appears increasingly that Th cells initiate the events of rejection; Tc/s, activated by Th derived factors, facilitate completion of the process.

The critical influence of cell products or mediators on other cell populations in the immunological cascade is also becoming increasingly appreciated. In particular, IL-2 has been shown both in vitro and in vivo to drive rejection forward. T and some B lymphocytes, as well as macrophages, express surface receptors for IL-2 (IL-2R) when activated, a discrete population which seems crucial in mediating the rejection process as shown by monoclonal antibodies (mAb) directed specifically against the receptors. Differential effects of anti-IL-2R mAb isotypes and IL-2R epitopes are under study. Gamma interferon (IFNγ) has been implicated in rejection. Transfer of this material to otherwise unresponsive recipients may produce acute rejection of their grafts; administration of anti-IFNγ mAb delays the rejection process. Although the function of tumour necrosis factor (TNF) in rejection is unknown, synergy between TNFα and IFNγ produces parenchymal injury.

An apparent common denominator of various states of host unresponsiveness involves cells with suppressor activity. It is becoming increasingly clear that no single cell is responsible for suppression; a cascade including at least three subpopulations and their individual products may sustain immunoregulation against the panoply of antigenic stimuli bombarding the host throughout life, as well as restoring immunological homeostasis following completion of rejection.

REFERENCES

Adams DO & Hamilton TA (1987) Molecular transduction mechanisms by which IFN-gamma and other signals regulate macrophage development. *Immunological Reviews* **97**: 5–27.

Araujo JL, Kupiec-Weglinski JW, Araneda D et al (1985) Phenotype, activation status, and suppressor activity of host lymphocytes during acute rejection and after cyclosporine induced unresponsiveness of rat cardiac allografts. *Transplantation* **40**: 278–284.

Austyn JM & Steinman TL (1988) Dendritic cells: A fresh view. In Morris PJ and Tilney NL (eds), *Transplant Reviews*, vol. 2, pp 139–176. Philadelphia: Grune and Stratton.

Austyn JM, Kupiec-Weglinski JW, Hawkins DF et al (1988) Migration patterns of dendritic cells in the mouse. Homing to T cell-dependent areas of spleen, and binding within marginal zone. *Journal of Experimental Medicine* **167**: 646–651.

Bach, FH, Bach MI & Sondel PM (1976) Differential function of major histocompatibility complex antigens in T-lymphocyte activation. *Nature* **259**: 273–281.

Bainbridge DR & Gowland G (1971) Studies on transplantation immunity: The nature of the response to allogeneic ⁵¹Cr labelled lymphoid cells and its relationship to homograft immunity. *Cellular Immunology* **2**: 115–127.

Baldwin WM III, Hendry W, Birinyi LK Jr & Tilney NL (1979) Immune responses to organ allografts. I. Intense B cell response to lymphoid tissue of unmodified rats to heart allografts. *Laboratory Investigation* **40**: 695–702.

Barker CF & Billingham RE (1977) Immunologically privileged sites. *Advances in Immunology* **25**: 1–54.

Billingham RW (1971) The passenger cell concept in transplantation immunology. *Cellular Immunology* **2**: 1–12.

Billingham RE, Brent L & Medawar PB (1954) Quantitation studies on tissue transplantation immunity. I. The survival times of skin homografts exchanged between members of different inbred strains of mice. *Proceedings of the Royal Society of London*, Series B. **143**: 43.

Cobbold, SP, Thierfelder S & Waldman H (1983) Immunosuppression with monoclonal antibodies. A model to determine the rules for effective serotherapy. *Molecular Biology and Medicine* **1**: 285.

Diamantstein T, Osawa H, Kirkman RL et al (1987) Interleukin 2 receptor – A target immunosuppressive therapy. In Morris PJ & Tilney NL (eds), *Transplant Reviews*, vol. I, pp 177–196. Orlando: Grune and Stratton.

Dorf ME & Benacerraf B (1984) Suppressor cells and immunoregulation. *Annual Reviews of Immunology* **2**: 127–158.

Faustman D, Stackman RM, Grebel H et al (1985) Prevention of rejection of murine islet allografts by pretreatment with anti-dendritic cell antibody. *Proceedings of the National Academy of Sciences USA*, **81**: 3864–3868.

Fuggle S, Errasti P, Daar A et al (1983) Localization of major histocompatibility complex (HLA-ABC and DR) antigens in 46 kidneys: differences in HLA-DR staining of tubules among kidneys. *Transplantation* **35**: 385–390.

Gowans JL, McGregor DD, Cowen DM & Ford CE (1962) Initiation of immune response by small lymphocytes. *Nature* **196**: 651–655.

Hall JS (1967) Studies of the cells in the afferent and efferent lymph of lymph nodes draining the site of skin homografts. *Journal of Experimental Medicine* **125**: 737–754.

Hancock WW, Lord RH, Colby AJ et al (1987) Identification of IL2R+ T cells and macrophages within rejecting rat cardiac allografts and comparison of the effects of treatment with anti-IL2R monoclonal antibody and cyclosporine. *Journal of Immunology* **138**: 164–170.

Häyry P, von Willebrand E, Parthenais E et al (1984) The inflammatory mechanisms of allograft rejection. *Immunological Reviews* **77**: 85–142.

Hendry WS, Tilney NL, Baldwin WM III et al (1979) Transfer of specific unresponsiveness to organ allografts by thymocytes. *Journal of Experimental Medicine* **149**: 1042–1055.

Heslop BF & Hardy BE (1971) The distribution of ^{51}Cr-labelled syngeneic and allogeneic lymph node cells in the rat. *Transplantation* **11**: 128–134.

Hume DM & Egdahl RH (1955) Progressive destruction of renal homografts isolated from the regional lymphatics of the host. *Surgery* **38**: 194–214.

Hutchinson IV (1986) Suppressor T cells in allogeneic models. *Transplantation* **41**: 547–555.

Jacob CO, van der Meide PH & McDevitt HO (1987) In vivo treatment of (NZB × NZW)F1 lupus-like nephritis with monoclonal antibody to gamma interferon. *Journal of Experimental Medicine* **66**: 798–803.

Kroczek RA, Black CDV, Barbet J et al (1978) Induction of IL-2 receptor expression in vivo. *Transplantation* **44**: 547–553.

Kupiec-Weglinski JW, Bordes-Aznar J, Clason AE et al (1982) Migration patterns of lymphocytes in untreated and immuologically manipulated recipients of organ allografts. *Transplantation* **33**: 593–598.

Kupiec-Weglinski JW, Filho MA, Strom TB et al (1984) Sparing of suppressor cells: a central action of cyclosporine. *Transplantation* **38**: 97–101.

Kupiec-Weglinski JW, Araujo JL, Towpik E, Araneda D & Tilney NL (1985) Host–graft relationships: the systemic nature of rejection. *Surgery* **98**: 254–265.

Lafferty KJ, Gill RJ, Babcock SK et al (1986) Activation and expression of allograft immunity. In Morris PJ and Tilney NL (eds), *Progress in Transplantation*, vol. 3, pp 55–84. Edinburgh: Churchill Livingstone.

Lechler RI & Batchelor JR (1982) Restoration of immunogenicity to passenger cell depleted kidney allografts by the addition of donor strain dendritic cells. *Journal of Experimental Medicine* **155**: 31–41.

Lowry RP & Blais D (1988) Tumor necrosis factor-alpha in rejecting rat cardiac allografts. *Transplantation Proceedings* **20**: 245–247.

Mason D W (1988) The roles of T cell subpopulations in allograft rejection *Transplantation Proceedings* **20**: 239–242.

Mason DW & Morris PJ (1986) Effector mechanisms in allograft rejection. *Annual Reviews of Immunology* **4**: 119–145.

Milton AD, Spencer SC & Fabre JW (1986) Detailed analysis and demonstration of differences in the kinetics of induction of class I and class II major histocompatibility complex antigens in rejecting cardiac and kidney allografts. *Transplantation* **41**: 499–508.

Mosmann TR & Coffman RL (1984) Two types of mouse helper T cell clone. Implications for murine regulation. *Immunology Today* **8**: 223–227.

Nathan CF, Murray HW & Cohn ZA (1980) The macrophage as an effector cell. *New England Journal of Medicine* **303**: 622–626.

Nemlander A, Saksela E & Häyry P (1983) Are 'natural killer' cells involved in allograft rejection? *European Journal of Immunology* **13**: 348–350.

Pedersen NC & Morris B (1970) The role of the lymphatic system in the rejection of homografts: A study of lymph from renal transplants. *Journal of Experimental Medicine* **131**: 936–969.

Peugh WN, Austyn JN, Carter NP et al (1987) The ability of dendritic cells to prevent the blood transfusion effect in a mouse cardiac allograft model. *Transplantation* **44**: 706–711.

Rygaard, J (1974) Thymus and Self. In Rygaard J and Povlsen CO (eds) *Proceedings of the First International Workshop on Nude Mice, Aarhus, Denmark, 1973.* Stuttgart: G. Fischer.

Scothorne RJ & MacGregor IA (1953) The vascularization of autografts and homografts of rabbit skin. *Journal of Anatomy* **87**: 379–386.

Sherwood RA, Brent L & Rayfield LS (1986) Presentation of alloantigens by host cells. *European Journal of Immunology* **16**: 569–574.

Snedire B & Schwartz R (1981) Antigen-specific proliferating T lymphocyte clones: methodology, specificity, MHC construction and alloreactivity. *Immunological Reviews* **54**: 187–224.

Smith KA (1984) Interleukin 2. *Annual Reviews of Immunology* **2**: 319–333.

Souther S G, Morris RE & Vistnes LM (1974) Prolongation of rat cardiac allograft survival by splenectomy following transplantation. *Transplantation* **17**: 317–319.

Stark RB, Dwyer EM & Forest MD (1960) Effect of surgical ablation of regional lymph nodes on survival of skin homografts. *Annals of the New York Academy of Sciences* **87**: 140–148.

Tilney NL, Strom TB, Macpherson SG & Carpenter CB (1975) Surface properties and functional characteristics of infiltrating cells harvested from acutely rejecting cardiac allografts in inbred rats. *Transplantation* **20**: 323–330.

Tilney, NL, McConarty JN & Strom TB (1978) Specificity of cellular migration into cardiac allografts in rats. *Transplantation* **26**: 181–186.

Tilney NL, Kupiec-Weglinski JW, Heidecke CD, Lear PA & Strom TB (1984) Mechanisms of rejection and prolongation of vascularized organ allografts. *Immunological Reviews* **77**: 185–216.

Tilney NL, Strom TB & Kupiec-Weglinski JW (1987) Humoral and cellular mechanisms in acute allograft injury. *Journal of Pediatrics* **111**: 1000–1003.

Wagner H, Hardt C & Heeg K (1980) T–T cell interactions during cytotoxic T lymphocyte (CTL) responses: T cell derived helper factor (interleukin 2) as a probe to analyze CTL responsiveness and thymic maturation of CTL progenitors. *Immunological Reviews* **51**: 215.

3 Immunosuppression in Tissue and Organ Transplantation

TERRY B. STROM

The success of organ transplantation, which is considered the treatment of choice in a variety of end-stage diseases, is limited primarily by allograft rejection. The immunological nature of allograft rejection was demonstrated as early as 1943 by Gibson and Medawar (see Appendix III). Medawar's group demonstrated in the early 1950s that the immune system could be modulated to prevent the rejection process, bringing about permanent skin graft survival in experimental animals (see Appendix III). Direct manipulation of the host's immune response provides a practical means of achieving success even when tissue matching of donor and recipient is less than optimal. However, although several highly efficacious immunosuppresive agents have been developed over 20 years, acute rejection occurring within days or months after a transplant operation is still a major obstacle to the success of organ replacement.

Immunosuppression in organ transplantation is in a state of flux. Although immunosuppression to abrogate host reactivity to allografts has been applied since the early days of clinical transplantation, immunosuppressive agents and protocols are constantly evolving. Treatment modalities may vary from organ to organ even though the same agents are used. No attempt will be made here to discuss the manifold protocols developed at different centres for a variety of transplanted organs.

During the early 1970s there was little improvement in graft survival, but a steady improvement in patient survival was seen as experience with monitoring and management of infectious complications improved. Clinical immunosuppression has advanced from the use of steroids and antimetabolites such as azathioprine, which provide a generalized modulation of the immune response, through the more finely targeted antilymphocyte sera, cyclosporin and, more recently, monoclonal antibodies.

Immunotherapy should, preferably, be donor-specific and targeted to minimize the risks of non-specific immunosuppression. An ideal immunosuppressant would specifically block the activities of only the small population of antigen-specific cells actually engaged in the events of rejection. Hence, a brief description of the molecular events of T cell activation and rejection follows (see also Chapter 2).

ORGAN TRANSPLANTATION: CURRENT CLINICAL AND
IMMUNOLOGICAL CONCEPTS   ISBN 0-7020-1393-5

T CELL ACTIVATION AND GRAFT REJECTION

Each of the agents used to suppress rejection blocks certain aspects of T cell activation. It is therefore important to understand the mechanisms of rejection in order to deduce the mode of action of immunosuppressive drugs. Cell-mediated rejection is effected by a diverse assembly of white blood cells, including CD8 + cytotoxic T cells, CD4 + helper T cells, antibody-forming B cells and macrophages. However, the rejection process is totally dependent upon a small population of T cells that bear recognition units, or receptors, for the histocompatibility antigens of the donor graft (Strom, 1984).

The T cell antigen recognition complex, which has been long postulated, but only recently defined in molecular tems, is a six-peptide chain structure that includes two immunoglobulin-like chains whose genes undergo recombination during T cell maturation, akin to the well described recombination events involved in the generation of antibody specificity in B cells (Kronenberg et al, 1986). These are the α and β T cell receptor chains. The other four chains, called CD3 proteins, are non-covalently linked to the α and β T cell receptor chains and are involved in the transmembrane signal produced by interaction of the α and β T cell receptor proteins with antigen (Weiss et al, 1986).

As a result of the encounter of donor-specific T cell clones with graft antigens, T cell activation and proliferation occur. The cascade of activation-associated events culminates in a remarkable amplification of immune activity by attracting a large number and wide variety of activated white blood cells into the graft. These events can now be described in a molecular context.

The cascade is initiated by the presentation of incompatible graft antigens to the host. Helper cells bearing the distinctive CD4 protein are not activated so much by donor HLA class I molecules of the HLA-A, B or C loci as by class II molecules such as HLA-DR. The CD4 protein binds to non-polymorphic region of HLA class II, thereby giving further strength to the attachment of the CD4 + T cell to the class II + donor cell. In contrast, cytotoxic T cells bearing the CD8 protein are activated primarily via recognition of HLA class I molecules of the graft.

T cell activation is initiated when those few clones of T cells bearing cell surface receptors specific for the graft antigens actively bind to these graft antigens. However, while antigen is the first external signal required for initiating T cell activation, antigen recognition is not itself sufficient to bring about T cell proliferation (Figure 1). Activated accessory cells, e.g., dendritic cells or macrophages, are likewise required. Direct cell–cell contact betwen T cells and macrophages, or stimulation of macrophages by soluble T cell products causes macrophage activation (Figure 2), which is required for support of full T cell activation (Williams et al, 1985). Engagement of T cell receptors with antigen causes the formation of intracellular second messengers that transduce signals from the cell membrane to the T cell nucleus (Figure 1) (Meuer et al, 1984; Weiss et al, 1985).

Investigations in several laboratories indicate that the cytoplasmic second messengers formed in T cells in response to antigen stimulation result from activation of phosphatidylinositol biphosphate to diacylglycerol, which activates protein kinase C, and inositol triphosphate which causes a precipitous rise in free cytosolic calcium (Figure 1). Some of the increased free cytosolic calcium may be mobilized from extracellular sources. In macrophages and other accessory cells activation by T cells or their products elicits the formation of second messengers which, in turn, activate the interleukin 1 (IL-1) gene. Transcription of messenger RNA encoding IL-1 proceeds, followed by translation of large α and β pro-IL-1 molecules (Figure 2) (Auron et al, 1987). Precursor molecules are cleaved intracellularly, and

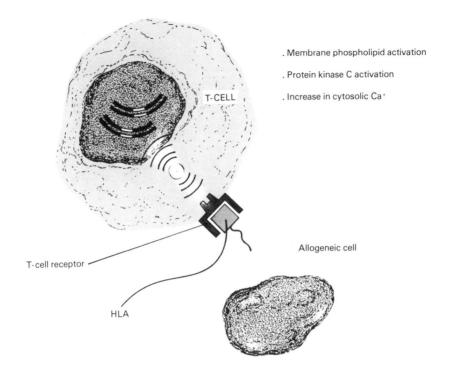

. Membrane phospholipid activation

. Protein kinase C activation

. Increase in cytosolic Ca$^+$

T-CELL

T-cell receptor

HLA

Allogeneic cell

Figure 1. The immune response to allogeneic tissues is initiated as T cells bearing antigen-specific receptor recognition units bind to alloantigen-bearing transplanted tissues. T cell activation signals initiated through engagement of antigen receptors are transduced via intra-cellular messengers.

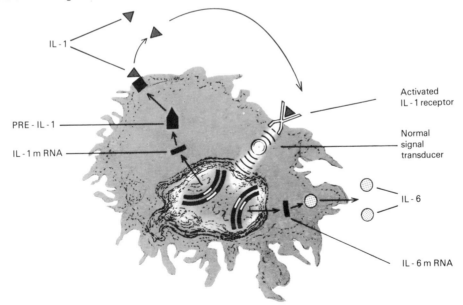

IL - 1

Activated
IL - 1 receptor

PRE - IL - 1

Normal
signal
transducer

IL - 1 m RNA

IL - 6

IL - 6 m RNA

Figure 2. Immune activation of alloantigen-specific T cells also results in activation of macrophages. Activated macrophages manufacture pro-inflammatory cytokines that support T cell activation.

the considerably smaller mature forms of IL-1 are secreted (Figure 2). IL-1 is an autocrine factor that activates transcription of the IL-6 gene in macrophages (Figure 2).

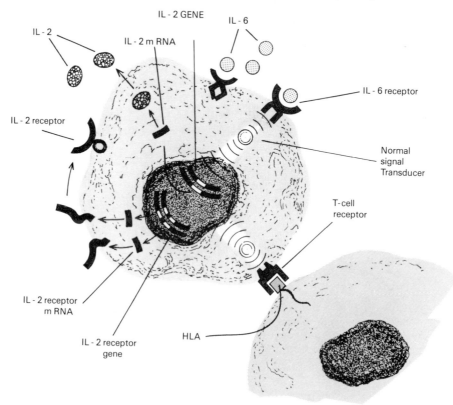

Figure 3.   At least two signals are required to stimulate T cell proliferation. Engagement of the T cell antigen receptor by antigen is necessary but not sufficient for T cell activation. Full T cell activation requires stimulation by antigen and accessory cells or their products.

T cells are stimulated by antigen and IL-6 to secrete the T cell growth factor, interleukin 2 (IL-2) (Pankewycz et al, 1989) and express de novo cell surface IL-2 receptors (Figure 3) (Cantrell and Smith, 1984; Williams et al, 1984; Weiss et al, 1986). This is of central importance in the events of T cell activation for several reasons (Weiss et al, 1985; Auron et al, 1987). IL-2 is not only a growth factor, but also stimulates antigen-activated T cells to release several other lymphokines that are critical to the events of rejection (Figure 4) (Howard et al, 1983; Inaba et al, 1983; Ythier et al, 1985). IL-2 serves a crucial role in eliciting the secretion of bioactive T cell-derived proteins called lymphokines that activate T cells, B cells and macrophages. Antigen-activated, IL-2-stimulated T cells release B cell activation factors (Inaba et al, 1983), such as IL-4 and IL-5, that enable antigen-activated B cells, to elaborate high-affinity, high-titre, anti-graft antibodies. IL-2 causes helper cells to release factors that permit the cytotoxic capacity of cytotoxic T cells to develop. It stimulates, too, the release of γ interferon (IFNγ) (Farrar et al, 1981) which in turn activates the cytodestructive activities of macrophages. Further, this lymphokine stimulates cells of the transplant that normally do not express class II HLA molecules to express such molecules (Pober et al, 1983; Kelley et al, 1984). The interaction of IL-2 and IL-2 receptors stimulates clonal proliferation (Figure 5) of both antigen-activated helper and cytotoxic T cells (Cantrell and Smith, 1984). IL-2 is also an anabolic factor essential for the viability of activated T cells (Maddock et al, 1985). Thus, IL-2-dependent mechanisms result in the activation of B cells, helper cells, cytotoxic cells and macrophages. Moreover, the allograft displays new HLA molecules induced by the actions of IL-2-dependent secretion of IFNγ, thus initiating a vicious circle of rejection-associated events. The initial response of a small number of donor-specific T cell clones, therefore, permits the activation of a critical mass of clonally expanded, antigen-activated T cells and other cells required for rejection.

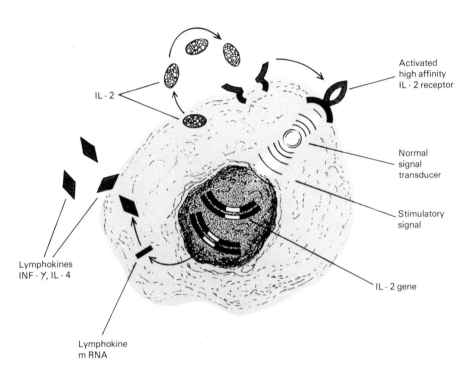

Figure 4. While activation of T cells by antigen and accessory cells initiated T cell activation, interleukin-2 plays a central role in T cell activation. IL-2 receptor-bearing, antigen-activated lymphocytes can be stimulated to secrete lymphokines by IL-2.

Nature has, fortunately, ensured that antigen-stimulated T cell lymphoproliferation can eventually be halted. As time passes following antigen activation, transcription of mRNA encoding lymphokine and IL-2 receptor slows down and the remaining transcripts, which are inherently labile molecules, degenerate. In the absence of IL-2 and IL-2 receptors, T cell proliferation ceases, and T cells revert, in the main, to the functional status of resting cells. Active intervention by suppressor cells may also contribute to regulation of the immune response.

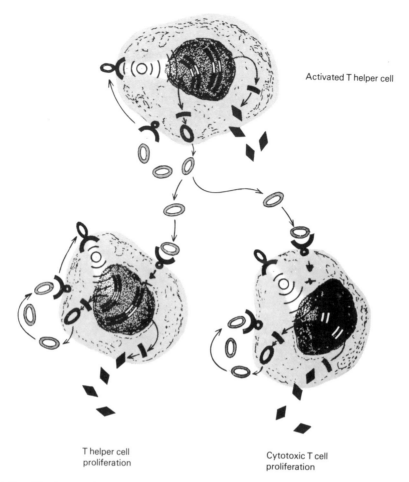

Activated T helper cell

T helper cell
proliferation

Cytotoxic T cell
proliferation

Figure 5.   The interaction of interleukin-2 (a T cell growth factor) with antigen-activated T cells bearing high affinity IL-2 receptors stimulates proliferation of these IL-2 receptor-responsive cells. The IL-2-responsive population includes cytotoxic T cells and lymphokine-secreting cells. As a consequence, the small population of donor-specific alloreactive cells propagates and becomes instrumental in rejecting the allograft.

IMMUNOSUPPRESSION IN GRAFT REJECTION

Immunosuppressive therapy to prevent or reverse acute rejection attempts to abrogate selectively the patient's reactivity to the allograft, while sparing as much as possible the immune response to other foreign antigens. Although this ideal immunosuppression has not been fully achieved, great strides have been made.

Three drugs have gained wide acceptance in the prevention of renal allograft rejection. The success of azathioprine and prednisone in the control of acute graft rejection was the breakthrough that allowed kidney transplantation to become a routinely applicable clinical reality. In 1983, somewhat belatedly, cyclosporin gained FDA approval in the United States and proved to be a boon to transplantation. One-year cadaver kidney graft survival improved by 15–20%; transplantation of other organs benefitted even more; heart–lung transplantation became possible, and both graft and patient survival improved in heart and liver transplants (see Appendix Ib & c). Each of these drugs blocks T cell proliferation, albeit at a slightly different step in the activation cascade. However, none of these agents inhibits the initial engagement of T cells by antigen.

Corticosteroids

Most immunosuppressive drug regimens employ an adrenal corticosteroid such as predni-sone in combination with other immunosuppressive agents. Corticosteroids provide the most proximal block in the T cell activation cascade; they interfere with T cell proliferation through their ability to block activation of the IL-1 and IL-6 genes (Figure 6) (Knudsen et al,

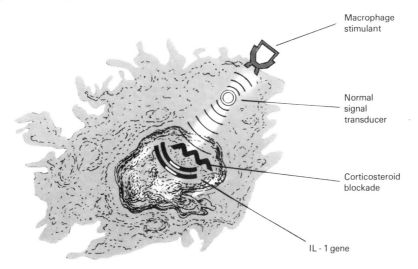

Macrophage
stimulant

Normal
signal
transducer

Corticosteroid
blockade

IL - 1 gene

Figure 6. Corticosteroids block activation of the IL-1 (and IL-6) genes.

unpublished data). Corticosteroid-treated macrophages do not produce IL-1-encoding mRNA, even when subsequently cultured in the presence of powerful macrophage stimu-lants. IL-1 was previously called endogenous pyrogen, because one of the major activities of this protein is to stimulate the thermoregulatory centres of the central nervous system and thereby to cause fever. The ability of steroids to prevent fever in septic states almost certainly derives from the blocking of IL-1 release. The fever associated with allograft rejection is probably caused by the secretion of IL-1. Febrile renal transplant recipients experiencing rejection generally do not improve their glomerular filtration rate unless steroid treatment first abolishes fever. Because IL-2 release is dependent upon IL-1-stimu-lated IL-6 release (see Figure 3), corticosteroids also indirectly block IL-2 (Table 1).

Conventional therapies for the treatment of acute renal allograft rejection include high-dose pulses of glucocorticoids. Glucocorticoids have broad, non-specific immunosuppres-sive and anti-inflammatory effects. Besides their effects on lymphokines, glucocorticoids reduce the migration of monocytes to sites of inflammation. A major drawback to the use of glucocorticoids in the treatment of acute rejection is that they inhibit the entire immune and inflammatory systems and alter many other steroid-responsive systems as well. The use of high doses of glucocorticoids can thus produce severe undesirable side-effects. These include decreased inflammatory and phagocytic capacity, resulting in increased susceptibility to infection, hyperglycaemia, hyperkalaemia, osteoporosis, increased capillary fragility, and growth suppression in children.

Table 1.   Steroids in immunosuppression.

Mode of action	Side-effects
Blocks IL-1 release directly	Increased susceptibility to infection
Blocks IL-6 release directly	
Blocks IL-2 release	Impaired wound healing
Non-specific immunosuppressive and anti-inflammatory effects	Growth suppression in children
	Aseptic necrosis of bone
Inhibits migration of immune cells to site of inflammation	Depression, sleep disturbances with high dose
	Hyperglycaemia
	Oedema
	Hypertension

Azathioprine

Although useful for inhibiting primary immune responses, azathioprine has little effect on secondary responses or in the reversal of acute allograft rejections. It blocks T cell activation at the most distal point compared with the other two drugs discussed here. This antimetabolite (Bach and Strom, 1986) is the imidazole derivative of 6-mercaptopurine and exerts its mode of action by blocking DNA synthesis. Azathioprine is catabolized in vivo to 6-mercaptopurine and other antimetabolites. It does not prevent initial gene activation, but instead powerfully inhibits gene replication and T cell activation (Figure 7; Table 2).

Further, azathioprine decreases the number of migratory mononuclear and granulocytic cells whilst inhibiting the proliferation of promyelocytes within bone marrow. As a result, the number of circulating monocytes capable of differentiating into macrophages is decreased. Among the possible deleterious effects of azathioprine administration are severe leukopenia and/or thrombocytopenia, gastrointestinal disturbances, fever, hepatotoxicity, and an increased risk of neoplasia.

Table 2.   Azathioprine in immunosuppression.

Mode of action	Side-effects
Inhibits DNA and RNA synthesis	Myelocyte suppression
Decreases the number of migratory mononuclear and granulocytic cells	Dose-related leukopenia, thrombocytopenia
	Gastrointestinal disturbances
Inhibits promyelocyte proliferation	Hepatotoxicity
	Increased risk of certain neoplasia
	Increased susceptibility to infection

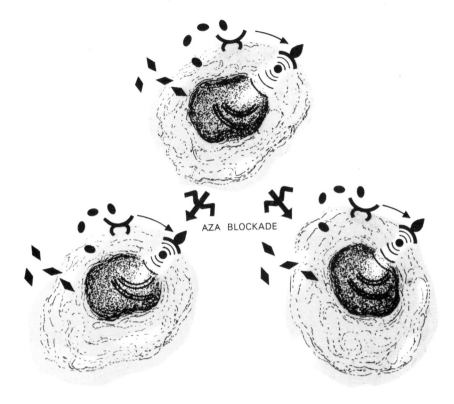

Figure 7.   Azathioprine is a classical antimetabolite and blocks cell proliferation.

Cyclosporin

The more recent introduction of cyclosporin, a small cyclic peptide of fungal origin, has played a major role in preventing the primary immunological reactions that endanger the success of organ and bone marrow transplants, and has resulted in improved graft survival rates in treated patients (see Appendix I). Due to its mode of action, cyclosporin (like azathioprine) is of limited value in the treatment of acute allograft rejection.

Cyclosporin blocks T cells at a slightly more distal step than corticosteroids. Elements of T cell activation proceed in an unimpeded fashion in the presence of cyclosporin, which does not totally prevent activation of the IL-2 receptor gene and which does not completely interfere with IL-2 receptor expression on the surface of antigen-stimulated T cells (Figure 8). Its primary action is to block the activation of the IL-2 and other lymphokine genes so that IL-2 encoding mRNA is not transcribed and IL-2 is not secreted (Granelli-Piperno et al, 1984). In the absence of IL-2, T cells do not proliferate, macrophage-activing IFNγ is not released, B cell activating factors are not released, and the events of T cell activation are sharply curtailed. Cyclosporin is probably the most powerful of the available drugs used to prevent rejection, with the best risk–benefit ratio.

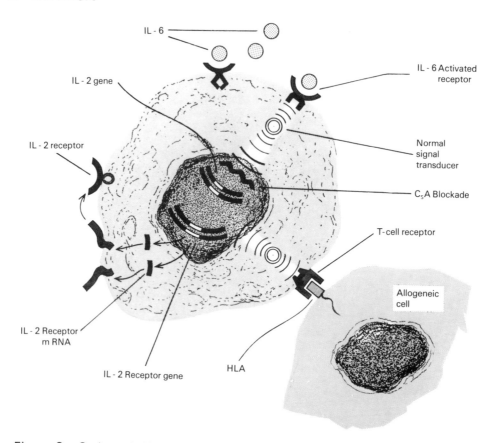

IL - 6

IL - 2 gene

IL - 2 receptor

IL - 2 Receptor
m RNA

IL - 2 Receptor gene

HLA

IL - 6 Activated
receptor

Normal
signal
transducer

C$_s$A Blockade

T-cell receptor

Allogeneic
cell

Figure 8.   Cyclosporin blocks activation of the IL-2 and other lymphokine genes. C$_s$A;
cyclosporin.

It is ironic that nephrotoxicity should be a major disadvantage of cyclosporin. This is of particular concern in renal transplantation because the features distinguishing cyclosporin toxicity from other causes of graft dysfunction are not clearly established. Signs of rejection such as an increase in serum creatinine level or oliguria may be due to cyclosporin toxicity, too, making the diagnosis more difficult, even with biopsy. Concern about the potentiation of early acute nephrotoxicity by cyclosporin has led to the development of regimens that avoid its use in the first few days after transplantation, and the use of other strong immunosuppressive agents such as monoclonal or polyclonal antithymocyte/lymphocyte globulin to supplement immunosuppression in the immediate post-transplant period (Hourmant et al, 1985).

Individual patients have remarkably different pharmacokinetic profiles after cyclosporin administration, with as many as 50% exhibiting a biphasic inhibition of mixed lymphocyte culture about 12 hours after a single dose; this suggests that cyclosporin should be given every 24 hours, rather than as the conventional 12-hour regimen (Kahan, 1984). Further definition of this variability, with the assessment of each patient's pharmacokinetic profile at the time of transplantation, might considerably improve this agent's risk–benefit ratio. A more fundamental hope is that a non-nephrotoxic derivative may soon be produced.

However, initial concern about the delayed severe kidney damage and extreme hypertension caused by cyclosporin has been largely alleviated by the gradual recognition that major reductions in cyclosporin dosage still provide excellent immunosuppression during the post-transplant months (Table 3).

Table 3.   Cyclosporin in immunosuppression.

Mode of action	Side-effects
Blocks activation of the IL-2 gene	Nephrotoxicity
Inhibits proliferation of T cells	Hepatotoxicity
	Hyperkalaemia
Prevents IFNγ release	Hypertension
Prevents release of B cell-activating factors	Hirsutism
	Breast fibroadenomas
	Gingival hypertrophy
	Increased susceptibility to infection
	Tremors or seizures

Multiple Drug Protocols

A regimen of azathioprine and prednisone in combination was the standard treatment for recipients of organ allografts prior to the introduction of cyclosporin. The widespread use of cyclosporin has significantly improved both patient and graft survival (see Appendix 1a); however, nephrotoxicity and the occurrence of rejection episodes remain drawbacks when cyclosporin is used as the sole drug. Although cyclosporin alone has been used with modest success in Europe, the results have not been as good in the United States. Accordingly, most European and North American transplant centres have evolved protocols using various combinations of drugs to reduce adverse drug reactions while maintaining improved patient and graft survival.

To date, almost all such protocols have included adjunctive steroid treatment. In the United States, studies in which patients were not splenectomized or extensively transfused prior to the transplantation, the addition of prednisone to the cyclosporin regimen improved graft survival. Prednisone appears to have a synergistic effect with cyclosporin, and this double drug regimen allows organ transplantation to patients who are HLA-mismatched, strong immune-responders, or those who have received no pre-transplantation transfusions.

Different schedules of cyclosporin, prednisone, and/or azathioprine have been adopted to reduce the potential cyclosporin-induced nephrotoxicity (Simmons et al, 1985). Each of the drugs blocks T cell proliferation, albeit at a slightly different step in the activation cascade. For that reason, triple drug therapy protocols may provide more effective immunosuppression. Further, the complications associated with any one drug could be minimized or even avoided in protocols employing lower doses of all three drugs. One practical advantage of triple drug therapy is that it permits more flexible immunosuppression. The dosage of the individual components can be altered to minimize complications or adverse effects (e.g. leukopenia, cyclosporin-induced nephrotoxicity, liver dysfunction) while maintaining adequate overall immunosuppression. However, the addition of a third drug to the immunosuppressive regimen can make patient management more difficult. Long-term results are needed to evaluate multiple drug protocols and to determine the optimal dosages.

Despite the encouraging results achieved thus far with multiple drug protocols, the shortcomings of current conventional immunosuppressive regimens cannot be ignored. These agents exert potent side-effects on non-lymphoid tissues. They impair the function of all T cells, not only the small proportion that mediate rejection; infection, therefore, remains a hazard. The well-documented modest increase in certain malignancies (Penn, 1978, 1987) remains a valid concern, but no one agent seems to produce a particular predisposition to malignancies.

TOWARDS SELECTIVE IMMUNOSUPPRESSION

Polyclonal Immune Globulins

Polyclonal antilymphocyte globulin (ALG) or antithymocyte globulin (ATG) preparations, available for use in organ transplantation since the 1970s, have proved to be more effective than steroids alone for reversing acute renal allograft rejection (Burdick, 1986; Cosimi and Delmonico, 1986). Such polyclonal immune globulins are obtained by injecting animals (e.g. horses, rabbits) with human lymphoid cells (e.g., B cell lymphoblasts, peripheral T cell lymphocytes, or thymus lymphocytes), and then separating the resulting immune sera to obtain purified γ globulin fractions.

Table 4.   Polyclonal immune globulins in immunosuppression.

Mode of action	Side-effects
Clearance of lymphocytes due to reticuloendothelial uptake	Thrombocytopenia, granulocytopenia
Complement-mediated lysis of lymphocytes	Antigen–antibody-induced glomerulonephritis
Blocking of lymphocyte function	Complex-mediated hypersensitivity (serum sickness)
Possible expansion of suppressor cell populations	Leukopenia
	Increased susceptibility to infection
	Fever, chills

Many types of cells have been evaluated as immunogens. Cultured lymphoblasts (to produce ALG) and human thymocytes (to produce ATG) are commonly used (Table 4). Cultured lymphoblasts are readily available, and are free of contaminating blood cells and stromal tissue, which could otherwise stimulate the production of unwanted antibodies. One possible disadvantage of cultured lymphoblasts arises from the fact that lymphoblasts are B cells rather than T cells (Burdick, 1986; Cosimi and Delmonico, 1986). Human thymus tissue, an excellent source of T cell antigens, may not always be available in adequate amounts. Absorption of antierythrocyte and antiplatelet antibodies is required with thymus cell preparations, yielding relatively pure antisera. Polyclonal immune globulins represent a heterogeneous group of antibodies, only a minority of which are specific to T cells. The irrelevant antibodies, in fact, account for the greatest binding activity of these preparations; some of them may react inappropriately with B cells and/or non-lymphoid tissue.

There are several possible mechanisms by which polyclonal immune globulin may exert its immunosuppressive effect. These include classic complement-mediated lysis of lymphocytes, clearance of lymphocytes due to reticuloendothelial uptake, expansion of suppressor cell populations, or the masking of T cell antigens, which may result in blocking of lymphocyte function. The specific antibodies bind to lymphocytes, and this usually results in a prompt and profound lymphopenia. The lymphopenia soon abates and the number of circulating T cells gradually increases, following cessation of treatment, although the proliferative response continues to be impaired. There is evidence that suggests that suppressor cells may be responsible for the prolonged immunosuppressive effect, after the resolution of lymphopenia. In short, the resolution of cell-mediated graft rejection results from the elimination of circulating T cells, and the subsequent positive inhibition of proliferative responses maintains the immunosuppressive effect (Burdick, 1986; Cosimi and Delmonico, 1986).

Each polyclonal immune globulin preparation varies in its constituent antibodies. Due to the unpredictable nature of the antibody mixture, treatment is associated with variable efficacy as well as with adverse reactions. Batch standardization and assessments of immunosuppressive potency are therefore difficult. Unwanted antibodies could cause thrombocytopenia, granulocytopenia, serum sickness, or glomerulonephritis. Owing to the development of host antibodies to the polyclonal immune globulin, anaphylactoid reactions are common (Burdick, 1986; Cosimi and Delmonico, 1986).

One early concern focuses on the potential for over-immunosuppression, not infrequently resulting in opportunistic infections. Caution is necessary when combining ATG with other immunosuppressive agents. Increased risk of over-immunosuppression has been related to the dosage and duration of therapy rather than the specific polyclonal immune globulin selected for treatment. If the effect on T cell levels is monitored, the dosage can be altered and the agent administered every other, or every third, day instead of daily, to achieve a level of T cells roughly 10% of that pre-treatment. The total treatment period for ATG is usually 10–14 days, antibody formation against the foreign protein being the limiting factor. It is generally necessary to administer polyclonal immune globulin through a central catheter because it tends to have an irritating sclerosing effect on peripheral veins. Intermittent fever, chills, and rash are ameliorated with administration of acetaminophen and diphenhydramine. Anaphylactic shock may have occurred in a few cases due to the formation of xenogeneic serum protein antibodies, but this is extremely rare.

Because initial clinical studies with polyclonal immune globulin as a prophylactic immunosuppressant showed conflicting results, it has not been universally used in this way. However, more recent studies have demonstrated a 10–15% improvement in renal graft survival with polyclonal immune globulin prophylaxis compared with steroid immunosuppression, that prophylactic use may reduce the number and severity of rejection episodes, and that those which do occur may be delayed and may be more easily reversible. In addition, polyclonal immune globulin is used at certain transplant centres during the initial period after allografting, before administration of cyclosporin is begun, in an effort to avoid early post-transplant nephrotoxicity without sacrificing protection from rejection (Hourmant et al, 1985).

Monoclonal Antibodies

These approaches hold great promise for a more sophisticated approach to immunosuppressive protocols. The constant domains of the T cell antigen receptor complex can now be directly targeted for therapy by the use of monoclonal antibodies. An early objective was to develop a pan-T cell monoclonal antibody that would function in the same way as a polyclonal antibody. However, this kind of antibody (OKT3) does not remove all T cells, although it has been found to block T cell function by specific interaction with molecules of the T cell receptor. OKT3 is, to date, the only commercially available monoclonal antibody for therapeutic use.

Six non-covalently linked T cell surface proteins constitute the T cell antigen recognition complex (Weiss et al, 1985, 1986; Kronenberg et al, 1986). These six proteins are expressed on essentially every functionally active T cell. The α and β chains are the antigen-binding proteins; their distal portions are unique and complementary for each antigen. As noted above, the other four CD3 proteins appear to play a key role in transducing signals from the antigen-binding α and β chains to the interior of the T cell (Weiss et al, 1985, 1986; Kronenberg et al, 1986). OKT3 antibody binds to CD3 at an antigenic site on the δ protein which is a 20 kDa molecule of the T lymphocyte-specific membrane protein. Hence, the monoclonal binds to a constant or non-varying component of the T cell antigen recognition complex. Immunosuppression with OKT3 monoclonal antibody blocks cytotoxic T lymphocyte-mediated cell lysis and other T cell functions (Van Wauwe et al, 1980; Landegran et al, 1982).

The clone that generated OKT3 was produced by sensitizing a mouse with human T lymphocytes, and then fusing the mouse's spleen cells with mouse myeloma cells to immortalize them. The resulting hybridomas were screened to select those producing the desired antibody – in this case, one uniquely reactive against a specific target site on human T cells. The hybridoma was then cloned to produce a strain of cells that produce a monoclonal antibody directed only against CD3. Because the stable hybridomas can provide a virtually limitless supply of specific antibodies that can be purified to complete homogeneity, the biological variability that complicates the use of polyclonal antibodies is eliminated.

Whenever allograft rejection occurs despite maintenance drug therapy, OKT3 is remarkably effective in reversing cellular rejection (Goldstein, 1987a). When this agent binds to the T cell antigen recognition complex, each of the latter's six proteins is stripped from the cell surface, either by shedding or internalization. OKT3-treated T cells therefore become literally blinded to the antigens of the allograft, and the rejection process comes to a halt. Although OKT3 is a potent T cell mitogen (Chang et al, 1981), in short-term cultures it blocks all known T cell functions in vivo. The advent of the pan-T cell monoclonal antibody OKT3 therefore represents an important refinement in therapy, the broad reactivity of conventional drugs with non-lymphoid tissues have been avoided.

Other monoclonal antibodies that react with T cells and cause their removal from the circulation have not yielded comparable rejection reversal rates (Goldstein, 1987b). This suggests that depletion of circulating T cells is not the sole mechanism by which OKT3 reverses rejection episodes (Table 5).

The efficacy and safety of OKT3 as therapy for acute renal allograft rejection is well substantiated by the results of controlled trials and widespread clinical experience. In a major, randomized, multicentre trial in the United States, it was shown that acute rejection episodes in cadaveric renal transplants were reversed in 94% of cases with OKT3, compared with 75% with conventional high-dose corticosteroid treatment ($p = 0.009$) (Ortho Multicenter Transplant Study Group, 1985). This difference in efficacy was reflected in a 17% greater graft survival 1 year after transplantation in patients treated with OKT3 than in those treated with high-dose steroids (Ortho Multicenter Transplant Study Group, 1985).

Table 5. OKT3 monoclonal antibody in immunosuppression.

Mode of action	Side-effects
Clearance of T lymphocytes due to reticuloendothelial uptake	Influenza-like symptoms following administration of first or second dose
Blocks T cell effector function	Fever, chills, tremors, headache
	Nausea, vomiting, diarrhoea
Modulation of antigen receptor/CD3 molecular complex	Respiratory symptoms (i.e. dyspnoea)
Postulated to block sessile T cells in the allograft	Increased susceptibility to infection
	Hypotension

OKT3 therapy is not without adverse effects (Table 5). Nearly all patients develop some severe flu-like symptoms following administration of the first or second dose, consisting of fever, shaking, chills and may include nausea, vomiting, diarrhoea, headache, anorexia, and weakness. These symptoms are likely to be due to an effect on T cells, for they are not seen once the CD3 antigen has been capped (Ortho Multicenter Transplant Study Group, 1985). It is now certain that these effects are linked to the transient mitogen-like properties of OKT3 and directly linked to the capacity of the agent to provoke cytokine release. Adverse reactions may be dampened by the administration of prednisone with the first dose, and this is now done routinely. However, because of the severity of these symptoms, and because some patients become hypotensive because of diarrhoea and vasodilation, patients should be monitored carefully in the hospital during the first 2 or 3 days of therapy. As for polyclonal antibody, the period of treatment is limited by the formation of neutralizing anti-mouse antibodies. One precaution that must be carefully observed is that the patient is not volume-overloaded prior to the initiation of OKT3 therapy. Severe pulmonary oedema has been reported in patients who were volume-overloaded prior to the first injection of OKT3.

Currently, there are multicentre trials underway to assess the use of OKT3 perioperatively. The objective of these studies is to determine whether OKT3 can be used prophylactically, instead of polyclonal ATG, to delay the initiation of cyclosporin therapy. The approach uses OKT3 to provide a window of immunosuppression until graft function is established, followed by the introduction of cyclosporin into the therapeutic protocol. The results of early trials in cardiac and hepatic allograft recipients are encouraging; however, long-term follow-up is needed.

Experimental Solutions

The ideal goal of blocking the activities of only those T cell clones that recognize the allograft could be realized by breaking the lock and key arrangement that intimately engages the graft antigens with those T cells bearing receptors that recognize them. This approach would be ideal because the overwhelming majority of immune cells involved in protective host defence mechanisms would not be targeted, and undesirable broad or pan-immunosuppression would be avoided. In theory, a perfect solution would be obtained by developing antibodies that react with the antigen-combining site of T cell antigen receptors for donor graft antigens. However, this has been confounded at least temporarily by the great genetic diversity of the HLA system, as well as by the substantive genetic repertoire of the T cell receptor for antigen. As predicted by knowledge of the extensive gene shuffling rearrangements of the T cell receptor, at least 1 million forms of this receptor exist. Clearly, too many reagents would be required to bring about clone-specific immunosuppressive therapy.

If the antigen-binding domains of individual T cell receptors cannot be easily targeted, can other structures be used to target selectively the small population of T cells actually engaged in rejection? Activated T cells express a variety of plasma membrane receptors that are absent from the surface of resting cells. One of these receptors, the IL-2 receptor, is not found on non-lymphoid tissues. One approach therefore being explored is to target IL-2R+ cells, as only newly activated cells bear this important protein. The IL-2 receptor is only transiently expressed during the brief proliferative burst of lymphocytes triggered in response to antigen. As the receptor is not expressed either resting or long-term memory cells, it was postulated that administration of anti-IL-2 receptor monoclonal antibodies in the early post-transplant period might provide selective immunosuppression. Could a single antibody directed against a receptor protein expressed in the common pathway of T cell activation be used in every recipient and donor combination?

In the mouse model, cardiac grafts transplanted across major transplantation barriers, are permanently engrafted following a 10-day course of rat anti-mouse anti-IL-2 receptor monoclonal antibody (Kirkman et al, 1985a). Even delayed application of the antibody can totally reverse ongoing cardiac graft rejection (Kirkman et al, 1985b). Dramatic effects have also been noted with mouse anti-rat antibodies in a rat heart transplant model (Kupiec-Weglinski et al, 1986). Despite cessation of therapy, graft rejection does not occur here, but this could be a peculiarity of the rat cardiac allograft model. Passive transfer experiments indicate that while donor-specific alloreactive helper cells are destroyed (Kupiec-Weglinski et al, 1989), donor-specific suppressor T cells (Kupiec-Weglinski et al, 1986) are spared the effects of anti-IL-2 receptor-directed therapy. These data demonstrate the significance of activated IL-2 receptor-bearing lymphocytes in graft rejection. In several models, the combined effects of anti-IL-2 receptor antibody and cyclosporin have been found to be synergistic. Early clinical experience with anti-IL-2 receptor monoclonal antibodies is highly promising (Soulillou et al, 1987; Cantorovich et al, 1989; Kirkman et al, 1989).

Other Future Prospects

It is to be hoped that the future of immunosuppressant therapy will include the development of additional monoclonal antibodies, or other T cell-specific magic bullets of low toxicity. The great variety of agents and of the antigens against which they can be directed, render this a promising but complex field for investigation over the next few years.

REFERENCES

Auron PE, Warner SN et al (1987) Studies on the molecular nature of human interleukin 2. *Journal of Immunology* **138**: 1447–1456.

Bach JF & Strom TB (1986) *The Mode of Action of Immunosuppressive Agents*, 2nd edn, pp 105–158. Amsterdam: Elsevier.

Burdick JF (1986) The biology of immunosuppression mediated by antilymphocyte antibodies, in Williams GM, Burdick JF & Solez K (eds) *Kidney Transplant Rejection: Diagnosis and Treatment*, pp 307–310. New York: Marcel Decker.

Cantorovich D, LeMauff J, Hourmant M et al (1989) Prophylactic use of a monoclonal antibody (33B3.1) directed against the interleukin-2 receptor following human renal transplantation. *Transplantation Proceedings*.

Cantrell PA & Smith KA (1984) The interleukin-2 T cell system. A new cell growth model. *Science* **224**: 1312.

Chang TW, Kung PC, Gingras SP et al (1981) Does OKT3 monoclonal antibody react with an antigen-recognition structure on human T cells? *Proceedings of the National Academy of Sciences, USA* **78**: 1805–1808.

Cosimi AB & Delmonico FL (1986) Antilymphocyte antibody immunosuppressive therapy, in Williams GM, Burdick JF & Solez K (eds) *Kidney Transplant Rejection: Diagnosis and Treatment*, pp 335–341. New York: Marcel Decker.

Farrar WL, Johnson HM & Farrar JJ (1981) Regulation of the production of immune interferon and cytotoxic T lymphocytes by interleukin 2. *Journal of Immunology* **126**: 1120–1125.

Goldstein G (ed) (1987a) Therapeutic use of the monoclonal antibody Orthoclone OKT3. *Transplantation Proceedings* **19** (supplement 1): 1–57.

Goldstein G (1987b) Overview of the development of Orthoclone OKT3: Monoclonal antibody for therapeutic use in transplantation. *Transplantation Proceedings* **19** (supplement 1): 1–6.

Granelli-Piperno A, Inaba K & Steinman RM (1984) Stimulation of lymphokine release from T lymphoblasts. Requirement for mRNA synthesis and inhibition by cyclosporine A. *Journal of Experimental Medicine*, **160**: 1792–1802.

Hourmant M, Soulillou JP, Remi JP et al (1985) Use of cyclosporin A after antilymphocyte serum in renal transplantation. *Presse Medicale*, **14**: 2093–2096.

Howard M, Matis L, Malek TR et al (1983) Interleukin 2 induces antigen-reactive T cell lines to secrete BCGF-1. *Journal of Experimental Medicine* **158**: 2024–2039.

Inaba K, Granelli-Piperno A & Steinman RM (1983) Dendritic cells induce T lymphocytes to release B cell-stimulating factors by an interleukin-2 dependent mechanism. *Journal of Experimental Medicine* **158**: 2040–2057.

Kahan BD (1984) Immunopharmacodynamic evaluation of cyclosporine-treated renal allograft recipients. *Transplantation* **38**: 657–664.

Kelley VE, Fiers W & Strom TB (1984) Cloned human interferon-gamma, but not interferon-beta or -alpha, induces expression of HLA-DR determinants by fetal monocytes and myeloid leukemic cell lines. *Journal of Immunology* **132**: 240–245.

Kirkman RL, Barret LV et al (1985a) Administration of an anti-interleukin-2 receptor monoclonal antibody prolongs cardiac allograft survival in mice. *Journal of Experimental Medicine*, **162**: 358–362.

Kirkman RL, Barret LV et al (1985b) The effect of anti-interleukin-2 receptor monoclonal antibody on allograft rejection. *Transplantation* **40**: 719–722.

Kirkman RL, Strom TB, Tilney NL et al (1989) Prophylactic use of anti-TAC, an anti-interleukin-2 receptor monoclonal antibody, following human cadaver donor kidney transplantation. *Transplantation,* in press.

Knudsen PJ, Dinarello CA & Strom TB (1987) Glucocorticoids inhibit transcription and post transcriptional expression of interleukin 1. *Journal of Immunology* **139**: 4129–4134.

Kronenberg M, Siu G, Hood LE et al (1986) The molecular genetics of the T cell antigen receptor and T cell antigen recognition. *Annual Reviews of Immunology* **4**: 593–621.

Kupiec-Weglinski JW, Diamantstein T, Tilney NL et al (1986) Therapy with monoclonal antibody to interleukin-2 receptor spares suppressor T cells and prevents or reverses acute allograft rejection in rats. *Proceedings of the National Academy of Sciences, USA* **83**: 2624–2627.

Kupiec-Weglinski JW, Padberg W et al (1987) Selective immunosuppression with anti-interleukin 2 receptor targeted therapy: Helper and suppressor cell activity in rat recipients of cardiac allografts. *European Journal of Immunology,* **17**: 313–320.

Landegran U, Ranstedt U, Axberg I et al (1982) Selective inhibition of human T cell cytotoxicity at levels of target recognition or initiation of lysis by monoclonal OKT3 and leu IIa antibodies. *Journal of Experimental Medicine* **155**: 1579–1684.

Maddock EO, Maddock SW, Kelley VE, et al (1985) Rapid stereospecific stimulation of lymphocyte metabolism by interleukin 2. *Journal of Immunology* **135**: 4004–4008.

Meuer SC, Hussey RE, Cantrell DA et al (1984) Triggering of the T3–T1 antigen-receptor complex results in clonal T cell proliferation through an interleukin-2 dependent autocrine pathway. *Proceedings of the National Academy of Sciences, USA* **81**: 1509–1513.

Ortho Multicenter Transplant Study Group (1985) A randomized clinical trial of Orthoclone OKT3 monoclonal antibody for acute rejection of cadaveric renal transplants. *New England Journal of Medicine* **313**: 337–342.

Pankewycz O, Kelley VE & Strom TB (1989) The cascading effects of IL-1, IL- and IL-2 in T-cell proliferation. *Clinical Immunology and Immunopathology* (in press).

Penn I (1978) Malignancies associated with immunosuppressive or cytotoxic therapy. *Surgery* **83**: 492.

Penn I (1987) Cancers following cyclosporine therapy. *Transplantation* **43**: 32–35.

Pober IS, Gimbrone MA, Cotran RS et al (1983) Ia expression by vascular endothelium is inducible by activated T cells and by human gamma interferon. *Journal of Experimental Medicine* **157**: 1339.

Simmons RL, Canafax DM, Strand M et al (1985) Management and prevention of cyclosporine nephrotoxicity after renal transplantation: use of low doses of cyclosporine, azathioprine, and prednisone. *Transplantation Proceedings* **17** (supplement 1): 266–275.

Soulillou JP, Peyronnet P, LeMauff J et al (1987) Prevention of rejection of kidney transplants by monoclonal antibody directed against interleukin-2 (receptors). *Lancet* **i**: 1339–1342.

Strom TB (1984) Immunosuppressive agents in renal transplantation. *Kidney International* **26**: 353–365.

Van Wauwe JP, DeMey JR & Grossend JG (1980) A monoclonal anti-human T lymphocyte antibody with potent mitogenic properties. *Journal of Immunology* **124**: 2708.

Weiss A, Imboden J et al (1985) The role of the T3 antigen/receptor complex in T cell activation. *Annual Reviews of Immunology* **4**: 593–620.

Weiss A, Imboden J. Hardy K et al (1986) The role of the antigen receptor complex in T-cell activation. *Annual Reviews of Immunology* **4**: 593–619.

Williams JM, Loertscher R, Cotner T et al (1984) Dual parameter flow cytometric analysis of DNA content, activation antigen expression, and T cell subset proliferation in the human mixed lymphocyte reaction. *Journal of Immunology* **132**: 2330–2337.

Williams JM, Deloria D, Hansen JA et al (1985) The events of primary T cell activation can be staged by use of Sepharose-bound anti T3 (64.1) monoclonal antibody and purified interleukin 1. *Journal of Immunology* **135**: 2249–2255.

Ythier AA, Abbud-Filho M, Williams JM, Loertscher R & Schuster MW (1985) Interleukin 2-dependent release of interleukin 3 activity by T4 + human T cell clones. *Proceedings of the National Academy of Sciences, USA* **82**: 7020–7024.

4 The Clinical and Laboratory Diagnosis of Graft Rejection

PETER J. MORRIS

The immune response to an allograft will almost invariably result in rejection if not prevented by appropriate treatment, and this response remains the major problem in organ transplantation (see Chapter 2). Not only are grafts lost in the early weeks or months after transplantation, but in surviving grafts the lesions frequently caused by early rejection reactions may lead to permanent damage and to a gradual deterioration of function, months to years later.

In organ transplants, a decline in function is usually the first sign of a rejection reaction. It is important to establish a prompt diagnosis either of rejection or of any unrelated complication that might be the cause of deteriorating function, so that prompt and appropriate treatment can be commenced to reverse the process. Much effort has been directed at the earlier diagnosis of rejection, before clinical signs become evident, in the expectation that treatment at a very early stage will prevent the full development of the immune reaction and so limit the resultant damage to the organ.

The principles of the diagnosis are essentially the same for all organ transplants, namely a deterioration of organ function accompanied by the appropriate histological changes of rejection. This review will be largely limited to the rejection of kidney transplants for which there is a wealth of clinical and laboratory data, but there will be brief comments on the approaches used for liver, heart, heart–lung and pancreas transplants.

KIDNEY

Several types of rejection have been recognized for many years, hyperacute, accelerated, acute and chronic. These descriptive terms are based on the timing of the rejection reaction and the postulated immunological mechanism causing rejection. Because the use of cyclosporin, either alone or in combination with other drugs, has become widespread, we have witnessed a change in the clinical features of acute rejection, and this will be discussed below.

ORGAN TRANSPLANTATION: CURRENT CLINICAL AND
IMMUNOLOGICAL CONCEPTS   ISBN 0-7020-1393-5

Hyperacute Rejection

If a renal transplant is performed in the presence of donor-specific HLA class I antibodies, the inevitable outcome is the immediate destruction of the graft. A graft that after revascularization is well perfused and may temporarily produce urine becomes flabby and blue, and urine output ceases abruptly. This usually occurs within an hour of revascularization, and if a biopsy is taken at this time it will show a widespread polymorphonuclear leucocyte infiltration and a little later glomerular and arteriolar thromboses (Williams et al, 1968). However, this classical presentation of hyperacute rejection is relatively rare today, for renal transplants are not performed in the presence of a positive antibody crossmatch due to HLA class I antibodies. Nevertheless, less florid examples of immunologically-mediated immediate graft rejection certainly do occur, for the incidence of non-functioning kidneys is still relatively high, and most of these non-functioning kidneys occur in patients who received a second graft. This suggests that lack of function is caused by an immunological reaction, although there is often little evidence in the shape of donor-specific antibody to support such a conclusion. In addition, the histology is not very revealing, at least in the very early stages, although after 24 hours or so arteriolar and glomerular thromboses become evident, followed by widespread infarction.

The most common cause of non-function immediately after transplantation is acute tubular necrosis (ATN), but technical complications such as ureteric obstruction or renal artery or venous thrombosis may also be responsible (Table 1). Thus the investigation of a non-functioning kidney would include a renogram to establish that the kidney is being perfused, and examination by ultrasound to exclude a diagnosis of ureteric obstruction. Finally a biopsy would distinguish between hyperacute rejection and ATN as the cause of non-function if there is still concern, a situation which might exist in the case of a retransplant or a transplant in a highly sensitized patient.

Table 1.   Conditions causing functional failure after renal transplantation.

Acute tubular necrosis
Hyperacute rejection
Ureteric obstruction
Renal artery thrombosis
Renal vein thrombosis

Accelerated Rejection

This type of rejection is the equivalent of second-set rejection in the experimental animal model and always occurs in a patient sensitized by a previous graft, blood transfusions or pregnancy. The reaction becomes evident between 2 and 4 days after transplantation, when the serum creatinine ceases to fall. This is followed by a rapid rise in creatinine, usually associated with a swollen and tender graft (difficult to evaluate in the first two days after surgery) and a moderate fever.

Biopsy of the kidney will reveal a dense mononuclear cell infiltrate and widespread oedema with or without vascular changes (Figure 1), the most florid of which are interstitial haemorrhage and fibrinoid necrosis of arteriolar walls. The presence of the latter vascular changes is a bad prognostic sign and there may be little response to treatment. In contrast, where there is only cellular infiltration and oedema, response to treatment is likely to be effective. This type of accelerated rejection is often seen in recipients of a one haplotype-disparate living related transplant, where the recipient has been prepared by transfusions from the kidney donor, and it almost certainly reflects a donor-specific response to the graft. It can occur despite a negative crossmatch, for this does not exclude the presence of pre-existing cellular sensitivity against, or memory for, donor histocompatibility antigen.

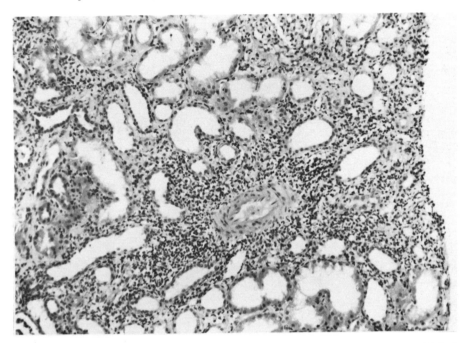

Figure 1. Biopsy of a cadaveric kidney allograft 4 days after transplantation, at which time the patient was febrile and had a tender swollen graft, showing a dense cellular infiltrate and oedema. (Haematoxylin and eosin stain, ×100.)

The diagnosis of accelerated rejection usually presents no problem in a patient with a kidney that functions immediately, but it may be less obvious in a patient with a poorly-functioning kidney due to acute tubular necrosis. The development of fever or a swollen tender kidney a few days after transplantation should give rise to suspicion, and once again the two most valuable investigations at this point are ultrasound to exclude ureteric obstruction or a urine leak, and a biopsy that will allow the diagnosis of a rejection reaction to be established. If fine needle aspiration cytology (FNAC) is used, the presence of lymphoblasts and macrophages in the aspirate allows a quick diagnosis.

Acute Rejection

This is the most frequent type of rejection seen after renal transplantation and the one that today causes most difficulty in diagnosis. Before the advent of cyclosporin this was not the case, for an acute rejection episode was classically associated with fever, a rise in serum creatinine, a fall in urine output, and a tender swollen kidney, just as seen in accelerated rejection. However, now that cyclosporin either alone or with other drugs is generally used for immunosuppression, at least in the early months after transplantation, the florid features of rejection described above are very uncommon, the clinical response being considerably muted.

An acute rejection episode usually occurs between 1 week and 2 months after transplantation. A delayed acute crisis can occur later still but it would generally be triggered by extraneous factors such as drug non-compliance. In the cyclosporin era such a reaction usually first occurs about 2–4 weeks after transplantation and is manifest by a moderate rise in serum creatinine and often, but not always, a moderate fever (perhaps up to 38.0 °C), usually with some swelling and tenderness of the kidney. This is a completely different picture from that of classical acute rejection described above and seen in the pre-cyclosporin era. What now complicates the diagnosis of rejection is the acute cyclosporin nephrotoxicity that can become evident at about the same time. Cyclosporin nephrotoxicity, too, is associated with a rising serum creatinine though without fever or graft swelling (Table 2).

Table 2. Some of the features which help to distinguish between acute rejection and cyclosporin nephrotoxicity as a cause of deterioration in graft function.

	Acute rejection	Acute cyclosporin toxicity
Serum creatinine	Elevated	Elevated
Urine output	Falling	Unchanged
Temperature	Elevated	Normal
Graft	Swollen and tender	Unchanged
Biopsy	Cellular infiltrate	Normal or minimal
	Oedema	cellular infiltrate
	Vascular changes	
	fibrinoid necrosis	Isometric vacuolization
	interstitial haem	of tubules
	thrombosis	
		Giant cell mitochondria
		Arteriolar thrombosis
Immunohistology	HLA class II induction	Normal expression of class II
Cyclosporin trough levels	Low	High

A biopsy is almost mandatory at this stage to establish the diagnosis. In the presence of acute rejection, one would expect to find a moderate to dense cellular infiltrate and widespread oedema, while in more severe cases there will also be interstitial haemorrhage, fibrinoid necrosis of arteriolar walls, and intimal fibrosis. Cyclosporin toxicity itself may be associated with a relatively normal histological appearance but a modest to moderate cellular infiltrate is often present. Sometimes changes are seen that are specifically associated with toxicity, such as giant cell mitochondria or isometric vacuolization in the tubular cells (Dunnill, 1988). There are, however, no histological features entirely characteristic of cyclosporin toxicity. Whole blood or serum levels of cyclosporin may be helpful, in that high levels are likely to be associated with toxicity and low levels with rejection (Morris, 1988).

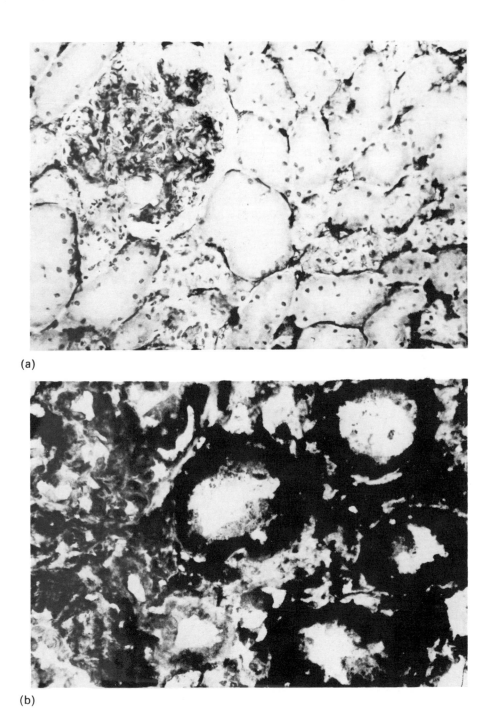

Figure 2. (a) Biopsy of a cadaveric kidney allograft at the time of transplantation, stained with a monoclonal antibody to HLA-DR (class II) using the immunoperoxidase technique. There is expression of class II only on mesangium, intertubular capillaries and dendritic cells (× 350). (b) The same kidney during an acute rejection showing extensive expression on tubules, previously negative (× 350).

Immunohistological examination of the kidney, too, may be helpful, for in an acute rejection episode there is induction of HLA class II antigens in cells (e.g. tubular cells) that do not constitutively express class II antigen, whereas this does not occur as a result of cyclosporin toxicity (Hall et al, 1984; Fuggle et al, 1986; Figure 2; see also Chapter 8b). Superficially this might appear to provide an accurate method for distinguishing between rejection and toxicity. However, we have demonstrated, using serial biopsies after transplantation, that if class II antigens appear at a very early stage then induction may continue for some time thereafter. Cyclosporin toxicity could therefore develop and co-exist in the presence of persisting class II antigen (Fuggle et al, 1989; Table 3). The identification of induced class II antigen expression nevertheless provides some help in distinguishing between rejection and cyclosporin toxicity as a cause of poor renal function.

Table 3.   Renal biopsies were examined for focal or generalized induction of HLA class II antigen in 14 instances of rejection, 9 of cyclosporin nephrotoxicity, and 9 of stable function. Although induction is common in the presence of rejection, it is also seen in grafts with stable function and nephrotoxicity (Fuggle et al, 1989).

Diagnosis	Induction of HLA class II antigen		
	Focal	Generalized	None
Rejection	3	7	4
Cyclosporin nephrotoxicity	2	3	4
Stable function	2	2	5

Cellular infiltration of the graft with leucocytes is a hallmark of rejection, but it can also occur in well functioning grafts, especially in the first few weeks after trai plantation (McWhinnie et al, 1985a). It is the *degree* of cellular infiltration that provides a diagnostic indication of rejection. The precise composition of the cellular infiltrate has attracted considerable attention since monoclonal antibodies detecting leucocyte subpopulations, and immunoperoxidase labelling techniques, have become available. The infiltrate in grafts undergoing rejection comprises around 60% macrophages, 35% T lymphocytes, and less than 10% NK/K cells (McWhinnie et al, 1986). Surprisingly, the composition of the infiltrate is much the same in grafts with stable function, although fewer cells are found. Furthermore, although it is still somewhat controversial, it would appear that there is no consistent change in the ratio of T helper to T cytotoxic/suppressor cells in grafts undergoing rejection compared with grafts with stable function, a point that has emerged from our studies involving serial biopsies (McWhinnie et al, 1985b).

Bearing in mind the cellular pattern of rejection in most cases, it is not surprising that FNAC, if used routinely (e.g. twice weekly) to monitor the graft, can pick up rejection at a relatively early stage, provided that the reaction is predominantly cellular rather than vascular (von Willebrand and Häyry, 1988). Increasing numbers of blast cells and macrophages suggest the onset of rejection, but they are not seen in the presence of cyclosporin toxicity (Figure 3). It is possible though, that vacuoles in tubular cells are indicative of drug-induced toxicity.

Because renal biopsies provide the diagnostic gold standard of rejection it is surprising that some units perform biopsies relatively infrequently, and then only when there is great uncertainty. Infrequent biopsies make it undoubtedly more difficult for the management team to interpret the histological picture. Nevertheless, there is justifiable concern that the risks associated with a Trucut needle biopsy are significant and that biopsies should therefore be restricted to situations in which the diagnosis cannot be established in any other way. However, Trucut needle biopsies can be performed with minimal morbidity, provided that their execution is restricted to two or three members of the management team. In our own unit, which carries out routine biopsies in the early weeks after transplantation (and which now number well over a 1000 biopsies), there have been no serious complications and no kidneys have been lost as a consequence. The recent introduction of the Biopty gun has simplified the procedure considerably and has decreased the incidence of post-biopsy haematuria. Although a slimmer core is obtained with the gun, this has proved satisfactory both with respect to routine histology and immunohistology.

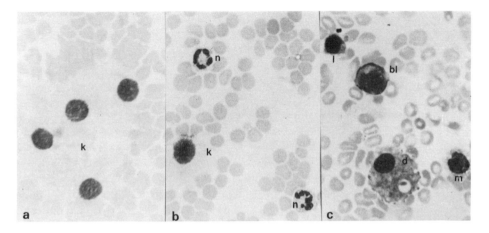

Figure 3. Fine-needle aspiration biopsies of human renal allografts with stable function (a and b) and undergoing cellular rejection (c). (Romanowsky stain, × 500). Key: normal (k) and damaged (d) renal parenchymal cells with neutrophils (n), a monocyte (m), a small lymphocyte (l) and a lymphoblast (bl).

Apart from the fears concerning the safety of the procedure, the infrequent use of biopsies is due to the assumption that a diagnosis of rejection can usually be made either clinically or by other less invasive techniques. Unfortunately this is not the case, especially with the use of cyclosporin, which reduces the clinical manifestations of rejection which may be associated with toxicity-induced deterioration in renal function. Although some units find isotope scans of value this has not been our experience, and we feel that their main value is in confirming that the kidney is being perfused. Ultrasound examination will confirm that a kidney is swollen, but its primary purpose is to exclude ureteric obstruction or a urine leak.

Over the years considerable efforts have been directed at detecting immunological changes in the recipient after transplantation, such as the appearance of anti-donor antibodies or donor-specific cytotoxic lymphocytes; and, indeed, a veritable industry in immunological monitoring has arisen. However, although changes can be detected in the blood in severe rejection crises or after rejected kidneys have been removed, immunological monitoring has not proved useful in detecting rejection at a stage before it becomes clinically evident, or in confirming that mild to moderate rejection is in progress.

This is perhaps not surprising, given that the immunological reaction occurs predominantly within the graft once it has been induced. For this reason FNAC is conceptually attractive, as it can be performed frequently, even daily. This technique is used routinely in many European transplant units but it has not yet achieved universal acceptance. In Oxford we have explored the technique for a number of years and still remain a little uncertain of its role in the absence of conventional histology, although our impression is that it has much the same accuracy as conventional biopsies and histology. For this reason we have embarked on a randomized prospective trial of patient management after transplantation by one of the three techniques: conventional histology, immunohistology and FNAC. All three assays are performed at the same time but only the results of the assay to which the patient has been randomly assigned are returned to the managing clinicians. The trial is still in progress but no problems have so far arisen in management with any of the three techniques. This should establish finally whether FNAC is an effective means of monitoring a graft after transplantation in comparison with conventional biopsy; it seems likely that it will prove to be so.

Chronic Rejection

Chronic rejection presents an insidious deterioration in renal function at any time from 6 months to many years after transplantation, and there is little or no response to additional treatment with high dose steroids. The histological picture shows interstitial fibrosis, marked intimal fibrosis of arteries and arterioles, glomerular hyalinization and a minimal to moderate cellular infiltration (Dunnill, 1988). The differential diagnosis (having excluded renal artery stenosis and ureteric obstruction as a cause of renal deterioration) lies between recurrent nephritis in the transplated kidney and chronic cyclosporin toxicity, and this distinction is often not easily made. This is particularly so in the case of cyclosporin toxicity, which is not associated with characteristic changes although striped interstitial fibrosis has been described as a common manifestation of this condition. Because of the relative absence of cellular infiltrates, and the widespread vascular changes in the graft, chronic rejection is considered to be due to a humoral response to the graft. There is, nevertheless, little convincing evidence to support the conclusion that chronic rejection is an ongoing immune response mediated by antibody, and it is likely that most of the changes of chronic rejection are the response to extensive immunological damage to the graft in the early months after transplantation and are essentially ischaemic in origin. The failure to respond to additional immunosuppressive treatment would be compatible with this suggestion.

It should not be forgotten that an acute rejection episode can occur years after transplantation, in both well-functioning kidneys and in kidneys suffering from chronic rejection. This is probably most often caused by drug non-compliance (though rarely admitted by patients), but it can also be triggered by infection or a blood transfusion, for example. A significant cellular infiltrate will be seen on biopsy, and this may be superimposed on changes associated with chronic rejection. In such cases there is often an improvement in renal function in response to treatment. For this reason a biopsy is advisable in any patient with a long-standing renal graft in which there is a rapid deterioration in function. Determination of cyclosporin levels is helpful, too, in revealing non-compliance.

LIVER

Deterioration in liver function, the hallmark of rejection, is not seen usually before the fifth day, and it generally occurs between 7 and 21 days after transplantation (Calne, 1987). Rejection of liver allografts was thought to occur rarely, the most frequent causes of deteriorating liver function being ischaemia, technical complications or sepsis. However, now that these problems have become less common due to better techniques of preservation and surgery, it is apparent that rejection occurs much more frequently than previously supposed and, in centres in which biopsies are performed routinely around the first week after transplantation, rejection is diagnosed in 50–70% of transplants (Williams et al, 1985).

Hyperacute Rejection

This is said not to occur in liver transplantation. Thus it is often possible to transplant livers successfully across major blood group barriers, e.g. A to O, or in the presence of a positive lymphocytotoxic crossmatch between donor and recipient. Even though the florid signs of classical hyperacute rejection are not seen, the success rate of liver grafting in the face of ABO incompatibility is less good than that of livers with ABO compatibility, and this suggests that pre-existing anti-erythrocyte antibody can cause liver injury (Gordon et al, 1987).

The outcome of liver transplantation in the presence of a positive lymphocytotoxic crossmatch must remain uncertain: Starzl's group has found no difference in survival (Gordon et al, 1986) whilst a recent report (see below) suggests that 'the vanishing bile duct syndrome' occurs frequently when the transplant is performed in the face of a positive crossmatch (Batts et al, 1988).

Furthermore, many of the data concerning the outcome of liver grafts performed in the presence of a positive crossmatch are unclear because of a failure to define the nature of the antibody causing the positive crossmatch. It is likely that in many instances the positive lymphocytotoxic crossmatch was due to autoantibodies or antibodies against donor class II HLA antigens (which are expressed only on the Kupffer and endothelial cells of the liver), rather than antibodies against class I HLA antigens, which are in any case only weakly expressed in the liver (Daar et al, 1984a). Thus, the failure of a liver to function normally from the time of transplantation, or the onset of an early rejection episode, should alert the physician to the possibility of antibody-mediated damage wherever the graft is ABO incompatible or it has been transplanted despite a positive crossmatch.

Acute Rejection

This generally occurs in the first or second weeks. In severe cases the patient will feel unwell and will have a fever associated with deterioration in liver function: serum bilirubin, alkaline phosphatase and aspartate transaminase will rise, and the prothrombin time will be increased. However, in less severe instances there may be little clinical evidence of rejection, at least in the first few days, despite deteriorating liver function.

Liver biopsies are extremely valuable in confirming the diagnosis, but hepatic artery or portal vein thrombosis should first be excluded by an isotope scan. The earliest change seen is a mononuclear cell infiltrate of the portal tracts, with infiltration and layering of the bile duct epithelium; later, focal necrosis of hepatocytes and intracanalicular cholestasis may be seen (Wight and Portmann, 1987).

In the normal human liver class I HLA antigens are weakly expressed on hepatocytes, moderately expressed on bile duct epithelium and strongly expressed on Kupffer cells, endothelium and interstitial cells; class II HLA antigens are absent on hepatocytes and bile duct epithelium but moderately or strongly expressed on Kupffer cells, endothelium and interstitial cells (Daar et al, 1984a,b; see also Chapter 8b). However, during acute rejection class I HLA antigens are strongly expressed on hepatocytes and bile duct epithelium, and class II HLA antigens on endothelium and bile duct epithelium, with expression by hepatocytes in many but not all instances (Steinhoff et al, 1988). It is worth noting that class II antigens were found on bile duct epithelium in apparently quiescent grafts, whereas they were present on hepatocytes only during rejection or viral infections such as cytomegalovirus.

Another attractive method of monitoring liver grafts is FNAC, again developed by the Helsinki group (Häyry et al, 1987). With liver transplants, frequent conventional core biopsies are unsafe because of the risk of haemorrhage and bile leakage, but FNAC is a safe procedure that can be performed frequently. Experience with this technique is as yet limited, but it may well be more valuable for the liver than for the kidney. Acute rejection may sometimes be irreversible and it is important to establish this diagnosis as soon as possible for, with the increasing supply of livers, retransplantation is now possible and should ideally be performed as soon as the irreversibility of rejection has been established.

Chronic Rejection

As more patients with liver allografts survive the perioperative period, loss of allografts caused by chronic rejection is becoming recognized more frequently and it is probably the major cause of graft failure after the first few months. The two major features recognized from biopsy or at autopsy are the occlusion of arteries with foam cells, and the disappearance of bile ducts. Chronic rejection is usually preceded by episodes of acute rejection in the early weeks after transplantation and it is associated with a steady deterioration of liver function that cannot be arrested or delayed by additional immunosuppressive treatment. Sometimes a micronodular cirrhosis develops, but fibrosis is not a feature of chronic rejection as in the case of the kidney (Wight and Portmann, 1987).

As mentioned above, the 'vanishing bile duct syndrome' has been described in livers transplanted in the presence of a positive lymphocytotoxic crossmatch and may be a manifestation of antibody-mediated liver damage (Batts et al, 1988).

PANCREAS

The pancreas, transplanted as a vascularized organ, has been considered to be relatively invulnerable to rejection, at least when given to uraemic patients concurrently with a kidney. However, now that many of the technical problems of pancreatic transplantation have been resolved and more sensitive methods of monitoring graft function have been developed, it has become clear that acute rejection is far more common than previously supposed (Tyden, 1988). When single pancreatic grafts are implanted into non-uraemic patients, acute rejection is common and to date the majority of technically successful single grafts have been lost from irreversible rejection. It is clear, however, that when a kidney and pancreas from the same donor are transplanted simultaneously, the pancreas is usually less susceptible to rejection than the kidney. There are many documented instances where a kidney has undergone acute rejection or even irreversible rejection without evidence of rejection of the pancreas.

In contrast to other organ transplants, a biopsy of the pancreas cannot be performed easily: most grafts are placed intraperitoneally and needle biopsies are too hazardous. If a biopsy is required a laparotomy is therefore obligatory. Nevertheless, the Minneapolis group has performed frequent 'mini-laparotomies' and biopsies, and this has provided invaluable information on the histological pattern of rejection in the pancreas (Sutherland et al, 1984). The predominant features are a mononuclear cellular infiltrate of the parenchyma, with intimal fibrosis of arteries. The islets themselves are often relatively free of cellular infiltrate, suggesting that the rejection response is mainly directed at the exocrine rather than the endocrine tissue. In contrast, biopsies performed in segmental pancreatic grafts between identical twins in the absence of immunosuppression in the recipient show a marked isletitis that is consistent with disease recurrence (see Chapter 7).

Because of the difficulties of regular biopsies much effort has been directed at other methods of diagnosing rejection (Tyden, 1988). A rise in the fasting blood glucose is not helpful as it is really an indication of irreversible rejection. Postprandial glucose elevations occur at an earlier stage of a rejection episode and are therefore a more useful indication. Nevertheless, as other factors influence glucose homeostasis, neither is an entirely reliable technique for defining rejection.

Bearing in mind the histological information that the exocrine part of the pancreas is more susceptible to rejection than the islets themselves, some measurement of exocrine function would appear to be a rational approach to monitoring. Serum amylase measurements have not proved useful, but the increasingly popular drainage of the pancreatic duct into the bladder allows the amylase content of the urine to be monitored; a fall in urine amylase has proved to be a relatively early and reliable indicator of rejection (Prieto et al, 1987). Similarly, the Stockholm group has shown that in pancreatic grafts in which the duct is drained into a Roux loop of small intestine, but with a catheter in the duct allowing collection of the exocrine juice, a decrease in the volume and amylase content of the exocrine secretion signifies rejection (Tyden, 1988). In addition, cytological examination of the secretion, which is normally devoid of cells, revealed the appearance of mononuclear cells during rejection episodes. These approaches are naturally not available if the blocked duct technique has been used (see Chapter 7).

Monitoring C-peptide levels could be useful if a rapid assay were available, for the levels are not influenced by steroid medication or by parenteral nutrition. However, levels may be artificially high when there is renal dysfunction. Isotope scans (with [75]seleniomethionine) showing a decreased uptake have been claimed to be useful, as has the increased uptake of [111]indium-labelled platelets in a rejecting pancreas.

Chronic rejection of pancreatic grafts undoubtedly occurs but it is an insidious process. A typical final event is the presentation at a follow-up clinic of a previously normoglycaemic patient with irreversible hyperglycaemia.

HEART AND HEART–LUNG

Electrocardiography was the only method of determining rejection in the early days of heart transplantation. The development of the endomyocardial biopsy technique by Caves et al (1973), performed via a percutaneous transvenous catheter, revolutionized the monitoring of cardiac transplant patients, for it could be performed frequently (e.g. weekly) and on an outpatient basis. Histological evidence of rejection was based on the presence of a mononuclear cellular infiltrate and myocyte necrosis, the latter being an indication of severe rejection requiring energetic treatment. Routine biopsies remain today the technique of choice in monitoring the course of a heart transplant.

Treatment for rejection is based on the histological findings and there are few significant clinical features of rejection, except in the later stages of irreversible rejection, when cardiac malfunction will be evident. Induction of class I and II HLA antigens on myocytes and endothelium may be a further early predictor of acute rejection, for this may occur quite early in the response before the cellular infiltrate is widespread (Rose et al, 1986).

In combined heart and lung transplants, routine biopsy of the heart using the percutaneous transvenous endomyocardial technique is used most commonly for monitoring the combined graft, based on the assumption that rejection of the heart is likely to be accompanied by rejection of the lungs. However, this is not always the case, and thus the recently described transbronchial lung biopsy technique is likely to prove a valuable monitor of rejection or infection in the lung (Higgenbottom et al, 1988). This will be an especially valuable method in the case of single or double lung transplants without an accompanying heart transplant.

SUMMARY

The diagnosis of rejection of an organ graft will reflect the systemic reaction of the immune response to the graft, namely fever and swelling of a graft that is palpable, accompanied by a deterioration in graft function as measured by biochemical or physiological tests. The gold standard of rejection of all organs is established by biopsy and the histological demonstration of a mononuclear cellular infiltrate and oedema, with varying degrees of arteriolar and arterial pathology and the later appearance of fibrosis. Immunohistology can be used to identify the phenotype of the cellular infiltrate, which comprises both CD4+ and CD8+ T lymphocytes, NK cells and macrophages, but no obvious pattern of rejection emerges other than an overall increase in the number of infiltrating cells. Induction of class I and class II HLA antigens is usually associated with rejection in most organs, but may occur in other inflammatory reactions; as such it can provide additional information of value in diagnosing rejection. Fine needle aspiration cytology is a newer technique that is applicable to kidney and liver transplants, and it seems likely to play an increasingly useful role in the diagnosis of rejection, particularly because it can be safely and frequently performed. The early diagnosis of rejection and the initiation of appropriate treatment may not only reverse the reaction but thereby diminish the resulting long-term damage to the organ.

REFERENCES

Batts KP, Moore SB, Perkins JD et al (1988) Influence of a positive lymphocyte crossmatch and HLA mismatching on vanishing bile duct syndrome in human liver allografts. *Transplantation* 45: 376–379.

Calne RY (1987) Diagnosis of rejection. In RY Calne (ed.), *Liver Transplantation*, 2nd edn, pp 301–304. London: Grune & Stratton.

Caves PK, Stinson EB, Billingham ME & Shumway NE (1973) Percutaneous transvenous endomyocardial biopsy in human heart recipients. *Annals of Thoracic Surgery* 16: 325–336.

Daar AS, Fuggle SV, Fabre JW, Ting A & Morris PJ (1984a) The detailed distribution of HLA-A, B, C antigens in normal human organs. *Transplantation* 38, 287–292.

Daar AS, Fuggle SV, Fabre JW, Ting A & Morris PJ (1984b) The detailed distribution of MHC class II antigens in normal human organs. *Transplantation* 38: 293–298.

Dunnill MS (1988) Histopathology of rejection in renal transplantation. In Morris PJ (ed.), *Kidney Transplantation: Principles and Practice*, 3rd edn, pp 439–472. Philadelphia: WB Saunders.

Fuggle SV, McWhinnie DL, Chapman JR, Taylor HM & Morris PJ (1986) Sequential analysis of HLA-Class II antigen expression in human renal allografts. *Transplantation* 42: 144–150.

Fuggle SV, McWhinnie DL & Morris PJ (1989) Immuno histological analysis of renal allograft biopsies from cyclosporine treated patients: induced HLA-class II antigen expression does not exclude a diagnosis of cyclosporine nephrotoxicity. *Transplantation International*, in press.

Gordon RD, Iwatsuki S, Esquivel CO et al (1986) Liver transplantation across ABO blood groups. *Surgery* 100: 342–348.

Gordon RD, Iwatsuki S, Tzakis SG et al (1987) The Denver–Pittsburg Liver Transplant Series. In PI Terasaki (ed.), *Clinical Transplants 1987*, pp 43–49. UCLA Tissue Typing Laboratory.

Hall BM, Bishop GA, Duggin GG et al (1984) Increased expression of HLA-DQ antigens on renal tubular cells in renal transplants, relevance to the rejection response. *Lancet* ii: 247–251.

Häyry P, von Willebrand E, Ahonen J. Lautenschlager I & Leskin R (1987) Aspiration cytology in organ transplantation. *Transplantation Reviews* 1: 133–158.

Higgenbottom TW, Stewart S & Wallwork J (1988) Transbronchial lung biopsy to diagnose lung rejection and infection in heart lung transplants. *Transplantation Proceedings* 20: 764–766.

McWhinnie DL, Thompson JF, Taylor HM et al (1985a) Leukocyte infiltration pattern in renal allografts assessed by immunoperoxidase staining of 245 sequential biopsies. *Transplantation Proceedings* 17: 560–561.

McWhinnie DL, Carter NP, Taylor HM et al (1985b) Is the T4/T8 ratio an irrelevance in renal transplantation monitoring? *Transplantation Proceedings* 17: 2548–2549.

McWhinnie DL, Thompson JF, Taylor HM et al (1986) Morphometric analysis of cellular infiltration assessed by monoclonal antibody labeling in sequential human renal allograft biopsies. *Transplantation* 42: 352–358.

Morris PJ (1988) Cyclosporine. In Morris PJ (ed.), *Kidney Transplantation: Principles and Practice*, 3rd edn, pp 439–472. Philadelphia: WB Saunders.

Prieto M, Sutherland DER, Goetz FC, Rosenberg J & Najarian JS (1987) Pancreas transplant results according to the technique of duct management: bladder versus enteric drainage. *Surgery* 192: 680–691.

Rose ML, Coles MI, Griffin RJ, Pomerance A & Yacoub MH (1986) Expression of class I and class II major histocompatibility antigens in normal and transplanted human hearts. *Transplantation* 41: 776–780.

Steinhoff G, Wonigest K & Pichlmayr R (1988) Analysis of sequential changes in major histocompatibility complex expression in human liver grafts after transplantation. *Transplantation* 45: 394–401.

Sutherland DER, Goetz FC & Najarian JS (1984) One hundred pancreas transplants at a single institution. *Annals of Surgery* 200: 414–440.

Tyden G (1988) Pancreatic graft rejection. In Groth CG (ed.), *Pancreatic Transplantation*, pp 249–267. Philadelphia: WB Saunders.

von Willebrand E & Häyry P (1988) Fine needle aspiration cytology of the transplanted kidney. In Morris PJ (ed.) *Kidney Transplantation: Principles and Practice*, 3rd edn. pp 491–510. Philadelphia: WB Saunders.

Wight DG & Portmann B (1987) Pathology of liver transplantation. In Calne RY (ed.), *Liver Transplantation*, 2nd edn, pp 385–435. London: Grune & Stratton.

Williams GM, Hume DM, Hudson RP et al (1968) 'Hyperacute' renal homograft rejection in man. *New Journal of Medicine* 279: 611–618.

Williams JW, Peters TG, Vera SR, Britt LG, van Voorst SJ & Haggitt RC (1985) Biopsy-directed immunosuppression following hepatic transplantation in man. *Transplantation* 39: 589–596.

5 Therapy, both Immunosuppressive and Antimicrobial, for the Transplant Patient in the 1990s

ROBERT H. RUBIN
A. BENEDICT COSIMI

The two most important barriers to successful organ transplantation are allograft rejection and life-threatening infection. These two processes are closely intertwined, the former necessitating immunosuppressive therapy and the latter made possible by such immunosuppressive therapy. An important truism of clinical transplantation may be summarized as follows: any intervention or modality that decreases the extent of rejection and thus permits the prescription of less intensive immunosuppressive therapy will result in a decrease in the incidence and severity of infection; conversely, any intervention or modality that decreases the risk of infection will permit the safer deployment of more intensive immunosuppressive therapy, thus resulting in the better control of the rejection process. In addition, it is now clear that certain infectious processes (particularly cytomegalovirus infection) that are themselves strongly influenced by the prescribed immunosuppressive therapy have significant immunomodulating effects (Rubin, 1988).

In addressing the question of determining the ideal regimen for immunosuppression for the next decade, we must look at the present and very considerable armamentarium of potential antirejection drugs, and decide (i) which agent or combination of agents permits the most reliable control of rejection, while (ii) minimizing the risk of infection. Other chapters in this book address the specific factors which are known to reduce the chances of graft rejection, such as histocompatibility matching, and pharmacological manipulation of immunobiological events which lead to rejection; but the choice of agents to maximize the therapeutic index of therapy, which tip the 'balance of survival' in favour of the patient and his graft, is a clinical choice, which can only be made rationally in the knowledge of potential complications in immunosuppressed graft recipients.

Here we will concentrate upon the problems of infection, and how immunosuppressive therapy might be modified or specific antimicrobial prophylaxis added so as to increase the chances of a positive outcome from organ transplantation. Eighty five per cent one-year graft survival following cadaveric renal transplantation and $> 95\%$ one-year patient survival is now being achieved regularly at many centres (and $> 75\%$ one-year survival

ORGAN TRANSPLANTATION: CURRENT CLINICAL AND
IMMUNOLOGICAL CONCEPTS   ISBN 0-7020-1393-5

for cardiac and liver transplantation). However, about 75% of these patients suffer at least one significant infection during this first year, and infection remains the major cause of death at all time points in the post-transplant period. Clearly, there is room for progress.

RISK OF INFECTION IN THE TRANSPLANT RECIPIENT

The infectious disease problems that occur following organ transplantation can be grouped into three categories: technical, epidemiological and viral infections, to which the transplant patient is uniquely susceptible (Table 1). Experience in the last 20 years has demonstrated that those problems of infectious disease which are related to technical errors in patients undergoing renal and cardiac transplantation can be virtually eliminated. Such technical errors resulting in significant infection in this circumstance include the following: undrained fluid collections, be they blood, urine, or lymphatic in origin, will invariably become secondarily infected; urine or other anastomotic leaks that require the insertion and the prolonged presence of drainage devices, nephrostomy tubes, etc., that traverse the primary cutaneous barrier to infection can be a source of localized Gram-negative bacterial or candidal superinfection that can disseminate in immunocompromised patients; and the prolonged presence of endotracheal tubes, central intravenous lines, and even intraarterial lines can lead to pneumonia or septicaemia, with dire consequences in this patient population. Prevention of these problems by exquisite attention to surgical technique, anaesthetic management, and prompt removal and frequent changing of vascular access sites rather than treatment of the secondary infections should be the primary emphasis and can be quite successful.

In contrast, the problems of viral infection and unsuspected epidemiological hazards are apt to remain for the foreseeable future. The risk of infection in the transplant patient is due to the interaction between two major factors: the *epidemiological exposures* encountered by the individual and the *net state of immunosuppression* (Rubin et al, 1981).

NOSOCOMIAL INFECTION

A wide range of infectious processes can affect transplant patients as a result of exposure to excessive numbers of organisms in the environment with the capacity to invade these altered hosts (Table 1). Of greatest concern are infections arising from exposure to the hospital environment. Although nosocomial infection is a problem of increasing concern for all hospitalized patients, the immunosuppressed patient population is at most risk. Any increase within the hospital environment of the level of *Aspergillus*, *Legionella*, or Gram-negative contamination of the air or potable water will constitute the highest risk to transplant patients with impaired host defences. Transplant patients serve as human sentinels of microbial contamination of the hospital environment. An analogy has been made between the immunocompromised patient within the hospital environment and the sentinel chickens that were formerly placed in swamps to monitor mosquito-borne arbovirus infection. Any excessive traffic in potential pathogens will be noted first and foremost in these individuals (Rubin, 1987).

Most epidemics of nosocomial opportunistic infection that have been documented thus far have been attributed to contamination of the air delivered to the patients' rooms

Table 1. Classification of infections of major importance in organ transplant patients (modified from Rubin, 1988).

A. *Infections related to technical implications**
    Transplantation of a contaminated allograft
    Anastomotic leaks or stenoses
    Wound haematoma
    Intravenous (and intra-arterial) line contamination
    Urinary or biliary catheter contamination
    Infected drainage system (i.e. chest tubes, intra-abdominal drains)
    Iatrogenic damage to the skin
    Wound infection

B. *Infections related to excessive nosocomial hazard*
    Aspergillus spp.
    Legionella spp.
    Pseudomonas aeruginosa and other Gram-negative bacilli
    Nocardia asteroides

C. *Infections related to particular exposures within the community*
    Mycobacterium tuberculosis
    Systemic mycotic infections in certain geographic areas
        Histoplasma capsulatum
        Coccidioides immitis
        Blastomyces dermatitides
    Community-acquired opportunistic infection due to ubiquitous saprophytes in the environment[+]
        Cryptococcus neoformans
        Aspergilllus spp.
        Nocardia asteroides
        Pneumocystis carinii
        Strongyloides stercoralis
    Respiratory infections circulating in the community
        Influenza
        Adenovirus
        Mycoplasma pneumoniae
    Infections acquired by the ingestion of contaminated food or water
        Salmonella spp.
        Listeria monocytogenes

D. *Viral infection of particular importance in the transplant patient*
    Herpes group viruses
    Hepatitis viruses
    Papovaviruses
    Human immunodeficiency virus
    Adenovirus

---

* All lead to infection with Gram-negative bacilli, *Staphylococcus* spp. and/or *Candida* spp.
[+] The incidence and severity of these infections and, to a lesser extent, the other infections listed are directly related to the net state of immunosuppression present in the individual patient.

('domiciliary' infections). Because these cases tend to occur in one ward, at around the same time, such epidemics are relatively easy to detect. They may be prevented effectively by the provision of an air supply that has been passed through properly functioning high efficiency particle air filters to the rooms of susceptible patients. Increasingly, however, 'non-domiciliary' epidemics of opportunistic infection are being discovered in immunocompromised patients. In these outbreaks, infection is acquired at a common site which provides essential services such as surgical or radiological procedures. Epidemics caused by contaminated air within operating rooms or radiology suites have now been documented in immunosuppressed patients who visit for tests or procedures. They are probably not uncommon, are more difficult to detect, and are not usually preventable because special air-processing units are restricted to the wards, and are not generally employed in the theatres or diagnostic suites. Because many epidemics, particularly those due to *Aspergillus* species, arise from dust produced by construction activities within the hospital, great care must be taken to coordinate such activities within the hospital, to protect the transplant patients during transportation through this environment, and to impose barrier containment on all such construction sites. During such building activities careful surveillance for opportunistic infection in the hospital as a whole must be carried out. It is likely that over the next decade this problem will receive increasing recognition (Allo et al, 1987; Rubin, 1987).

REDUCING THE HAZARDS OF IMMUNOSUPPRESSION

The net state of immunosuppression is determined by a complex array of events: the nature, dose, and duration of the immunosuppressive therapy being administered; the presence or absence of granulocytopenia or lymphopenia; technical factors that could compromise the primary mucocutaneous barrier to infection such as surgical wounds, nasogastric tubes, intravenous lines, and urinary catheters; metabolic factors such as uraemia, hyperglycaemia, and the state of nutrition; and finally, the immunomodulating effects of such viruses as cytomegalovirus, the hepatitis viruses, and the human immunodeficiency virus (Rubin et al, 1981).

Certain clinical precepts concerning the minimization of the risk of infection derive from these considerations, which should be borne in mind when choosing an immunosuppressive regimen for a particular patient.

1. The greater the state of immunosuppression the greater is the need for protection from even the most non-virulent of micro-organisms in the patient's environment; conversely, the greater the environmental hazard, the more limitations must be placed on the immunosuppressive therapy prescribed. Accordingly, the prompt identification and correction of any excessive infectious hazard from infected patients on the ward, and from contaminated air will contribute greatly to the safety of an immunosuppressive programme.
2. Because the net state of immunosuppression varies at different points in the post-transplant period, more than one form of environmental protection and anti-infection prophylaxis must be applied at different stages during pre-transplant work-up, and after transplant surgery.
3. The different immunosuppressives currently used generate different qualitative and quantitative degrees of susceptibility to infection, due to the wide range of their specific and non-specific action on the immune system. Different regimens therefore generate differing patterns of clinical susceptibility to viruses and bacteria. On the one hand, such knowledge will lead to the more rational prescription of such immunosuppressive therapies; on the other hand, specific antimicrobial prophylaxis administered as an adjunct to immunosuppression may contribute to prevention of both rejection and infection.

TIMETABLE FOR THE OCCURRENCE OF INFECTION IN THE ORGAN TRANSPLANT RECIPIENT

One of the most important developments of the past two decades is the recognition that different types of infections commonly occur at different times after the commencement of immunosuppression; the risk of a particular infection at any time is, to some extent, predictable. The dose of immunosuppressive drugs administered on a given day is not all that important; rather, it is the cumulative effect of therapy that has been given over several weeks which determines the net risk; it is how such therapy interacts with the other factors that contributes to the degree of hazard to the patient from infection. This fact creates perhaps the most deceptive aspect of the care of transplant patients: whereas, increasing the dose of immunosuppressives often rapidly improves allograft function, the life-threatening infection engendered may not be manifest for several weeks.

The fact that immunosuppressive drugs are prescribed from the day of transplant surgery has allowed us to study the incidence of infection with various microbial agents at various times during the first few months of anti-rejection therapy. Perhaps not surprisingly, there is an expected predictable pattern or timetable for particular infections which are apt to occur and cause clinical disease (Figure 1). Thus, three time periods can be identified (Rubin et al, 1981).

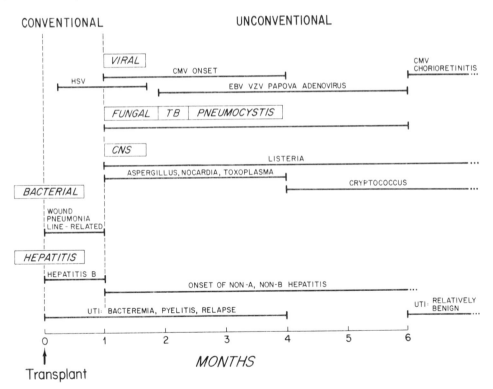

Figure 1. Timetable for the occurrence of infections in the organ transplant patient. Exceptions to this timetable should initiate a search for an unusual environmental hazard. CMV, cytomegalovirus; HSV, herpes simplex virus; EBV, Epstein–Barr virus; VZV, varicella-zoster virus; CNS, central nervous system; UTI, urinary tract infection. Modified from Rubin et al (1981).

Infection in the First Month Post-transplant

During this period, there are three major forms of infection that may become clinically manifest:

1. Infection that was present prior to transplantation and which continues or is exacerbated by immunosuppressive therapy after transplantation; the major examples of this category of infection are: hepatitis (both hepatitis B and non-A, non-B hepatitis), smouldering bacterial infection such as tuberculosis, the parasitic infection strongyloidiasis, and the geographically restricted systemic mycoses (blastomycosis, coccidioidomycosis, and histoplasmosis).
2. Infection transmitted via a contaminated allograft.
3. The routine bacterial infections of the surgical wound, lungs, intravenous lines, and bladder catheters found in non-immunosuppressed patients undergoing comparable types of surgery.

The last group constitute more than 90% of the infections occurring in this time period.

During this first month we would *not* expect to see opportunistic infections due to such organisms as *Aspergillus*, *Nocardia*, or *Legionella* species. In the rare instances when such infections are documented, they have invariably been associated with excessive epidemiological hazards within the hospital environment.

Infection 1–6 Months After Transplantation

This is the critical time period for the transplant patient when the risk of serious infectious disease is maximal. There are two reasons for this – the preceeding month's course of immunosuppressive therapy is long enough to depress significantly host defences against infection, and a variety of viral infections that are ubiquitous among transplant patients, and that contribute significantly to the net state of immunosuppression, are now present. There are two major groups of infectious disease which predominate during this period:

1. Viral infections, including those due to the hepatitis viruses, Epstein–Barr virus (EBV), the human immunodeficiency virus (HIV) and, most especially, cytomegalovirus (CMV).
2. Infection caused by a variety of opportunistic pathogens, such as *Pneumocystis carinii*, the fungi, and *Listeria*.

Viral reactivation can now occur; some of these viruses individually cause bone-marrow suppression and debility effects which can be synergistic with immunosuppressive therapy. Thus there is a high risk that opportunistic infection will occur if the appropriate epidemiological exposure takes place. Figure 2 illustrates this phenomenon with the presentation of a case of a renal transplant patient with *Pneumocystis carinii* pneumonia superimposed on symptomatic CMV infection. In the absence of viral infection, only an unusual epidemiological exposure will normally result in opportunistic infection. Figure 3 illustrates this occurrence with the presentation of a case of invasive pulmonary aspergillosis occurring 2 weeks post-renal transplant due to excessive amounts of *Aspergillus* spores in the air, related to construction activities.

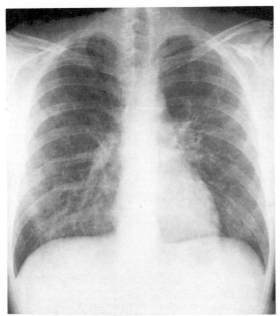

Figure 2. Chest X-ray of a renal transplant patient with biopsy-proven *Pneumocystis carinii* pneumonia occurring 6 weeks post-transplant. The patient had had an uncomplicated clinical course until 4 weeks post-transplant when unexplained fevers and then leukopenia and mild abnormalities in liver function tests developed. Cytomegalovirus was grown from the blood, urine, and saliva. Over the 4 days prior to this X-ray, non-productive cough and increasing shortness of breath were noted and arterial blood gases drawn on room air revealed a pO_2 of 58 mmHg, pCO_2 of 28 mmHg and a pH of 7.52. This case is an example of opportunistic pneumonia occurring in a patient with active CMV infection.

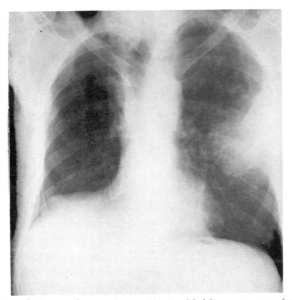

Figure 3. Chest X-ray of a renal transplant patient with biopsy-proven invasive pulmonary aspergillosis developing 2 weeks post-transplant. The patient was free of viral infection and had only received conventional doses of cyclosporin and prednisone. Epidemiological investigation revealed that this patient was one of five immunocompromised patients who developed invasive pulmonary aspergillosis due to exposure to a radiological suite undergoing extensive remodelling and construction.

Infection in the Late Period, More Than 6 Months After Transplantation

Infections at this stage can be divided into three categories:

1. Chronic viral infection plus chronic immunosuppressive therapy will lead in approximately 10% of individuals to the following progressive diseases: chorioretinitis due to CMV, progressive liver disease caused by the hepatitis viruses, hepatocellular carcinoma due to hepatitis B virus or B cell lymphoproliferative disease due to EBV.
2. The community-acquired infections such as urinary tract infection, influenza, and pneumocococcal pneumonia; these occur predominantly in individuals with a good clinical outcome from transplantation who have good allograft function, are receiving minimal immunosuppressive therapy, and who do not suffer chronic viral infection.
3. The life-threatening opportunistic infections with such pathogens as *Pneumocystis carinii*, *Cryptococcus neoformans*, *Listeria monocytogenes* and *Nocardia asteroides*; these diseases occur particularly in individuals with a relatively poor outcome of transplantation who suffer from poor allograft function, who have been prescribed too much acute and chronic immunosuppressive therapy, and who harbour chronic CMV and/or hepatitis virus infection.

It would therefore appear that advances in therapy for transplant patients over the next decade should be focused on the following issues: (i) the continuing refinement of technical approaches to limit the surgical complications that are the prime cause of infection in the first month post-transplant and the deployment of specific antimicrobial prophylactic measures during the pre- and postoperative periods aimed at preventing wound and urinary tract infection; (ii) the use of immunosuppressive therapies and antiviral strategies that will minimize the extent and the effects of the viral infections (CMV, EBV and hepatitis) that appear to play such a dominant role in the pathogenesis of most infections in the transplant patient. In addition, when a patient develops an excessive risk of infection, or if those strategies fail, specific manipulations of the environment and antibiotic prophylaxis should be considered to provide particular protection during the period of excessive risk.

CYTOMEGALOVIRUS

Cytomegalovirus (CMV) is the single most important cause of infection in the transplant patient, with some evidence of CMV infection being demonstrable in about 75% of transplant recipients. CMV shares with the other members of the herpes virus group (EBV, varicella-zoster virus [VZV], and herpes simplex virus [HSV]) three important characteristics that cause these viruses to have a major impact on transplant recipients: *latency* – primary infection results in life-long dormant infection of a variety of cell types, including leukocytes, and renal, hepatic, and cardiac tissue. Such dormant infections are subject to reactivation by such factors as immunosuppressive therapy and allograft rejection; *cell association* – spread of the virus occurs from cell to cell, thus rendering humoral immunity inefficient and cell-mediated immunity paramount in terms of host defences against the virus; *oncogenicity* – all members of the herpes virus group should be considered potentially oncogenic (Ho, 1977).

Three epidemiologic patterns of CMV infection have been observed in transplant recipients, each with its own risk of clinically significant disease (Rubin, 1988):

Primary CMV infection. This occurs when donor tissue or cells latently infected with CMV are placed from a CMV-seropositive donor into a seronegative recipient, with subsequent reactivation of the latent virus and dissemination in the CMV naive host. All individuals who have antibody to CMV (and hence are seropositive) harbour latent virus in a variety of cells and tissues. In 85–95% of cases, the latently infected cells are within the transplanted allograft; in the remaining 5–15% of cases the infection is transmitted in viable leukocytes administered with blood products donated by a seropositive donor. Approximately 60% of individuals at risk for primary CMV infection develop symptomatic CMV disease (Betts et al, 1975; Ho et al, 1975).

Reactivation CMV infection. This occurs when endogenous, latent virus within a transplant patient who is seropositive for CMV prior to transplantation is reactivated after transplantation. Although laboratory evidence of viral reactivation can be found in virtually every sero-positive individual only a minority (< 20%), become symptomatic (Ho, 1982).

Superinfection due to CMV. This occurs when a seropositive individual reactivates during the post-transplant period latent virus that had been present in cells present in an allograft (or blood product) derived from a seropositive donor, rather than his own endogenous virus. Studies performed in kidney allograft recipients suggest that this happens in about 50% of such cases, and that as many as half of these individuals become ill (Chou, 1986; Grundy et al, 1987).

Whichever form of CMV infection occurs in a transplant recipient, the peak activity of this virus occurs 1–4 months following transplantation, although there are rare, documented cases of either primary acquisition of the virus or superinfection due to community-based acquisition of the infection many months later. The clinical effects of the virus may be grouped into four general categories: the first two of these are regarded as proven, the third likely, and the last speculative (Rubin, 1988):

1. The direct causation of a variety of 'infectious disease syndromes' by the virus itself (Table 2).
2. The production of a generalized state of immunosuppression by the virus that is additional to that produced by pharmacological immunosuppression and which renders the patient susceptible to secondary infection with such opportunistic pathogens as *Pneumocystis carinii*, *Listeria monocytogenes*, and *Aspergillus* species (see above).
3. The causation of allograft injury by a process that is somewhat different from classical rejection. There is now a body of circumstantial evidence potentially linking CMV with a form of glomerular injury in renal transplant recipients, with an increased incidence of accelerated coronary artery atherosclerosis similar to chronic rejection and with the so-called 'disappearing bile duct syndrome' as a manifestation of chronic rejection in liver transplant recipients. This immunomodulatory effect of CMV appears to be an indirect rather than a direct one. Current evidence favours the hypothesis that

CMV infection results in the elaboration of a variety of cytokines, particularly α- and γ-interferon, which, under certain circumstances, can cause an upregulation of the expression of HLA antigens on allografted tissue. This results in greater immune injury to the allograft (O'Grady et al, 1988; Rubin, 1988).

4. The participation of the virus in the pathogenetic processes that result in the development of malignancies.

Table 2.   Clinical syndromes caused directly by cytomegalovirus in the organ transplant patient.

Early (1–4 months post-transplant)
   Fever of unknown origin
   Mononucleosis-like syndrome
   Pneumonia
   Leukopenia and/or thrombocytopenia

   Gastrointestinal tract inflammation
   Hepatitis
   ? Neurological syndromes

Late (after 4 months post-transplant)
   Progressive chorioretinitis
   ? Chronic liver dysfunction

The most important exogenous factor influencing the course of CMV infection is the immunosuppressive therapy that is administered (Rubin, 1988). A number of studies over the past two decades have demonstrated that: corticosteroids on their own have little effect on the course of CMV infection, and do not reactivate latent virus; and that cytotoxic drugs such as azathioprine or cyclophosphamide, are not only capable of reactivation but can also increase the susceptibility to active virus and, perhaps, extend the spectrum of tissue damage induced by the virus (Dowling et al, 1976). Of all the immunosuppressive agents used in transplant patients, antilymphocyte antibodies have had the greatest CMV-promoting effect. Thus, when antithymocyte globulin (ATG) is added to conventional azathioprine and prednisone regimens, there is a higher rate of viraemia and symptomatic disease in the ATG group as well as an attenuation of the beneficial effects of prophylactic α-interferon on CMV observed compared with the non-ATG treated patients. Evidently this is an effect attributable to the addition of ATG to other immunosuppressive regimens. In a subsequent study the ATG treated patients received approximately 50% as much azathioprine and prednisone as the group of patients who received only these latter drugs. No difference was found in either the incidence or clinical severity of CMV between the two groups, suggesting that it is the net immunosuppressive effect or net cytotoxic (? lymphocytotoxic) effect that is important in determining the effects of CMV on the transplant patient. Similar observations have been made in patients treated with the pan-T-cell monoclonal antibody OKT3 (Rubin and Tolkoff Rubin, 1984).

The practical impact of different immunosuppressive regimens on the outcome of CMV infection was emphasized by a multicentre study of CMV infection in more than 1200 transplant recipients. In this study, patients at risk of primary CMV treated with conventional immunosuppression (azathioprine and prednisone) had a similar rate of survival with a functioning allograft at 6 months as those without CMV infection. In contrast, patients at risk for primary CMV who had been treated with antilymphocyte antibodies (ATG or antilymphocyte globulin) in addition to conventional therapy showed a significant decrease in the percentage of individuals surviving with functioning grafts (53.1% v. 70.8%, $p = 0.05$). Conversely, patients at high risk of reactivation disease had a markedly improved graft survival if treated with antilymphocyte antibody therapy (71% survival with a functioning graft at 6 months v. 61%, $p = 0.003$) (Rubin et al, 1985).

Less complete information is available on the impact of cyclosporin on the course of CMV infection in human transplant recipients. At present, the following observations appear to be valid: (i) cyclosporin therapy, with or without low-dose prednisone, is associated with a lower incidence of infection than conventional azathioprine–prednisone therapy, combined with antilymphocyte antibody treatment (given prophylactically or as an acute rejection treatment); (ii) cyclosporin therapy and conventional azathioprine–prednisone therapy without antilymphocyte antibody treatment are associated with similar rates of infection; (iii) overall, because cyclosporin is associated with decreased allograft rejection, and a lesser need for adjunctive antilymphocyte treatment, its use may be associated with a lower incidence of symptomatic CMV infection for a given rate of allograft survival (Bia et al, 1985; Najarian et al, 1985).

In devising the optimal immunosuppressive programme for the 1990s an important issue is what can be done to diminish the impact of CMV. Two different strategies appear to be possible: changes in the immunosuppressive therapy itself and antiviral strategies.

Changes in Immunosuppression to Reduce the Impact of CMV

As discussed above, there are at least two stages of CMV infection that might be influenced by immunosuppressive therapy – the reactivation of latent virus and the weakening of host defences against active, replicating virus. The first question that might be asked is what effects do each of the various components of immunosuppressive therapy have on these two stages. In order to analyse this question we have turned to a murine system. Dosage schedules of immunosuppressive therapy have been devised so as to produce equal anti-rejection effects, as defined by an equal potency in prolonging skin graft survival times. When the effects of equivalent ATG and cyclosporin regimens on CMV infection are compared, striking differences are noted. Whereas ATG has a striking ability to reactivate latent virus, cyclosporin is essentially unable to do so. In contrast, ATG has only minimal effects on the course of active infection, whereas cyclosporin is a major influence in promoting active infection. For example, a lethal intraperitoneal dose of murine CMV in BALB/c mice was approximately 10^6 plaque-forming units (pfu); when ATG was administered, the lethal dose was about 10^5 pfu; and when a schedule of cyclosporin with comparable anti-rejection effects to that of the ATG regimen was administered, the lethal dose was 10^2 pfu (Auchincloss and Rubin, unpublished data).

The implications of these findings are important. First, in these experiments we have, for the first time, demonstrated that the anti-rejection effects can be separated from their direct effects on viral infection. Second, it would suggest that early in the post-transplant course, before viral reactivation has occurred, that cyclosporin is the safest form of immunosuppression in terms of CMV infection, and that ATG usage (and, by inference, perhaps the use of other forms of lymphocytotoxic therapy such as anti-T cell monoclonal antibodies, azathioprine, and cyclophosphamide) should be avoided or minimized during this time. In contrast, in patients with active CMV infection, it might be reasonable to minimize cyclosporin use and base anti-rejection therapy more on ATG and/or corticosteroids. We suggest that this type of analysis, i.e. the determination of the effects on both reactivation of latent virus and on active viral infection, should be part of the evaluation of any new immunosuppressive drug or programme, at least until specific non-responsiveness to transplanted tissues without the need for generalized immuno-suppression becomes a clinical reality.

Immunosuppressive therapies that result in cytotoxicity, particularly lymphocytotoxi-city, have the most potent CMV reactivating effects. Thus, immunosuppressive strategies that do not have such effects would have great appeal, particularly in the first few weeks post-transplant. An example of one such approach that merits attention is that which inhibits intercellular adhesion molecules that appear to be critical in many inflammatory and immunological reactions. A glycoprotein present on the surface of leukocytes, the lymphocyte-function-associated antigen-1 (LFA-1) appears to be essential to lymphocyte functions that require cell-to-cell contact. LFA-1 binds to another intercellular adhesion molecule (ICAM-1) which is present on the surface of a variety of cells when inflammation is present, including fibroblasts and endothelial cells. The expression of ICAM-1 on these cells is stimulated by mediators of inflammation such as interleukin 1, tumour necrosis factor, and γ-interferon. Antibodies to either LFA-1 or ICAM-1 can block inflammatory processes. Because ICAM-1 is only expressed during the course of inflammation and in tissues that are undergoing inflammatory reactions, it is a particularly attractive specific target for anti-rejection therapy. Preliminary studies of the action of monoclonal antibodies to such intercellular adhesion molecules in a primate transplan-tation model appear very promising. Because of the lack of cytotoxicity associated with the use of such an 'inflammation blocking' strategy, anti-rejection therapy based on this approach might be postulated to have a lesser ability to reactivate latent virus (Leading Article, 1988; Cosimi, unpublished data).

Specific Antiviral Measures

The most obvious antiviral strategy against CMV is to avoid the transplantation of organs from seropositive donors into seronegative recipients, so called 'protective matching'. This will effectively prevent more than 85% of primary CMV disease. However, since approximately 50% of potential donors are CMV seropositive, this would greatly limit the availability of organs for seronegative patients at a time when there is already a shortage of organs for transplantation (Rubin and Tolkoff-Rubin, 1984). A different approach to limiting the effects of CMV infection on the organ transplant recipient is the addition of antiviral agents to current immunosuppressive regimens. There are three possible components to this antiviral strategy.

Prophylactic. At present, the most promising prophylactic treatment is the administration of hyperimmune anti-CMV immunoglobulin during the first 2–4 months after transplantation. Studies in a murine model, in renal transplant recipients at risk for primary infection (the group of renal transplant patients at greatest risk for significant consequences of CMV infection), and in bone marrow transplant recipients show considerable benefits for this approach (Rubin, 1988). Recently, acyclovir administered orally in very high doses has been reported to have comparable prophylactic benefit in preventing CMV infection (Balfour et al, 1987).

Active therapy. In those patients developing symptomatic CMV infection as a conse-quence of immunosuppressive therapy, the antiviral drug ganciclovir (DHPG) has been shown to have beneficial effects. In addition, there is an increasing body of evidence in both animal models and in transplant patients that the combination of ganciclovir with hyperimmune anti-CMV globulin is even more effective therapeutically than either agent alone, particularly in immunosuppressed individuals (Rubin, 1988).

Prevention of superinfection with other micro-organisms. Because one of the major effects of CMV infection on the transplant patient is its immunosuppressing effect, it would seem reasonable to take steps to limit the chances of opportunistic superinfection during the time of active CMV infection. Such attempts should include protection against potential environmental hazards (for example, if the patient is hospitalized, providing care in rooms in which the air has been specially filtered) and the prescription of specific antimicrobial prophylaxis. For the latter, we have found that low-dose trimethoprim–sulphamethoxa-zole therapy (one single strength tablet containing 80 mg trimethoprim and 400 mg sulphamethoxazole) is well-tolerated and provides effective prophylaxis against *Pneumo-cystis carinii*, *Nocardia asteroides*, and *Listeria monocytogenes* superinfection (Rubin, 1988).

EPSTEIN–BARR VIRUS

A complete summary of the clinical effects of Epstein–Barr virus (EBV) infection in the transplant patient has been very difficult to compile. The clinical effects of EBV and CMV are probably very similar, and the ubiquity of CMV makes the recognition of EBV-specific clinical syndromes in the individual patient virtually impossible. Evidence of active EBV infection, primarily reactivation infection, can be found in 40–70% of transplant recipients, with immunosuppressive therapy having similar modulating effects as with CMV infection. However, one particular aspect of EBV infection in transplant patients bears special attention – the EBV-associated lymphoproliferative syndromes (Rubin, 1988).

Approximately 10–15% of the malignancies observed in organ transplant recipients are a form of lymphoma known as immunoblastic sarcoma (formerly called reticulum cell sarcoma). In these individuals, a polymorphic B cell lymphoma invades the central nervous system, nasopharynx, liver, small bowel, heart, and/or allograft. It is currently believed that these B cell proliferations evolve from a benign EBV-dependent polyclonal B cell hyperplasia to a malignant, EBV-independent monoclonal B cell lymphoma (Hanto et al, 1983).

The pathogenesis of this process is thought to be as follows: In immunologically normal individuals previously infected with EBV (and who are therefore antibody-positive and latently infected with this virus), circulating cytotoxic T lymphocytes specific for EBV-induced antigens on the surface of infected B lymphocytes act as a surveillance mechanism in preventing the outgrowth of virally-induced, transformed cells that are thought to initiate the oncogenic process which culminates in lymphoprolifera-tive disease. In immunosuppressed patients, this system of protection is defective, with the greatest impairment being observed with cyclosporin administration (Bird et al, 1981; Crawford et al, 1981; Yao et al, 1985).

This cyclosporin-induced suppression of the surveillance function of cytotoxic T lymphocytes against the outgrowth of EBV-transformed B lymphocytes is a dose-related phenomenon. Its incidence has decreased in recent years with adjustments in the dosage of cyclosporin achieved by the widespread practice of monitoring the blood concentration of this drug. In addition, in the early stages of this process, when the lymphoproliferation is still polyclonal in character, regression occurs when the cyclosporin is discontinued and/or acyclovir (an antiviral drug with activity against EBV) is administered (Starzl et al, 1984). However, even with low doses of cyclosporin, this process can occur (Bia and Flye, 1985). Because other components of the immunosuppressive regimen can have similar effects, particularly anti-T lymphocyte antibody, an additive or net suppressive effect on immune surveillance must be considered as likely.

Before new forms of immunosuppressive therapy are applied, therefore, the effects of the regimen on the cytotoxic T lymphocyte surveillance function against EBV-induced oncogenesis must be considered and, if possible, measured. As with CMV infection, the therapeutic programmes of the future should feature one or probably both of two strategies already mentioned above; an ideal immunosuppressive protocol should leave immunological surveillance intact while still preventing allograft rejection. Strategies based on the induction of specific tolerance or the deployment of therapies aimed at inhibiting the intercellular adhesion molecules appear particularly appealing: also it would be useful to develop an antiviral agent such as acyclovir that could be given either prophylactically or therapeutically to prevent this aspect of EBV infection, even when the normal cytotoxic T lymphocyte mechanism is impaired.

BACTERIAL INFECTION

As discussed previously, the majority of bacterial infections in transplant patients relate to surgical complications which are usually caused by technical problems incurred in the management of the patient in the perioperative period (see Table 1). Such technical problems result either from the bypassing of normal mucocutaneous barriers to infection (as with the introduction of bacteria via the endotracheal tube, intravenous lines, or bladder catheter) or result from tissue injury which will lead to infection. Immunosuppression, particularly the steroid component, then plays a secondary role in increasing the impact of such infections and in promoting opportunistic superinfection. Therapeutic programmes of the 1990s that will limit the impact of such infections, should therefore include the following (Rubin, 1988):

1. Surgical technique must be scrupulous, to minimize tissue necrosis, postoperative lacerations, and leakage from suture-lines involving the urinary or gastrointestinal tract. Closed drainage of wounds should be used judiciously. The insertion of intravenous lines and catheters must be done using aseptic techniques by trained staff. It is essential to eradicate all foci of active infection before commencing a transplant operation and immunosuppression.
2. A major theme of modern immunosuppressive therapy is the development of anti-rejection programmes that are steroid-sparing. Corticosteroids have the broadest depressing effect on host defences: the deployment of more specific drugs that permit the use of smaller doses of corticosteroid, or even their complete elimination, results in a decreased risk of infection in general, and of bacterial and fungal infection in particular.

3. Cytotoxic drugs such as azathioprine and cyclophosphamide have been used to great advantage in the management of allograft rejection. Their major side-effect is bone marrow toxicity, with the development of granulocytopenia being particularly ominous. Granulocytopenia carries a major risk of bacterial invasion, and regimens that avoid bone marrow toxicity therefore remain a priority. There are at least two potential approaches to accomplishing this task in the future — the use of cyclosporin which reduces the need for bone marrow-toxic immunosuppressive regimens, and the addition of such bone marrow stimulating agents as the newly available haematopoietic hormones (e.g., erythropoietin and the bone marrow colony stimulating factors) to bone marrow-toxic regimens.

4. Antibacterial prophylaxis should be used routinely during all transplant procedures. Wound infections can be almost eradicated in renal transplant recipients with 24 hours of antimicrobial therapy beginning just before surgery. Low-dose trimethoprim-sulphamethoxazole (one single strength tablet at bedtime) or ciprofloxacin (250 mg at bedtime) can essentially eradicate urinary tract infection.

One particular form of bacterial infection that merits special attention is tuberculosis, as reactivation tuberculosis occurs at a rate approximately 100 times that of the general population and both prophylaxis and treatment of tuberculosis in transplant patients can be difficult (Rubin, 1988). One year of isoniazid (INH) prophylaxis following transplantation is effective prophylaxis, but can be difficult to accomplish because of concerns regarding INH hepatotoxicity in a population receiving other potentially hepatotoxic drugs and with a significant incidence of viral hepatitis. Because of these factors and because the rate of activation of dormant tuberculosis in tuberculin-positive organ transplant recipients has been remarkably low, we and other transplant groups (Thomas et al, 1979) have reserved INH prophylaxis for particular groups of patients felt to be at higher risk. One year of INH prophylaxis is instituted in the following groups of patients: recent tuberculin converters; those with a history of untreated or suboptimally treated tuberculosis in the past decade; those with significant abnormalities on chest radiography; those with histories of genitourinary tuberculosis; those who possess other risk factors, such as malnutrition (Rubin, 1988).

One other aspect of antituberculosis therapy in transplant patients meriting attention is that antituberculous drugs can have an adverse effect on allograft survival through their effects on the metabolism of immunosuppressive drugs. Rifampicin, and probably other antituberculous drugs as well, will stimulate hepatic enzymes responsible for the catabolism of immunosuppressive drugs. Thus, a given dose of prednisone can have less anti-rejection effects because of this increased rate of drug breakdown and rejection can ensue (Buffington et al, 1976). This phenomenon is particularly important with cyclosporin-based immunosuppressive regimens, as the increased metabolism of cyclosporin caused by increased activity of the hepatic cytochrome p450 enzyme system has resulted in severe rejection due to inadvertent under-immunosuppression. Such effects can be looked for beginning 1–2 weeks after the initiation of rifampicin therapy, with peak effects observed after 1–2 months. Thus, patients must be closely monitored and their immunosuppressive regimen increased when rifampicin and probably any antituberculosis drug, is employed (Langhoff and Madsen, 1983; Modry et al, 1985; Rubin, 1988).

FUNGAL INFECTION

Fungal infection in the transplant recipient is of two types: reactivation of latent infection that had been acquired by residence in areas endemic for these agents prior to transplantation, with reactivation and dissemination caused by the immunosuppressive therapy; and new opportunistic infections acquired after transplantation. In the first category belong reactivation histoplasmosis, coccidioidomycosis, and blastomycosis (as does the non-fungal but pathogenetically similar entity, reactivation tuberculosis). The major factor involved in such reactivation infections, with subsequent dissemination, is impaired cell-mediated immunity, with the net state of immunosuppression being the major determinant of risk of reactivation. As antifungal prophylaxis in patients with dormant infection (similar to isoniazid prophylaxis in tuberculin-positive individuals who are immunosuppressed) is not yet feasible, we must devise immunosuppressive regimens that produce less generalized suppression of cell-mediated immunity before we can hope to control this problem (Rubin, 1988).

A more common problem is the acquisition of more opportunistic fungal infection following transplantation. This form of infection is perhaps the most clear-cut example of how clinically significant infection can be the result of an interaction between epidemiological exposures and the net state of immunosuppression. If the intensity of exposure is great enough, then any patient is likely to develop infection; if immunosuppression is strong enough, even trivial exposures can lead to life-threatening infection. These infections can be grouped into three general categories: primary disseminated infection caused by *Histoplasma capsulatum*, *Coccidioides immitis*, *Blastomyces dermatididis*, and other geographically restricted mycotic agents; primary infection, usually of the lungs, occasionally of the nasal sinuses, most commonly by *Cryptococcus neoformans* or *Aspergillus* species (the opportunistic bacterial organism *Nocardia asteroides* too, belongs here); and sequential and concurrent secondary infection, either of the lungs or via infected intravenous lines, by *Candida* species, *Aspergillus* species, or *Torulopsis glabrata*. Two strategies can prevent these infections: protection against environmental exposure (particularly, in the hospital setting, the provision of filtered air); and, again, the use of immunosuppressive programmes that will provide a less profound generalized state of immunosuppression. The same principles discussed previously for CMV infection are operative here (Rubin, 1988).

PROTOZOAN INFECTION

There are three protozoan infections of importance in the transplant patient – those due to *Pneumocystis carinii*, *Toxoplasma gondii*, and *Strongyloides stercoralis*. All three are seen particularly in individuals with profound depression of cell-mediated immunity, with the highest attack rates being observed in individuals 1–4 months post-transplant with viral infection (and hence a greatly increased net state of immunosuppression). *Pneumocystis carinii* appears to be primarily a reactivation infection, and this can be effectively prevented with the use of prophylactic agents such as low-dose trimethoprim–sulphamethoxazole prophylaxis or weekly pentamidine administration by aerosol.

Toxoplasmosis occurs most commonly when an individual who has had no past experience with this organism receives an allograft that harbours dormant *Toxoplasma gondii.* This is a significant concern mainly in cardiac allograft recipients, in whom the transplantation of a heart from a seropositive donor into a seronegative recipient carries a significant risk of causing a disseminated toxoplasmosis syndrome with particular impact on the central nervous system. Fortunately, effective prophylaxis in this situation is available, with pyrimethamine and sulphasoxazole (or other sulphonamides) providing excellent prevention not only against toxoplasmosis but also *Pneumocystis.*

Strongyloides stercoralis occurs when an individual harbours asymptomatic gastrointestinal infection before transplantation, with subsequent dissemination when the net state of immunosuppression is at its greatest. With this organism, the strategy is treatment and eradication with thiabendazole prior to transplantation. Thus, all individuals with a history of travelling or residence in areas of the world with endemic strongyloidiasis should be carefully screened before transplantation (Rubin, 1988).

Thus, when considering future prevention of parasitic infection in transplant recipients, it is quite clear that the intensity of the immunosuppressive therapy administered will have an impact on the occurrence of such infections. However, even without modifying present immunosuppressive regimens, the incidence of these infections can be markedly reduced with practical antimicrobial agents that are already available.

SUMMARY

This chapter has two major themes: infection and rejection are closely linked in the transplant patient, with the common link being the immunosuppressive therapy that is administered; and the risk of infection is due to an interaction between the net state of immunosuppression and the epidemiological exposures. In developing therapeutic regimens for the transplant patient in the 1990s, we should think in terms of three different components:

Immunosuppressive therapy. Clearly, the main thrust must be towards the development of steroid-sparing, immunosuppressive programmes, with specific unresponsiveness to the allografted organ being the ultimate goal. Short of this, the immunosuppressive programmes of the future will be more specific and non-toxic for the bone marrow. Because of the importance of viral infections, the assessment of such programmes in terms of their effects on viral reactivation and dissemination will be highly desirable. Special emphasis must be given to the potential of a given agent for reactivating latent CMV infection or for blocking the cell-mediated immune response to CMV and EBV. Especially promising in this area are strategies based on blockage of the intercellular adhesion molecules that are restricted to inflamed or immunologically active tissue.

Specific antimicrobial prophylaxis. The addition of certain antimicrobial agents to immunosuppressive regimens in use now could play a significant role in the prevention of life-threatening infection, and should be regarded as important parts of therapy. Prime examples of this approach are the efficacy of trimethoprim–sulphamethoxazole, trimethoprim, and ciprofloxacin in the prevention of urosepsis in renal transplant recipients; trimethoprim–sulphamethoxazole in the prevention of *Pneumocystis carinii*, and probably *Listeria monocytogenes* and *Nocardia asteroides* infection; and pyrimethamine and sulphasoxazole in the prevention of toxoplasmosis in patients at risk for this.

Environmental protection. As described above, there is a timetable that derives from the time course of the development of immunosuppression and which allows the prediction of clinical susceptibility to opportunistic infections. Protecting the patient from excessive exposure to potential pathogens during the period of maximal immunosuppression (for instance by air infiltration) can markedly diminish the rate of infection.

REFERENCES

Allo MD, Miller J, Townsend T & Tan C (1987) Primary cutaneous aspergillosis associated with Hickman intravenous catheters. *New England Journal of Medicine* **317**: 1105–1108.

Auchincloss H Jr & Rubin RH: The differential effects of equi-anti-rejection dose of ATG and cyclosporine on the course of murine cytomegalovirus infection, manuscript in preparation.

Balfour HH, Chace BA, Spaleton JT, Simmons RL & Fryd, DS (1989) A randomized, placebo-controlled trial of oral acyclovir for the prevention of cytomegalovirus disease in recipients of renal allografts. *New England Journal of Medicine* **320**: 1381–1387.

Betts RF, Freeman RB, Douglas RG Jr et al (1975) Transmission of cytomegalovirus infection with renal allograft. *Kidney International* **8**: 385–392.

Bia MJ & Flye MW (1985) Immunoblastic lymphoma in a cyclopsorine-treated renal transplant recipient. *Transplantation* **39**: 673–674.

Bia MJ, Andiman W, Gaudio K et al (1985) Effects of treatment with cyclosporine versus azathioprine on incidence and severity of cytomegalovirus infection posttransplantation. *Transplantation* **40**: 610–614.

Bird AG, McLaughlin SM & Britton S (1981) Cyclosporin A promotes spontaneous outgrowth *in vitro* of Epstein–Barr virus-induced B-cell lines. *Nature* **289**: 300–301.

Buffington GA, Dominguez JH, Piering WF et al (1976) Interaction of rifampin and glucorticoids – adverse effect on renal allograft function. *Journal of the American Medical Association* **236**: 1958–1960.

Chou S (1986) Acquisition of donor strains of cytomegalovirus by renal-transplant recipients. *New England Journal of Medicine* **314**: 1418–1423.

Crawford DH, Swany P, Edwards JMB et al (1981) Long-term T-cell mediated immunity for Epstein–Barr virus in renal allograft recipients receiving cyclosporin A. *Lancet* **i**: 10–12.

Dowling JN, Saslow AR, Armstrong JA & Ho M (1976) Cytomegalovirus infection in patients recovering from immunosuppressive therapy for rheumatologic disorders. *Journal of Infectious Disease* **133**: 399–408.

Grundy JE, Super M, Lui S et al (1987) The source of cytomegalovirus infection in seropositive renal allograft recipients is frequently the donor kidney. *Transplantation Proceedings* **19**: 2126–2128.

Hanto DW, Gajl-Peczalska KJ, Frizzera G et al (1983) Epstein–Barr virus (EBV) induced polyclonal and monoclonal B-cell lymphoproliferative disease occurring after renal transplantation. Clinical, pathologic, and virologic findings and implications for therapy. *Annals of Surgery* **198**: 356–369.

Ho M (1977) Virus infections after transplantation in man; brief review. *Archives of Virology* **55**: 1–24.

Ho M (1982) *Cytomegalovirus, Biology and Infection.* New York: Plenum Medical.

Ho M, Suwansirikul S, Dowling JN et al (1987) The transplanted kidney as a source of cytomegalovirus infection. *New England Journal of Medicine* **293**: 1109–1112.

Langhoff E & Madsen S (1983) Rapid metabolism of cyclosporine and prednisone on kidney transplant patients receiving tuberculostatic therapy. *Lancet* **ii**: 1031–1034.

Leading Article (1988) Intercellular adhesion molecules and recurrent infection. *Lancet* **ii**: 831–832.

Modry DL, Stinson EB, Oyer PE et al (1985) Acute rejection and massive cyclosporine requirements in heart transplant recipients treated with rifampin. *Transplantation* **39**: 313–314.

Najarian JS, Fryd DS, Strand M et al (1985) A single institution, randomized, prospective trial of cyclosporine versus azathioprine–antithymocyte globulin for immunosuppression in renal allograft recipients. *Annals of Surgery* **201**: 142–157.

O'Grady JG, Alexander GJM, Sutherland S et al (1988) Cytomegalovirus infection and donor/recipient HLA antigens: interdependent co-factors in pathogenesis of vanishing bileduct syndrome after liver transplantation. *Lancet* **ii**: 302–305.

Rubin RH (1987) The compromised host as sentinel chicken. *New England Journal of Medicine* **317**: 1151–1153.

Rubin RH (1988) Infection in the renal and liver transplant patient. In Rubin RH & Young LS (eds) *Clinical Approach to Infection in the Compromised Host*, 2nd edn, pp 57–621. New York: Plenum Medical.

Rubin RH & Tolkoff-Rubin NE (1984) The problem of cytomegalovirus infection in transplantation. In PJ Morris & NL Tilney (eds) *Progress in Transplantation*, vol. 1, pp 89–114. Edinburgh: Churchill Livingstone.

Rubin RH, Wolfson JS, Cosimi AB et al (1981) Infection in the renal transplant recipient. *American Journal of Medicine* **70**: 405–411.

Rubin RH, Tolkoff-Rubin NE, Oliver D et al (1985) Multicenter seroepidemiologic study of the impact of cytomegalovirus infection on renal transplantation. *Transplantation* **40**: 243–249.

Starzl TE, Nalesnik MA, Porter LA et al (1984) Reversibility of lymphomas and lymphoproliferative lesions developing under cyclosporine–steroid therapy. *Lancet* **i**: 583–587.

Thomas PA Jr, Mozes MF & Jonasson O (1979) Hepatic dysfunction during isoniazid chemoprophylaxis in renal allograft recipients. *Archives of Surgery* **114**: 597–599.

Yao QY, Rickinson AB, Gastron JS et al (1985) In vitro analysis of the Epstein–Barr virus: Host balance in long-term renal allograft recipients. *International Journal of Cancer* **35**: 43–49.

6 Bone Marrow Transplantation and Graft-versus-host Disease

KEITH M. SULLIVAN
RAINER STORB

More than 30 years have passed since experiments first demonstrated that mice could be protected from otherwise lethal irradiation by splenic shielding or marrow infusions (Jacobson et al, 1950; Lorenz et al, 1951). The first successful human bone marrow transplants were carried out in the 1950s from identical twin donors (Thomas et al, 1959). Since then, progress in key areas in transplantation biology has made transplantation more widely applicable; marrow transplantation is now a worldwide activity involving nearly 200 transplant centres. The International Bone Marrow Transplant Registry estimates that between 1955 and 1985, 9445 patients received marrow transplants (Bortin and Rimm, 1986). As of 1 February 1988, 3000 marrow transplants (2498 allogeneic, 317 autologous, and 185 syngeneic) have been carried out by the Seattle Marrow Transplant Team alone.

Initially considered highly experimental and used only as a last resort, clinical results have improved as marrow transplantation is performed earlier in the course of disease. In patients with haematological malignancies, maximal tumour destruction is afforded by pre-transplant preparation with supralethal doses of total body irradiation (TBI) and high-dose chemotherapy. Antineoplastic treatment can be administered in doses restricted only by the limits of extramedullary toxicity. Marrow grafting is used to restore immune function in patients with immunological deficiencies and can usually be performed without preparative immunosuppression. In contrast, patients with severe aplastic anaemia must have host immune function ablated with immunosuppressive drugs to prevent marrow graft rejection. The so-called inborn error diseases also require prepara-tive conditioning, after which transplantation of donor monocytes and macrophages allows correction of the functional or enzymatic defect.

Marrow transplantation differs from solid organ transplantation in that donor bone marrow contains immunocompetent T lymphocytes capable of responding, once engrafted, in an allogeneic reaction against disparate histocompatibility antigens located on host tissues, thereby producing a graft-versus-host reaction. Thus, the allogeneic marrow transplant procedure requires both pre-transplant immunosuppressive condition-ing to facilitate engraftment and post-transplant methods to prevent graft-versus-host

ORGAN TRANSPLANTATION: CURRENT CLINICAL AND
IMMUNOLOGICAL CONCEPTS   ISBN 0-7020-1393-5

disease (GVHD). With time, specific donor–host immunological non-reactivity (i.e. graft-specific tolerance) develops and long-term immunosuppressive treatment is discontinued in most patients within 3–6 months of transplant.

This chapter will review current clinical results and highlight problems and progress in our understanding of the biology of bone marrow transplantation.

TECHNIQUES OF TRANSPLANTATION

Marrow Source

Allogeneic marrow grafts are usually performed from genotypically human leukocyte antigen (HLA)-identical sibling donors. The HLA complex, coded for by genes located on the sixth human chromosome, is a heterogenous region on cell surfaces with several major loci of transplantation importance (Hansen and Thomas, 1983; see also Chapter 6). HLA-A, -B, and -DR alleles are detected by serological microcytotoxicity assay. HLA-D alleles are determined by mixed leukocyte reactivity. Other genetic determinants outside the currently known HLA system govern the so-called 'minor' transplantation antigens. Individuals inherit one HLA haplotype from each parent, and within any given family there are four HLA haplotypes giving approximately a 25% chance of having a genotypically HLA-identical sibling. Most allogeneic transplants are from HLA-identical siblings but recently HLA-nonidentical family members have been used who are genotypically identical for one shared haplotype but differ for 0, 1, 2, or 3 loci on the other. This increases the pool of possible related donors by about 10%. As discussed below, recent clinical studies have shown encouraging results using phenotypically HLA-identical unrelated marrow donors. With registries containing 1000, 10 000 or 100 000 volunteer marrow donors, the average probability of finding an HLA-A, -B, or -DR match are 3.8, 14, and 32.2%, respectively (Beatty et al, 1988).

Syngeneic transplants are performed from identical twin donors who represent an ideal source of bone marrow. Graft-versus-host disease and graft rejection are rarely, if ever, observed in syngeneic transplants, and the marrow inoculum is free of contaminating tumour cells.

In autologous transplantation, marrow is harvested while the patient is in chemo-therapy-induced remission (Dicke et al, 1984). Before cryopreservation, the marrow may be treated ex vivo with antineoplastic agents in an attempt to remove clonogenic tumour cells (Santos and Colvin, 1986; Yeager et al, 1986; Auber et al, 1988). If stored for more than one day, the marrow requires freezing to preserve stem cell viability. Cryopreservation is carried out in the presence of a cryoprotective agent, such as dimethylsulphoxide and hydroxyethyl starch (Stiff et al, 1987). Pluripotent haematopoietic stem cells stored at ultra-low temperature can be thawed years later and used for successful engraftment.

Haematopoietic stem cells obtained from peripheral blood are occasionally used for autologous transplantation (Kessinger et al, 1988). Peripheral blood can be collected during multiple pheresis procedures allowing stem cell transplantation of patients who are ineligible for autologous marrow harvest due to anaesthetic risk or prior pelvic irradiation. Another rich source of stem cells is fetal liver (Prummer and Fliedner, 1986). Severe combined immunodeficiency can be corrected with infusion of fetal liver cells, but because of a variety of practical and ethical considerations, few such transplants have been performed.

More recently, autologous bone marrow harvested during leukaemic relapse has been grown in long-term culture conditions that appear to favour selective survival of normal stem cells over that of the malignant cells (Chang et al, 1986). Problems relating to the efficiency of the technique and the perpetuation of long-term cultures are considerable. The use of haematopoietic growth factors may be of benefit in the application of this technology.

Donor Selection

In an attempt to increase the number of potential marrow donors, the Seattle group has performed transplants from HLA-nonidentical family members (Beatty et al, 1985). Results from over 200 such transplants to date indicate that, within each disease category, survival after phenotypically-identical and one-antigen-mismatched marrow grafts is equivalent to results obtained with HLA-identical transplants. However, delayed or failed marrow engraftment, infection and acute GVHD are more common. Surprisingly, despite the higher incidence of GVHD, survival of phenotypically HLA-identical or one locus mismatched patients is not significantly different from that of patients given genotypically HLA-identical marrow grafts. However, results in patients given two- or three-locus-mismatched grafts are considerably worse, and long-term survival is only 10–20%.

Another alternative might be to consider transplantation from an HLA-identical, unrelated donor (O'Reilly et al, 1977; Hansen et al, 1980; Hows et al, 1986; McGlave et al, 1987). Although the clinical experience to date is small, results with phenotypically-identical, unrelated donors are encouraging. The experience with mismatched, unrelated donors is less satisfactory, with a high mortality from infectious complications (Gingrich et al, 1988). One possible explanation for this is that fully-allogeneic (donor-derived) T lymphocytes may not function effectively in an immunological response if mismatched for major histocompatibility complex antigens with the host (Rayfield and Brent, 1983).

While the expanding availability of alternative donors is encouraging, donor selection criteria become more complex. In some families, several HLA-identical siblings may be identified as potential donors. In general, selection of donors is based upon the health of the donor with regard to anaesthesia and marrow harvest. Blood group incompatibility does not influence donor selection because of the ease of preventing ABO-incompatible transfusion reactions by the use of plasma exchange or immunoabsorption to remove anti-A or anti-B antibodies (Bensinger et al, 1982). Because of the importance of preventing GVHD and cytomegalovirus (CMV) infection after transplantation, other criteria should be considered for selection of a matched donor from among several candidates. Data from the International Bone Marrow Transplant Registry indicate that the incidence of acute GVHD is increased when the donor and patient are sex-mismatched (Gale et al, 1987). This is especially true when alloimmunized parous females donate marrow to male recipients. This could be caused by immunization against the human H-Y (minor) antigen (see Chapter 1). Thus, sex matching or selection of a non-parous female might reduce the risk of GVHD. Transplant-related mortality can also be reduced by selection of a donor who is CMV antibody-seronegative, if the marrow graft recipient is likewise CMV-seronegative. Previous studies have shown that primary CMV infection in seronegative patients with seronegative marrow donors can be prevented by exclusive use of CMV-seronegative blood products (Bowden et al, 1986). Finally, the age of the donor may be a factor. Because of anaesthetic risk and changes in blood volume, marrow donors under 60 years of age are preferred. Children under 2 years of age may also safely donate marrow (Sanders et al, 1987). The volume of marrow obtained from very young children ranges from 15–19 ml/kg weight and contains 2.5–10.4 × 10^8 nucleated cells/kg donor weight. Among both children and adults, the incidence of major life-threatening complications (such as bacteraemia or cardiovascular collapse) during or after the marrow harvest is exceedingly small (0.27% or less) (Bortin and Buckner, 1983; Buckner et al, 1984).

If an identical twin or a genotypically HLA-identical sibling is not available, searches of extended family members, including parents and cousins, should be conducted to locate a suitable mismatched family donor. Because of an increased risk of GVHD, patients who are more than 50 years of age or who have no better than a two- or three-antigen HLA-nonidentical putative marrow donor, should be considered for an autologous marrow transplant. Bilateral marrow aspirates from the iliac crests (with cytogenetics if there was a prior clonal marker of malignancy) should be performed before marrow harvest to ensure continued remission. For patients in bone marrow relapse, or those who prefer an allogeneic marrow donor, the search for an unrelated donor can be started. National registries in the United States and the United Kingdom have tens of thousands of volunteer donor records on file, and a search for an HLA-A and -B locus match can be made quickly. Thereafter, potential donors would be called in for additional DR typing and mixed leukocyte culture testing with cells from the patient. In addition, the volunteer donor should have a physical examination with CMV, ABO and HIV testing as well as counselling concerning the risk. On average, these procedures require 2–3 months for completion, making the search for unrelated donors for patients with rapidly progressive malignancy ill-advised.

Marrow Harvest

Multiple marrow aspirations from the iliac crests are sterilely performed under general anaesthesia to obtain between 400 and 1000 ml of marrow yielding 2–6 × 10^8 nucleated cells/kg recipient weight. Details of the marrow harvest have been previously reported (Thomas and Storb, 1970). Bone marrow is placed into heparinized tissue culture, passed through wire mesh to remove aggregates, and infused intravenously. Haematopoietic stem cells circulate through the lungs and home to the marrow cavities, and within 2–4 weeks marrow cellularity and peripheral blood counts increase as the graft becomes functional.

Preparation for Transplantation

The marrow is infused on the last day of the pre-transplant preparative conditioning. The conditioning regimen is used to ablate the host immune response so that the graft will not be rejected. Additionally, in patients with haematological malignancy, the preparative conditioning serves as a supralethal antineoplastic treatment, from which the patient is 'rescued' by the transplant. The first transplants in patients with leukaemia were carried out with only chemotherapy or only single-dose TBI (Thomas et al, 1975). Recurrent leukaemia was seen in almost all of these early patients, and, to increase the leukaemic cell kill, cyclophosphamide (60 mg/kg) was given on each of two days before irradiation. TBI dose rates range from 2.5–85 cGy per minute delivered by opposing cobalt-60 sources or linear accelerators (Lam et al, 1980). Fractionation of TBI has recently been used to decrease toxicity and increase malignant cell destruction. Fractionated doses range from

1.25 to 3.3 Gy, and fraction intervals range from 3 to 24 hours with total TBI doses ranging from 5 to 15.75 Gy. A regimen of hyperfractionated TBI followed by cyclophosphamide in children with acute leukaemia appears encouraging (Brochstein et al, 1987) but the results require confirmation. It is unclear whether the inversion of the chemoradiotherapy sequence or the dose schedule of TBI contributes to the improved survival.

The possible number of combinations of TBI dose, fraction and schedule is limitless. While intensifying the dose or schedule of chemoradiotherapy might reduce rates of recurrent leukaemia, overall survival may not improve due to increased morbidity and mortality from regimen-related toxicities (UCLA Team, 1977; Bearman et al, 1988). Phase I/II reports of new regimens of high-dose etoposide (Blume et al, 1987), high-dose cytarabine (Riddell et al, 1988), cyclophosphamide/BCNU(carmustine)/etoposide (Jagannath et al, 1986; Zander et al, 1987) and busulphan/cyclophosphamide (Santos et al, 1983; Tutschka et al, 1987) appear of great interest, but require Phase III testing to confirm any apparent improvement in long-term survival.

Toxicity of Conditioning

Damage to normal rapidly dividing tissue is an unavoidable consequence of high-dose chemoradiotherapy. During the first month post-transplant, painful oral mucositis is observed, which generally improves upon recovery of adequate nuetrophil counts. Oral mucositis pain may be relieved by patient-controlled analgesia coupled with delivery of intravenous opioids tailored to blood concentrations. Fractionation of TBI has apparently lessened damage to normal lung tissues, as evidenced by a reduction in the rate of 'idiopathic' interstitial pneumonia (Meyers et al, 1983). Older patient age, presence of severe GVHD, high dose rate of TBI, prior mediastinal irradiation, and prolonged use of methotrexate appear to increase the risk for interstitial pneumonitis (Weiner et al, 1986; Appelbaum et al, 1987). Liver disorders, especially veno-occlusive disease (VOD), appear to be increasing in frequency, perhaps due to an increase in the incidence of prior non-A, non-B hepatitis (McDonald et al, 1986). The clinical course of VOD is well characterized with a case fatality rate as high as 30%. In some centres hepatic VOD is the third major cause of death in allogeneic graft recipients and the second in autologous graft recipients (McDonald et al, 1985, 1987; Jones et al, 1987). This and other toxicities may be amplified by post-transplant immunosuppression with methotrexate or cyclosporin. Other acute toxicities are less common. Neurotoxicty may be an immediate or delayed complication of the preparative regimen, but fortunately this is an infrequent occurrence (Sullivan et al, 1982; Thompson et al, 1986).

Long-term side-effects of high-dose chemoradiotherapy have been described (Sullivan et al, 1984): impairment of growth and sexual development has been observed in children (Sanders et al, 1986) and TBI prevents recovery of normal gonadal function in the majority of patients (Sanders et al, 1983); cataracts have been observed in 80% of patients given single-dose TBI, but the incidence may be reduced to 20% in patients given fractionated TBI (Deeg et al, 1984, 1986).

In an attempt to decrease toxicity and increase anti-tumour therapy, novel methods of radiation delivery are being explored in preclinical and clinical studies (Appelbaum et al, 1986; Macklis et al, 1988). Monoclonal antibodies homing to antigens on haematopoietic and tumour cells have been conjugated with radio-isotopes to deliver irradiation to

Table 1. HLA-identical marrow transplantation for severe aplastic anaemia.

Centre	Reference	Study year	Number of patients	Graft rejection (%)	Actuarial survival (%)		
					CY	CY + TAI/TLI	CY + TBI
Seattle*	Anasetti et al, 1986	1972–84	50	10	82		
Seattle	Storb, 1987	1978–85	138	11	73		
IBMTR	Gluckman, 1988	1988		11	52–70	64	54
IBMTR	Champlin, 1986	1978–86	455	17	55	65	46
EBMTR	Bacigalupo et al, 1985	1980–83	165	17	62	70	40

* Untransfused patients only.
CY, cyclophosphamide; EBMTR, European Bone Marrow Transplant Registry; IBMTR, International Bone Marrow Transplant Registry; TAI, thoraco-abdominal irradiation; TBI, total body irradiation; TLI, total lymphoid irradiation.

marrow, spleen, and lymph nodes with greater selectivity and less damage than external beam irradiation. Such radio-immunotherapy may bring about a substantial improvement in the results of transplantation for malignant disease.

RESULTS OF TRANSPLANTATION

Non-malignant Disorders

Within the non-malignant diseases, the largest transplant experience has been with patients suffering from severe aplastic anaemia. Although some patients with severe marrow failure may respond to treatment with antithymocyte globulin or immunosuppressive agents, responses may be incomplete or transient, and marrow grafting is generally considered the treatment of choice for patients less than 40 years of age who have an HLA-identical sibling. A commonly used preparative regimen for allogeneic transplants includes cyclophosphamide (50 mg/kg on each of four successive days) followed by marrow transplantation (Storb et al, 1984). Other preparative regimens have combined high-dose cyclophosphamide with total lymphoid irradiation (TLI), thoracoabdominal irradiation (TAI), or TBI.

Table 1 summarizes long-term results after HLA-identical marrow transplantation for the treatment of severe aplastic anaemia. Marrow grafting before transfusion of blood products avoids transfusion-induced sensitization, lowers the likelihood of marrow graft rejection, and results in 10-year survival in more than 80% of patients (Anasetti et al, 1986). For repeatedly transfused patients conditioned with cyclophosphamide alone, results obtained before 1976 showed a marrow graft rejection rate of 30%. Increasing bone marrow cell dose and infusion of viable donor buffy coat cells decrease the incidence of graft rejection (Storb et al, 1982; Niederwieser et al, 1988). Other approaches to reduce rejection of the graft call for more intense pre-transplant immunosuppression to destroy residual host cells by combining cyclophosphamide with TAI, TLI or TBI (Ramsay et al, 1983; Bacigalupo et al, 1985; Champlin, 1986; Storb 1987; Gluckman, 1988). Any gains in decreased rates of graft rejection appear to have been offset by more frequent irradiation-related toxicity. Furthermore, the incidence of graft rejection in the current decade appears to be declining for other reasons, perhaps due to decreased sensitization by more widespread use of leukocyte-depleted blood products (Deeg et al, 1986).

Table 2.   HLA-nonidentical marrow transplantation for severe aplastic anaemia.

| Centre | Reference | Study year | Number of patients | Graft rejection (%) | Actuarial survival (%) | |
					CY	CY + TBI
Seattle	Beatty et al, 1987	1970–85	24	43	32	50
EBMTR	Bacigalupo et al, 1987	1987	46	33	15	30

CY, cyclophosphamide; EBMTR, European Bone Marrow Transplant Registry.

Table 2 summarizes results obtained in patients with severe aplastic anaemia who received marrow grafts form HLA-nonidentical donors. More intensive preparative conditioning with cyclophosphamide and by TBI is required to facilitate engraftment of histoincompatible marrow (Bacigalupo et al, 1987; Beatty et al, 1987). Long-term survival decreases with an increasing degree of genetic disparity between donor and recipient, due to the greater likelihood of graft failure and GVHD.

Marrow transplantation has been applied successfully to a long list of genetic diseases of lymphohaematopoietic cells (Hobbs, 1985; Thomas, 1985; Parkman, 1986). Disorders corrected by marrow grafting include severe combined immunodeficiency disease, Wiskott–Aldrich syndrome, osteopetrosis, Gaucher's disease, adenosine deaminase deficiency, mucopolysaccharidoses, sickle cell anaemia, Fanconi's anaemia, and thalassaemia. Timing of the transplant appears to be critical, for results are less satisfactory when vital organs have been damaged by advanced disease. In children less than 15 years of age with homozygous β-thalassaemia, disease-free survival of approximately 75% has been reported after HLA-identical marrow transplantation (Lucarelli et al, 1987). Allogeneic transplantation for Fanconi's anaemia has resulted in long-term survival of 50–70% (Deeg et al, 1983; Gluckman, 1988). The intensity of the pre-transplant conditioning regimen in patients with Fanconi's anaemia should be lessened because of constitutional defects in DNA repair, leading to increased toxicity from the preparative regimen (Gluckman et al, 1983, 1984). Recent studies report a 40–50% leukaemia-free survival in patients with myelodysplastic or preleukaemic syndromes transplanted before the development of overt leukaemia (Appelbaum et al, 1987; O'Donnell et al, 1987).

Malignant Disorders

For malignant diseases, TBI (9.2–10.0 Gy in a single fraction, or 12.0–15,75 Gy in multiple fractions) has been combined with cyclophosphamide (60 mg/kg × 2) to facilitate marrow engraftment and destroy host malignant cells (Thomas, 1983). Until 1975, marrow grafting was carried out only in leukaemia patients whose conventional treatment had failed (Thomas et al, 1977). Although mortality and post-transplant relapse rates were high, approximately 15% of patients with otherwise end-stage leukaemia became long-term survivors (Thomas, 1983).

Tables 3–5 summarize results in patients transplanted during advanced stages of leukaemia (Sanders et al, 1985, 1987; Goldman, 1986; Thomas et al, 1986; Clift et al, 1987; Storb, 1987; Gratwohl et al, 1988). In general, actuarial estimates of post-transplant relapse exceed 50% in patients with acute leukaemia transplanted during refractory relapse or chronic myelogenous leukaemia in blast crisis. For patients in early first relapse, transplantation during untreated recurrence offers improved survival and a lower probability of relapse than results in transplantation during second remission (Appelbaum et al, 1983; Clift et al, 1987).

Significant improvement is observed when marrow grafting is employed in earlier stages of leukaemia (Thomas et al, 1979). As shown in Table 6, most teams report 45–55% long-term, disease-free survival in patients with acute non-lymphoblastic leukaemia transplanted during first remission (Clift et al, 1987; Gratwohl et al, 1988). Similar results have been seen in patients with acute lymphoblastic leukaemia in first remission, although there is controversy as to the criteria for selection of patients (Blume et al, 1987; Doney et al, 1987; Herzig et al, 1987; Gratwohl et al, 1988; Hoelzer et al, 1988). As shown in Table 7, 50–60% of long-term, disease-free survival has been reported after allogeneic transplantation for chronic myelogenous leukaemia in chronic phase (Goldman, 1986;

Table 3. HLA-identical marrow transplantation for advanced-stage acute non-lymphoblastic leukaemia.

Centre	Reference	Disease stage	Study year	Number of patients	Probability of relapse (%)	Actuarial survival (%)
Seattle	Clift et al, 1987	ANL resistant, 1st relapse	1973–85	29	56	21
Seattle	Clift et al, 1987	ANL untreated, 1st relapse	1973–85	54	36	30
Seattle	Clift et al, 1987	ANL ≥ 2nd remission	1973–85	49	37	28
EBMTR	Gratwohl et al, 1988	ANL ≥ 2nd remission	1979–86	149	47	25

ANL, acute non-lymphoblastic leukaemia; EBMTR, European Bone Marrow Transplant Registry.

Table 4. HLA-identical marrow transplantation for advanced-stage acute lymphoblastic leukaemia.

Centre	Reference	Disease stage	Study year	Number of patients	Probability of relapse (%)	Actuarial survival (%)
Seattle	Storb, 1987	ALL relapse	1976–85	192	75	18
Seattle	Sanders et al, 1987	ALL 2nd remission < 18 y.o.	1973–85	57	42	40
Seattle	Storb, 1987	ALL 2nd remission ≥ 18 y.o.	1976–85	30	45	20
Seattle	Storb, 1987	ALL ≥ 3rd remission	1976–85	58	58	30
EBMTR	Gratwohl et al, 1988	ALL ≥ 2nd remission	1979–86	360	50	28

ALL, acute lymphoblastic leukaemia; EBMTR, European Bone Marrow Transplant Registry; y.o., year old.

Table 5. HLA-identical marrow transplantation for advanced-stage chronic myelogenous leukaemia.

Centre	Reference	Disease stage	Study year	Number of patients	Probability of relapse (%)	Actuarial survival (%)
Seattle	Thomas et al, 1986	CML blast crisis	1970–84	42	80	14
Seattle	Thomas et al, 1986	CML accelerated phase	1970–84	46	38	15
IBMTR	Goldman, 1986	CML blast crisis	1978–85	54	45	16
IBMTR	Goldman, 1986	CML accelerated phase	1978–85	203	54	29

CML, chronic myelogenous leukaemia; IBMTR, International Bone Marrow Transplant Registry.

Table 6. HLA-identical marrow transplantation for acute leukaemia in first remission.

Centre	Reference	Disease stage	Study year	Number of patients	Probability of relapse (%)	Actuarial survival (%)
Seattle	Clift et al, 1987	ANL 1st remission	1973–85	231	25	46
Seattle	Doney et al, 1987	ALL 1st remission	1976–85	46	41	28
EBMTR	Gratwohl et al, 1988	ANL 1st remission	1979–86	578	20	50
EBMTR	Gratwohl et al, 1988	ALL 1st remission	1979–86	260	25	50

ALL, acute lymphoblastic leukaemia; ANL, acute non-lymphoblastic leukaemia; EBMTR, European Bone Marrow Transplant Registry.

Table 7. HLA-identical marrow transplantation for chronic myelogenous leukaemia in chronic phase.

Centre	Reference	Disease stage	Study year	Number of patients	Probability of relapse (%)	Actuarial survival (%)
Seattle	Thomas et al, 1986	CML chronic phase	1970–84	67	22	49
EBMTR	Gratwohl et al, 1988	CML chronic phase	1979–86	454	22	44
IBMTR	Goldman et al, 1988	CML chronic phase	1978–85	405	19	55

CML, chronic myelogenous leukaemia; EBMTR, European Bone Marrow Transplant Registry; IBMTR, International Bone Marrow Transplant Registry.

Thomas et al, 1986; Goldman et al, 1988; Gratwohl et al, 1988). Data from the Seattle team indicate an actuarial survival of almost 80% in patients with chronic myelogenous leukaemia in chronic phase, transplanted within 1 year of diagnosis (Thomas and Clift, 1989).

Approximately 15–20% of patients with end-stage lymphoma survive free of disease for more than 5 years after allogeneic transplantation (Sullivan et al, 1986; Appelbaum et al, 1987). Preliminary results suggest that up to 40% cure may be possible if marrow transplantation is offered in early first relapse or second remission. Recent reports also suggest curative potential after allogeneic transplantation for multiple myeloma (Gahrton et al, 1987).

The above results were obtained with allogeneic transplantation. Recent studies suggest up to 45% actuarial survival 2 years after autologous marrow transplantation for acute non-lymphoblastic leukaemia in first remission, and 30% for patients transplanted in second remission (Linch and Burnett, 1986; Dicke et al, 1987). In acute lymphoblastic leukaemia, European data with autologous transplantation in second or subsequent remission are also encouraging (Gorin and Aegerter, 1987). Nevertheless, the follow-up periods are short and patient selection and treatment has varied. It is not clear whether ex vivo treatments designed to rid the marrow of contaminating leukaemia cells are beneficial.

Finally, for the rare patient with an identical twin, syngeneic marrow transplantation should be offered as the 'ideal autologous transplant'. Identical twin transplants have been carried out in acute leukaemias, chronic myelogenous leukaemia, and non-Hodgkin's lymphomas (Fefer et al, 1977, 1982; Appelbaum et al, 1981).

Timing of Transplantation

Among patients with acute lymphoblastic leukaemia in second or subsequent remission, prior studies have shown a significant survival advantage of bone marrow transplantation compared to results obtained with continued conventional chemotherapy (Johnson et al, 1981). Among patients with acute non-lymphoblastic leukaemia, there is little doubt that continued conventional chemotherapy offers little chance for cure after first marrow relapse. Long-term results are now available from a prospective study comparing marrow transplantation of patients with acute non-lymphoblastic leukaemia in first remission with continued chemotherapy (Appelbaum et al, 1988). Five-year disease-free survival for the chemotherapy group was 21%, compared to 48% for the transplant group ($p = 0.004$). However, risks of marrow transplantation increase with patient age due to increased frequency of GVHD and infectious complications (Thomas et al, 1982). For patients of more than 40 years of age, one approach might be to delay allogeneic marrow transplantation until early first relapse (Appelbaum et al, 1983).

Issues of timing of transplantation may be equally critical in chronic myelogenous leukaemia, a disease which cannot be cured by any treatment other than marrow transplantation, but which has an indolent chronic phase of unpredictable length (mean duration approximately 36 months). Some investigators have created mathematical models and computer programs of the course of disease to address this complex issue (Segel et al, 1986). Seattle data suggest that the clinical outcome of transplantation is best when performed in the chronic phase within 1 year of diagnosis (Thomas and Clift, 1989). These findings require confirmation but suggest an advantage for early transplantation.

BIOLOGY OF TRANSPLANTATION

Haematopoietic Reconstitution

In a normal marrow transplant, granulocyte and platelet counts recover by day 40–50, and erythrocyte transfusions are discontinued by day 60–90 post-transplant. In most cases haemopoiesis is entirely of donor origin, although some patients show persistent chimeric mixtures of donor and host cells (Hill et al, 1986; Petz et al, 1987; Bertheas et al, 1988). Recovery of monocytes as well as hepatic and bronchoalveolar macrophages is likewise of donor derivation. Platelet recovery may be delayed in recipients of autologous transplants, even in the absence of in vitro marrow treatment (Hill et al, 1989). Haematological recovery may also be slower in patients with severe marrow fibrosis (Rajantie et al, 1986).

Failure of marrow engraftment occurs in less than 1% of leukaemia patients prepared with TBI who receive unmodified HLA-identical sibling transplants (Beatty et al, 1985). Occasionally, graft function may be affected by myelosuppressive drugs, viral infection, damage to the marrow microenvironment, or a graft-versus-host stromal effect (Deeg et al, 1979; Emerson and Gale, 1987; Peralvo et al, 1987; Torok-Storb et al, 1987).

Among patients with aplastic anaemia prepared with only cyclophosphamide and given unmodifed HLA-identical marrow, factors associated with graft rejection include previous blood-product transfusions, a positive relative response in mixed leukocyte culture against the donor, a low marrow cell dose, marrow grafts from male donors (see Chapter 1), and lack of infusion of viable donor buffy coat cells in addition to the marrow (Storb et al, 1983).

Among patients prepared for transplantation with TBI, failure of marrow engraftment occurs in primarily two settings. In recipients of unmodified HLA-nonidentical marrow grafts, failure of sustained engraftment is seen in 5% of phenotypically-identical, 7–10% of one-locus mismatched, and 15–25% of two- or three-loci mismatched recipients (Beatty et al, 1985). For both HLA-identical and HLA-nonidentical transplant recipients, there is an increased rate of graft failure after in vitro T-cell depletion used to prevent GVHD (Martin et al, 1985; Kernan et al, 1987). Presumably, donor T cells are needed to destroy host cells which mediate graft rejection. Patients with haematological malignancy given T-depleted marrow grafts after a preparative regimen of cyclophosphamide (120 mg/kg) and 15.75 Gy fractionated TBI have a 27% cumulative incidence of graft failure, while for those prepared with cyclophosphamide and 12.0 Gy it is as high as 69% graft failure ($p < 0.05$) (Martin et al, 1988). It appears that the more complete the T cell depletion and the less intensive the pre-transplant conditioning, the greater the likelihood of graft failure. Current studies are aimed at augmenting immunosuppression before transplantation (with increased doses of TBI, total lymphoid irradiation, anti-Ia or anti-LFA-1 monoclonal antibodies) or using more 'selective' T cell-depletion techniques in an attempt to retain T cell subsets needed for engraftment (Ganem et al, 1988; Martin et al, 1988).

Delayed or failed marrow engraftment is a serious event, and fatal infectious complications are frequently observed (Pirsch and Maki, 1986). Attempts at a second marrow infusion of donor origin to correct poor graft function (Bolger et al, 1986), or a second preparation of the recipient followed by a second transplant after rejection of the first donor marrow (Storb et al, 1987), may achieve self-sustaining haematopoiesis, but long-term survival is poor because of intercurrent infection and toxicity.

Considerable attention has been given to the administration of haematopoietic growth factors to speed marrow graft recovery. Recombinant human granulocyte–macrophage colony-stimulating factor (GM-CSF) can accelerate myeloid recovery after autologous marrow transplantation (Brandt et al, 1988). This could lead to a reduction in the cost of transplantation thanks to earlier discharge from hospital. Current studies are aimed at enhancing the effectiveness of haematopoietic growth factors when combined with other lymphokines.

Immunological Reconstitution

Following intensive pre-transplant conditioning, severe immunodeficiency is demonstrated in autologous, syngeneic and allogeneic transplant recipients. Although some functional components of the immune system return within weeks of transplantation, most assays and functions remain impaired for 9–12 months after marrow grafting (Witherspoon et al, 1984; Lum, 1987; Martin et al, 1987). Apart from the risk of varicella zoster virus (VZV) infection within the first year, patients free of chronic GVHD are, in general, remarkably free of infection. However, patients developing chronic GVHD have multiple B- and T-cell abnormalities that persist for as long as GVHD remains active (Lum, 1987). In a multivariant analysis of infections in patients surviving more than 6 months after transplantation, only chronic GVHD was found to be associated with late non-VZV infections (Atkinson et al, 1982). HLA-nonidentity of the marrow graft increased the risk of late infections beyond that caused by chronic GVHD alone, and this suggests that full genotypic identity for HLA may be required for optimal immune reconstitution.

Attempts have been made to accelerate immune recovery after marrow grafting. Use of thymic epithelial grafts or administration of thymic hormone such as thymopentin or thymosin fraction 5 do not hasten recovery of T cell function (Witherspoon et al, 1988). Passive antibody prophylaxis with high-dose intravenous γ globulin appears promising (Sullivan, 1987). In five controlled studies, infection developed in 30% of immunoglobulin recipients and in 43% of controls. In four controlled trials, interstitial pneumonia developed in 17% of immunoglobulin recipients and in 43% of control patients. However, methods of immunoglobulin preparation, antibody titre, dose and schedule of prophylaxis varied widely in these studies, as did other critical patient, transplant regimen, and supportive care factors, and the data need to be interpreted with caution.

PROBLEMS OF TRANSPLANTATION

Infectious Complications

There is an inter-related and time-dependent relationship between opportunistic infections, recovery of immune function, and GVHD (Sullivan, 1986). Despite supportive care including antibiotic and antifungal therapy and, in some cases, protective isolation environments, 5% of HLA-identical marrow graft recipients die of bacterial or fungal infections during the early period of granulocytopenia (Navari et al, 1984; Meyers, 1986). Mortality is further increased in recipients of HLA-nonidentical marrow. During the second and third month after transplant, interstitial pneumonia may develop, and approximately half of these are due to CMV (Meyers et al, 1982). CMV pneumonia is observed in about 15% of patients with haematological malignancy receiving HLA-identical marrow transplants, and it has a fatality rate of 85%. CMV infection occurs more frequently in CMV antibody-seropositive patients, in older patients, and in those developing acute GVHD (Meyers et al, 1986). There is no effective therapy for this disorder, although recent investigations suggest that a combination for ganciclovir and CMV hyperimmune globulin may benefit some patients.

Prevention of CMV pneumonia is of paramount importance. Although 50% of the North American population harbours latent virus as evidenced by CMV-antibody seropositivity, CMV-seronegative patients with seronegative marrow donors can be protected effectively from serious CMV infection by the exclusive use throughout the transplant of screened blood products from CMV-seronegative donors (Bowden et al, 1986). In a prospective randomized study, 1 of 32 seronegative patients developed CMV infection after seronegative blood support compared to 8 of 25 seronegative patients receiving unscreened blood ($p < 0.007$) (Bowden et al, 1986).

Other prophylactic regimens include the use of intravenous immune globulin to prevent CMV infection and interstitial pneumonia (Sullivan, 1987; Winston et al, 1987). Intravenous immunoglobulin has been shown to reduce the incidence of septicaemia in marrow transplant recipients, especially in the post-engraftment period (Petersen et al, 1987).

Acute GVHD

The immunopathogenesis of GVHD is reviewed elsewhere (Tsoi, 1982; Sullivan, 1986). This disorder is presumably a consequence of engrafted immunocompetent donor lymphoid cells reacting with transplantation antigens located in the skin, liver, and gastrointestinal tract of an immunoincompetent host. It is one of the major and unique complications of allogeneic marrow transplantation.

Between 20 and 50% of patients given marrow from HLA-identical siblings develop significant acute GVHD. Death is often due to infectious complications that are increased by GVHD-associated immunodeficiency and by damage to portals of entry through the skin and intestinal tract. Treatment of established severe disease is often ineffective (Deeg et al, 1985; Kennedy et al, 1985) and emphasis is placed on prevention.

Table 8 outlines methods used to prevent GVHD. In vivo prophylaxis with immunosuppressive agents is of key importance. Single-institution and transplant registry experience suggests a 70–100% incidence of grade II–IV (moderate–severe) acute GVHD when post-transplant immunosuppression is not used after unmodifed allogeneic transplants (Sullivan et al, 1986; Gale et al, 1987). Methotrexate and cyclosporin appear to be equally effective in preventing GVHD when used as single-agent prophylaxis (Deeg et al, 1985; Storb et al, 1988). In contrast to patients with solid organ transplants, marrow graft recipients do not need immunosuppression for indefinite periods. In most cases, immuno-suppression can be discontinued 3–6 months after grafting, when stable graft–host tolerance is achieved. Although the mechanisms of graft tolerance are still incompletely understood, certain data suggest that specific suppressor T cells of donor origin mediate graft tolerance (Tsoi, 1982).

A combination of methotrexate given intermittently for 11 days after transplantation along with cyclosporin given for 180 days, is superior to either drug alone in preventing acute GVHD and leads to improved survival (Storb et al, 1986). While these results are very encouraging, renal and hepatic toxicity may limit drug dose or schedule and impair the efficacy of prophylaxis (Yee et al, 1988). Moreover, even though the incidence of acute GVHD is reduced, there is no apparent alteration in the incidence of chronic GVHD (Sullivan et al, 1987).

Table 8.   Prevention of graft-versus-host disease.

Histocompatibility matching of donor and recipient
In vivo prophylaxis
   Methotrexate (MTX)
   Cyclophosphamide (CY)
   Antithymocyte globulin (ATG)
   Cyclosporin (CsA)
   MTX + CsA
   MTX + Prednisone
   MTX + ATG + Prednisone
   MTX + CsA + Prednisone
Sterile environment and gut decontamination
Total lymphoid irradiation
Thymic transplantation
In vitro marrow treatment
   Monoclonal anti-T cell antibody ± complement
   Monoclonal anti-T cell antibody coupled with ricin
   E-rosette depletion
   ATG + complement
   Elutriation
   Soybean lectin agglutination
   Immunoadsorbent column

In experimental studies, germ-free mice receiving H-2-incompatible marrow have diminished mortality and a lessened incidence of enteric GVHD compared to conventionally housed animals (van Bekkum and Knaan, 1977). Micro-organisms could act as triggers for GVHD, perhaps by sharing antigenic epitopes with gut epithelial cells. Alternatively, reactivation of latent virus could induce virus-associated antigens on cell surfaces to become targets for alloreactivity. Of 130 patients with aplastic anaemia, patients treated in laminar airflow room isolation had a 23% incidence of grade II–IV acute GVHD compared to a 39% incidence in patients in conventional rooms ($p = 0.05$) (Storb et al, 1983). Survival was also improved (87% v. 69%, $p = 0.03$).

T lymphocytes appear vital for the genesis of GVHD and provide the rationale for in vitro depletion of marrow T cells in an attempt to prevent GVHD (Table 8). Numerous depletion techniques have been employed, but at present no compelling evidence favours one over another. With any of these techniques there is a decrease in the number of infused T cells, somewhere in the order of 1–3 log reduction. As discussed earlier, graft failure has been observed with most of these depletion techniques. However, GVHD is also reduced when at least 1.5 log T cells are removed (Kernan et al, 1986). Significant GVHD is seen in only 11% of HLA-identical, and in 28% of HLA-nonidentical, recipients of T cell-depleted marrow grafts (Reisner et al, 1981; Filipovich et al, 1982; Prentice et al, 1982; Bozdech et al, 1985; de Witte et al, 1986; Herve et al, 1987; Racadot et al, 1987; Hale et al, 1988). However, the incidence of graft rejection among HLA-identical transplants increases from less than 1% in unmodified marrow transplants to 10–20% in T cell-depleted transplants. Among HLA-nonidentical recipients, graft failure increases from 10–20% with unmodified transplants to 35% with T cell removal. Moreover, recurrent leukaemia is more frequent after T cell depletion (Mitsuyasu et al, 1986; Goldman et al, 1988). This is presumed to be due to a loss of a graft-versus-leukaemia effect associated with GVHD.

Chronic GVHD

Chronic GVHD is a protean disorder with a spectrum of clinical findings resembling several naturally occurring autoimmune diseases such as systemic lupus erythematosus, lichen planus, scleroderma, primary biliary cirrhosis, Sjögren's syndrome, and eosinophilic fasciitis (Shulman et al, 1980; Sullivan et al, 1981; Schubert et al, 1984). Chronic GVHD develops between 100 and 400 days post-transplant. Overall, 25–50% of long-term survivors of allogeneic marrow transplants develop this disorder. Risk factors for its development include increasing patient age, prior acute GVHD, and viable donor buffy coat cell infusions (Sullivan et al, 1981; Storb et al, 1983). The immunopathology and clinical features have been described (Sullivan and Parkman, 1983). With the use of early immunosuppressive treatment, the incidence of disabling scleroderma and joint contractures has fallen from 40–50% to 5–10%. Obliterative bronchiolitis, however, is now recognized in 10–20% of patients with chronic GVHD (Clark et al, 1987).

Encapsulated bacterial organisms are the most frequent cause of late infection in patients with chronic GVHD. Decreased serum opsonic activity for S. pneumoniae has been reported in these patients (Winston et al, 1979). Bacterial pneumonia, septicaemia, and sinusitis are the major types of infection. Interstitial pneumonia developing after day 100 is observed predominantly in patients with chronic GVHD (Sullivan et al, 1986). Among 198 patients with extensive chronic GVHD, 3 of 20 (15%) untreated patients (i.e. no immunosuppressive therapy and no antibiotic prophylaxis) developed late interstitial pneumonia. Among 124 patients given immunosuppressive treatment with prednisone ± azathioprine and prophylaxis with trimethoprim–sulphamethoxazole (TMP–SMX) the figure was 8%, and for 54 patients with chronic GVHD given immunosuppressive treatment without TMP–SMX prophylaxis it was 28% ($p = 0.001$). It appears reasonable to provide TMP–SMX prophylaxis during the therapy of chronic GVHD.

Without immunosuppressive treatment, <20% of patients with extensive chronic GVHD survive with Karnofsky performance scores of >70%. Autoimmune-like abnormalities, weight loss, pulmonary complications, and contractures contribute to the morbidity of untreated disease. We conducted a double-blind randomized trial comparing prednisone and placebo (group I, $n = 63$) to azathioprine (1.5 mg/kg/day) and prednisone (group II, $n = 63$) given as early treatment of extensive chronic GVHD (Sullivan et al, 1988). Patients with platelet counts <100 000/μl received prednisone alone (group III, $n = 38$). All three groups received doses of prednisone (1 mg/kg every other day) and prophylactic TMP–SMX (one double-strength tablet twice daily). The double-blind nature of the study allowed analysis of the contribution of cytotoxic treatment to the frequency of late infections to chronic GVHD. For groups I, II and III, the respective incidence of infection was: disseminated VZV, 11%, 24%, 34%; bacteraemia, 6%, 11%, 34%; interstitial pneumonia, 5%, 14%, 18%. Non-relapse mortality estimates were: 21% in group I, 40% in group II, and 58% in group III (I v. II, $p = 0.003$; I v. III, $p = 0.001$).

Actuarial survival five years after transplant was 61% in group I, 47% in group II, and 26% in group III (I v. II, $p = 0.03$; I v. III, $p = 0.0001$). Thus, treatment with prednisone alone resulted in fewer infections and better survival than prednisone and azathioprine in standard-risk chronic GVHD. Treatment with prednisone alone was less effective in high-risk patients with thrombocytopenia. The reason for the increased risk of infection in patients with thrombocytopenia was unclear, since their granulocyte counts were normal.

We reasoned that GVHD-associated immunosuppression was the cause of increased infection in high-risk patients. In patients with high-risk chronic GVHD who had persisting thrombocytopenia we next studied oral cyclosporin (6 mg/kg every 12 h every other day) combined in an alternating-day regimen with prednisone (1 mg/kg every other day) and daily TMP–SMX (Sullivan et al, 1988). After 9 months of therapy, a good response to treatment (i.e. normal skin and oral biopsies and no evidence of clinical GVHD) with this combination regimen was twofold higher than with previous treatment using prednisone alone. Moreover, long-term survival improved to over 50% in patients with thrombocytopenia.

Recurrence of Malignant Disease

Recurrence of malignancy is a major cause of transplant failure. Actuarial estimates of post-transplant relapse range from 20–80%. Most (95%) of the recurrences are in host-type cells, demonstrating the inability of the conditioning regimen to destroy all clonogenic malignant cells. A small number of recurrences have been in cells of donor origin (Schubach et al, 1982; Deeg et al, 1984; Witherspoon et al, 1985). There may be an increased risk for development of secondary malignancies in patients given T-depleted marrow grafts or in patients treated with monoclonal antibodies for steroid-resistant GVHD (Martin et al, 1984). Some of these secondary tumours have detectable Epstein–Barr virus.

In general, syngeneic and autologous transplant recipients have higher relapse rates than allogeneic transplant recipients who develop GVHD (Weiden et al, 1981; Kersey et al, 1987; Apperley et al, 1988). This graft-versus-leukaemia effect of allogeneic donor cells is called adoptive immunotherapy and has been studied in a variety of transplantable tumour models (Greenberg et al, 1981; Okunewick and Meredith, 1981). Recent analyses of the Seattle experience confirm a graft-versus-leukaemia effect in man (Sullivan et al, 1987, 1989). Figure 1 depicts the probability of relapse in 154 patients with acute non-lymphoblastic leukaemia and acute lymphoblastic leukaemia transplanted during relapse. Patients were selected who survived 150 days after unmodified HLA-identical marrow grafts (to be at risk to develop chronic GVHD) and were analysed according to the presence or absence of grade II–IV acute and/or chronic GVHD. Those who had no acute and no chronic GVHD demonstrated a higher probability of relapse (75% v. 40%, $p = 0.0001$). As shown in Figure 2, patients free of GVHD had a lower long-term survival (20% v. 37%, $p = 0.0023$). Current studies are aimed at manipulating a graft-versus-leukaemia effect to improve long-term, disease-free survival in patients with advanced-stage malignancies.

FUTURE OF TRANSPLANTATION

The ability of pluripotent stem cells to self-renew and differentiate into various

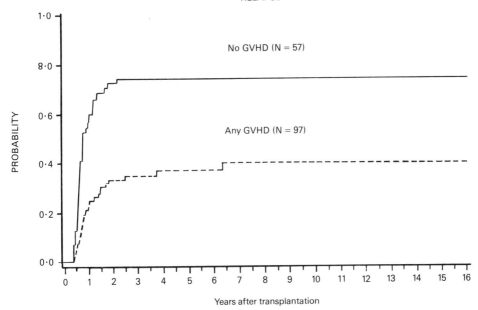

Figure 1. Kaplan–Meier estimates of the probability of relapse of leukaemia in 154 patients with acute non-lymphoblastic leukaemia and acute lymphoblastic leukaemia transplanted during relapse, grouped by the presence or absence of graft-versus-host disease (GVHD). Patients were alive in remission 150 days after unmodified HLA-identical marrow transplantation in Seattle.

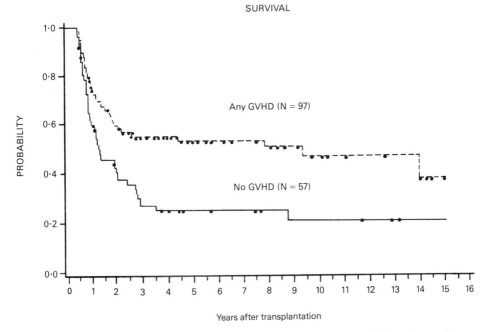

Figure 2. Kaplan–Meier estimates of the probability of survival in 154 patients with acute non-lymphoblastic leukaemia and actue lymphoblastic leukaemia transplanted during relapse, grouped by the presence or absence of graft-versus-host disease (GVHD). Patients were alive in remission 150 days after unmodified HLA-identical marrow transplantation in Seattle.

haematopoietic precursors has made them potential targets for somatic gene therapy (Parkman, 1986; Cline, 1987; Lehn, 1987). Gene cloning and transfer could be used to replace defective genes in haematopoietic tissue to cure otherwise lethal hereditary diseases. Techniques of gene transfection and the future for gene transfer in haematopoietic stem cells are discussed in detail in Chapter 8.

SUMMARY

It is now nearly two decades after the first successful human marrow transplants from HLA-identical siblings for the treatment of life-threatening haematological disorders. Initially considered only in patients with refractory end-stage disease, techniques have proven to be curative for patients with many different haematological disorders. Results in the treatment of thalassaemia and aplastic anaemia are superior to any other form of available therapy. In younger patients, transplantation appears the treatment of choice for chronic myelogenous leukaemia, for acute non-lymphocytic leukaemia in first remission, and for any acute leukaemia that has relapsed. For older patients with acute non-lymphoblastic leukaemia in first remission and chronic myelogenous leukaemia in chronic phase, the risk of immediate complications from marrow grafting must be weighed against the potential for long-term cure.

Despite this progress in transplantation, major problems remain. More effective and less toxic conditioning regimens must be developed, and novel approaches such as monoclonal antibodies linked to radio-isotopes or bone-seeking isotopes hold promise. Marrow graft failure in patients receiving T cell-depleted grafts or in recipients of HLA-nonidentical marrow is a frustrating impediment to the broader application of marrow transplantation. Better understanding of the regulation of haematopoiesis and its acceleration by recombinant growth factors may overcome these obstacles. Similarly, preclinical studies of interleukins hold promise for accelerating immune reconstitution after transplantation and decreasing the infectious morbidity. As our understanding of gene transfer techniques improves, transplantation programs with molecular medicine for the treatment of haemopoietic disorders may one day become a reality.

REFERENCES

Anasetti C, Doney KC, Storb R et al (1986) Marrow transplantation for severe aplastic anemia: Long term outcome in 50 'untransfused' patients. *Annals of Internal Medicine* **104**: 461–466.
Appelbaum FR, Fefer A, Cheever MA et al (1981) Treatment of non-Hodgkin's lymphoma with marrow transplantation in identical twins. *Blood* **58**: 509–513.
Appelbaum FR, Clift, RA, Buckner CD et al (1983) Allogeneic marrow transplantation for acute non-lymphoblastic leukaemia after first relapse. *Blood* **61**: 949–953.
Appelbaum FR, Badger C, Nelp WB et al (1986) Labeled monoclonal antibodies as a preparative regimen for marrow transplantation: Initial dosimetry *Experimental Hematoloty* **14** (abstract): 456.
Appelbaum FR, Sullivan KM, Buckner CD et al (1987) Treatment of malignant lymphoma in 100 patients with chemotherapy, total body irradiation and marrow transplantation. *Journal of Clinical Oncology* **5**: 1340–1347.
Appelbaum FR, Storb R, Ramberg RE et al (1987) Treatment of preleukemic syndromes with marrow transplantation. *Blood* **69**: 92–96.

Appelbaum FR, Fisher L & Thomas ED, for the Seattle Bone Marrow Transplant Team (1988) Chemotherapy versus marrow transplantation for adults with acute nonlymphocytic leukemia: A five-year follow-up. *Blood* **72**: 179–184.

Apperley JF, Mauro FR, Goldman JM et al (1988) Bone marrow transplantation for chronic myeloid leukaemia in first chronic phase: importance of a graft-versus-leukaemia effect. *British Journal of Haematology* **68**: 239–245.

Atkinson K, Farewell V, Storb R et al (1982) Analysis of late infections after human bone marrow transplantation: Role of genotypic nonidentity between marrow donor and recipient and of nonspecific suppressor cells in patients with chronic graft-versus-host disease. *Blood* **60**: 714–720.

Auber ML, Horwitz LJ, Blaauw A et al (1988) Evaluation of drugs for elimination of leukemic cells from the bone marrow of patients with acute leukemia. *Blood* **71**: 166–172.

Bacigalupo A, DiGiorgio F, Congiu M et al (1985) Treatment of severe aplastic anemia in Europe 1970–1983: A report of the EBMT SAA Working Party. *Experimental Hematology* **13** (supplement 17): 56–57.

Bacigalupo A, Hows J, Gordon-Smith EC et al (1987) Bone marrow transplantation for severe aplastic anemia (SAA) from donors other than HLA identical siblings: A report of the EBMT working party. *Experimental Hematology* **15** (abstract 419): 613.

Bearman SI, Appelbaum FR, Buckner CD et al (1988) Regimen-related toxicity in patients undergoing bone marrow transplantation. *Journal of Clinical Oncology* **6**: 1562–1568.

Beatty PG, Clift RA, Mickelson EM et al (1985) Marrow transplantation from related donors other than HLA-identical siblings. *New England Journal of Medicine* **313**: 765–771.

Beatty PG, Di Bartolomeo P, Storb R et al (1987) Treatment of aplastic anemia with marrow grafts from related donors other than HLA genotypically matched siblings. *Clinical Transplantation* **1**: 117–124.

Beatty PG, Dahlberg S, Mickelson EM et al (1988) Probability of finding HLA-matched unrelated marrow donors. *Transplantation* **45**: 714–718.

Bensinger WI, Buckner CD, Thomas ED & Clift RA (1982) ABO-incompatible marrow transplants. *Transplantation* **33**: 427–429.

Bertheas MF, Maraninchi D, Lafage M et al (1988) Partial chimerism after T-cell-depleted allogeneic bone marrow transplantation in leukemic HLA-matched patients: A cytogenetic documentation. *Blood* **72**: 89–93.

Blume KG, Forman SJ, O'Donnell MR et al (1987) Total body irradiation and high-dose etoposide: A new preparatory regimen for bone marrow transplantation in patients with advanced hematologic malignancies. *Blood* **69**: 1015–1020.

Blume KG, Forman SJ, Snyder DS et al (1987) Allogeneic bone marrow transplantation for acute lymphoblastic leukemia during first complete remission. *Transplantation* **43**: 389–392.

Bolger GB, Sullivan KM, Storb R et al (1986) Second marrow infusion for poor graft function following allogeneic marrow transplantation. *Bone Marrow Transplantation* **1**: 21–30.

Bortin MM, for the Advisory Committee of the International Bone Marrow Transplant Registry (IBMTR), and Buckner CD, for the Seattle Bone Marrow Transplant Team (SMTT) (1983) Major complications of marrow harvesting for transplantation. *Experimental Hematology* **11**: 916–921.

Bortin MM & Rimm AA (1986) Increasing utilization of bone marrow transplantation. *Transplantation* **42**: 229–234.

Bowden RA, Sayers M, Flournoy N et al (1986) Cytomegalovirus immune globulin and seronegative blood products to prevent primary cytomegalovirus infection after marrow transplant. *New England Journal of Medicine* **314**: 1006–1010.

Bozdech MJ, Sondel PM, Trigg ME et al (1985) Transplantation of HLA-identical T-cell-depleted marrow for leukemia: Addition of cytosine arabinoside to the pretransplant conditioning prevents rejection. *Experimental Hematology* **13**: 1201–1210.

Brandt SJ, Peters WP, Atwater SK et al (1988) Effect of recombinant human granulocyte-macrophage colony-stimulating factor on hematopoietic reconstitution after high-dose chemotherapy and autologous bone marrow transplantation. *New England Journal of Medicine* **318**: 869–876.

Brochstein JA, Kernan NA, Groshen S et al (1987) Allogeneic bone marrow transplantation after hyper-fractionated total-body irradiation and cyclophosphamide in children with acute leukemia. *New England Journal of Medicine* **317**: 1618–1624.

Buckner CD, Clift RA, Sanders JE et al (1984) Marrow harvesting from normal donors. *Blood* **64**: 630–634.

Champlin RE for the Advisory Committee of the IBMTR (1986) Current status of bone marrow transplantation for severe aplastic anemia *Experimental Hematology* **14** (abstract 831): 552.

Chang J, Morgenstern G, Deakin D et al (1986) Reconstitution of haemopoietic system with autologous marrow taken during relapse of acute myeloblastic leukaemia and grown in long-term culture. *Lancet* i: 294–295.

Clark JG, Schwartz DA, Flournoy N et al (1987) Risk factors for airflow obstruction in recipients of bone marrow transplants. *Annals of Internal Medicine* 107: 648–656.

Clift RA, Buckner CD, Thomas ED et al (1987) The treatment of acute nonlymphoblastic leukemia by allogeneic marrow transplantation. *Bone Marrow Transplantation* 2: 243–258.

Cline MJ (1987) Gene therapy: Current status. *American Journal of Medicine* 83: 291–297.

Deeg HJ, Meyers JD, Storb R, Graham TC & Weiden PL (1979) Effect of trimethoprim–sulfamethoxazole on hematological recovery after total body irradiation and autologous marrow infusion in dogs. *Transplantation* 28: 243–246.

Deeg HJ, Storb R, Thomas ED et al (1983) Fanconi's anemia treated by allogeneic marrow transplantation. *Blood* 61: 954–959.

Deeg HJ, Flournoy N, Sullivan KM et al (1984) Cataracts after total body irradiation and marrow transplantation: A sparing effect of dose fractionation. *International Journal of Radiation Oncology Biology Physics* 10: 957–964.

Deeg HJ, Sanders J, Martin P et al (1984) Secondary malignancies after marrow transplantation. *Experimental Hematology* 12: 660–666.

Deeg HJ, Loughran TP, Storb R et al (1985) Treatment of human acute graft-versus-host disease with antithymocyte globulin and cyclosporine with or without methylprednisolone. *Transplantation* 40: 162–166.

Deeg HJ, Storb R, Thomas ED et al (1985) Cyclosporine as prophylaxis for graft-versus-host disease: A randomized study in patients undergoing marrow transplantation for acute nonlymphoblastic leukemia. *Blood* 65: 1325–1334.

Deeg HJ, Sullivan KM, Buckner CD et al (1986) Marrow transplantation for acute nonlymphoblastic leukemia in first remission: Toxicity and long-term follow-up of patients conditioned with single dose or fractionated total body irradiation. *Bone Marrow Transplantation* 1: 151–157.

Deeg HJ, Self, S, Storb R et al (1986) Decreased incidence of marrow graft rejection in patients with severe aplastic anemia: Changing impact of risk factors. *Blood* 68: 1363–1368.

de Witte T, Hoogenhout J, de Pauw B et al (1986) Depletion of donor lymphocytes by counterflow centrifugation successfully prevents acute graft-versus-host disease in matched allogeneic marrow transplantation. *Blood* 67: 1302–1308.

Dicke KA, Jagannath S, Spitzer G et al (1984) The role of autologous bone marrow transplantation in various malignancies. *Seminars in Hematology* 21: 109–122.

Dicke KA, Spitzer G & Jagannath S (eds) (1987) *Autologous Bone Marrow Transplantation*. Proceedings of the Third International Symposium on Autologous Transplantation. Houston: The University of Texas Press.

Doney KC, Buckner CD, Kopecky KJ et al (1987) Marrow transplantation for patients with acute lymphoblastic leukemia in first marrow remission. *Bone Marrow Transplantation* 2: 355–363.

Emerson SG & Gale RP (1987) The regulation of hematopoiesis following bone marrow transplantation. *International Journal of Cell Cloning* 5: 432–449.

Fefer A, Buckner CD, Thomas ED et al (1977) Cure of hematologic neoplasia with transplantation of marrow from identical twins. *New England Journal of Medicine* 297: 146–148.

Fefer A, Cheever MA, Greenburg PD et al (1982) Treatment of chronic granulocytic leukemia with chemoradiotherapy and transplantation of marrow from identical twins. *New England Journal of Medicine* 306: 63–68.

Filipovich AH, Ramsay NKC, Warkentin PI et al (1982) Pretreatment of donor bone marrow with monoclonal antibody OKT3 for prevention of acute graft-versus-host disease in allogeneic histocompatible bone marrow transplantation. *Lancet* i: 1266–1269.

Gahrton G, Tura S, Flesch M et al (1987) Bone marrow transplantation in multiple myeloma: Report from the European Cooperative Group for Bone Marrow Transplantation. *Blood* 69: 1262–1264.

Gale RP, Bortin MM, van Bekkum DW et al (1987) Risk factors for acute graft-versus-host disease. *British Journal of Haematology* 67: 397–406.

Ganem G, Kuentz M, Beaujean F et al (1988) Additional total-lymphoid irradiation in preventing graft failure of T-cell-depleted bone marrow transplantation from HLA-identical siblings: Results of a prospective randomized study. *Transplantation* 45: 243–248.

Gingrich RD, Ginder GD, Goeken NE et al (1988) Allogeneic marrow grafting with partially mismatched, unrelated marrow donors. *Blood* **71**: 1375–1381.

Gluckman E (1988) Impact of the conditioning regimen on the outcome of bone marrow transplantation for severe aplastic anemia. *Journal of Cellular Biochemistry* **Supplement 12C**: 70 (abstract K017).

Gluckman E, Devergie A & Dutreix J (1983) Radiosensitivity in Fanconi anaemia: Application to the conditioning regimen for bone marrow transplantation. *British Journal of Haematology* **54**: 431–440.

Gluckman E, Berger R & Dutreix J (1984) Bone marrow transplantation for Fanconi anemia. *Seminars in Hematology* **21**: 20–26.

Goldman JM, for the Advisory Committee of the IBMTR (1986) Current status of bone marrow transplantation for chronic myelogenous leukemia. *Experimental Hematology* **14**: 486.

Goldman JM, Gale RP, Horowitz MM et al (1988) Bone marrow transplantation for chronic myelogenous leukemia in chronic phase: Increased risk for relapse associated with T-cell depletion. *Annals of Internal Medicine* **108**: 806–814.

Gorin NC & Aegerter P (1987) Autologous bone marrow transplantation for acute leukemia in remission: Fourth EBMTR survey. *Bone Marrow Transplantation* **2** (supplement 1): 320–323.

Gratwohl A, Hermans J, Barrett AJ et al (1988) Allogeneic bone marrow transplantation for leukaemia in Europe: Report from the Working Party on Leukaemia, European Group for Bone Marrow Transplantation. *Lancet* i: 1379–1382.

Greenberg PD, Cheever MA & Fefer A (1981) Eradication of disseminated murine leukemia by chemoimmunotherapy with cyclophosphamide and adoptively transferred immune syngeneic Lyt-1$^+$ 2$^-$ lymphocytes. *Journal of Experimental Medicine* **154**: 952–963.

Hale G, Cobbold S & Waldmann H for CAMPATH-1 users (1988) T cell depletion with CAMPATH-1 in allogeneic bone marrow transplantation. *Transplantation* **45**: 753–759.

Hansen JA & Thomas ED (1983) The immunogenetics of clinical bone marrow transplantation. In RS Weiner, E Hackel, CA Schiffer, (eds) *Bone marrow transplantation: A technical workshop.* Arlington, VA: American Association of Blood Banks, 23–47.

Hansen JA, Clift RA, Thomas ED et al (1980) Transplantation of marrow from an unrelated donor to a patient with acute leukemia. *New England Journal of Medicine* **303**: 565–567.

Herve P, Cahn JY, Flesch M et al (1987) Successful graft-versus-host disease prevention without graft failure in 32 HLA-identical allogeneic bone marrow transplantations with marrow depleted of T cells by monoclonal antibodies and complement. *Blood* **69**: 388–393.

Herzig RH, Barrett AJ, Gluckman E et al (1987) Bone marrow transplantation in high-risk acute lymphoblastic leukaemia in first and second remission. *Lancet* i: 786–789.

Hill RS, Petersen FB, Storb R et al (1986) Mixed hematologic chimerism after allogeneic marrow transplantation for severe aplastic anemia is associated with a higher risk of graft rejection and a lessened incidence of acute graft-versus-host disease. *Blood* **67**: 811–816.

Hill RS, Mazza P, Amos D et al (1989) Engraftment in 86 patients with lymphoid malignancy after autologous marrow transplantation. *Bone Marrow Transplantation* **4**: 69–74.

Hobbs JR (1985) Correction of 34 genetic diseases by displacement bone marrow transplantation. *Plasma Therapy and Transfusion Technology* **6**: 221–246.

Hoelzer D, Thiel E, Loffler H et al (1988) Prognostic factors in a multicenter study for treatment of acute lymphoblastic leukemia in adults. *Blood* **71**: 123–131.

Hows JM, Yin JL, Marsh J et al (1986) Histocompatible unrelated volunteer donors compared with HLA nonidentical family donors in marrow transplantation for aplastic anemia and leukemia. *Blood* **68**: 1322–1328.

Jacobson LO, Simmons EL, Marks EK et al (1950) The role of the spleen in radiation injury and recovery. *Journal of Laboratory and Clinical Medicine* **35**: 746–770.

Jagannath S, Dicke KA, Armitage JO et al (1986) High-dose cyclophosphamide, carmustine, and etoposide and autologous bone marrow transplantation for relapsed Hodgkin's disease. *Annals of Internal Medicine* **104**: 163–168.

Johnson FL, Thomas ED, Clark BS et al (1981) A comparison of marrow transplantation with chemotherapy for children with acute lymphoblastic leukemia in second or subsequent remission. *New England Journal of Medicine* **305**: 846–851.

Jones RJ, Lee KSK, Beschorner WE et al (1987) Venoocclusive disease of the liver following bone marrow transplantation. *Transplantation* **44**: 778–783.

Kennedy MS, Deeg HJ, Storb R et al (1985) Treatment of acute graft-versus-host disease after allogeneic marrow transplantation: A randomized study comparing corticosteroids and cyclosporine. *American Journal of Medicine* **78**: 978–983.

Kernan NA, Collins NH, Juliano L et al (1986) Clonable T lymphocytes in T cell-depleted bone marrow transplants correlate with development of graft-v-host disease. *Blood* **68**: 770–773.

Kernan NA, Flomenberg N, Dupont B & O'Reilly RJ (1987) Graft rejection in recipients of T-cell-depleted HLA-nonidentical marrow transplants for leukemia. *Transplantation* **43**: 843–847.

Kersey JH, Weisdorf D, Nesbit ME et al (1987) Comparison of autologous and allogeneic bone marrow transplantation for treatment of high-risk refractory acute lymphoblastic leukemia. *New England Journal of Medicine* **317**: 461–467.

Kessinger A, Armitage JO, Landmark JD, Smith DM & Weisenburger DD (1988) Autologous peripheral hematopoietic stem cell transplantation restores hematopoietic function following marrow ablative therapy. *Blood* **71**: 723–727.

Lam W-C, Order SE & Thomas ED (1980) Uniformity and standardization of single and opposing cobalt 60 sources for total body irradiation. *International Journal of Radiation Oncology Biology Physics* **6**: 245–250.

Lehn PM (1987) Gene therapy using bone marrow transplantation. *Bone Marrow Transplantation* **1**: 243–258.

Linch DC & Burnett AK (1986) Clinical studies of ABMT in acute myeloid leukemia. *Clinical Hematology* **15**: 167–186.

Lorenz E, Uphoff D, Reid TR & Shelton E (1951) Modification of irradiation injury in mice and guinea pigs by bone marrow injections. *Journal of the National Cancer Institute* **12**: 197–201.

Lucarelli G, Galimberti M, Polchi P et al (1987) Marrow transplantation in patients with advanced thalassemia. *New England Journal of Medicine* **316**: 1050–1055.

Lum LG, (1987) A review: The kinetics of immune reconstitution after human marrow transplantation. *Blood* **69**: 369–380.

Macklis RM, Kinsey BM, Kassis AI et al (1988) Radioimmunotherapy with alpha-particle-emitting immunoconjugates. *Science* **240**: 1024–1026.

Martin PJ, Shulman HM, Schubach WH et al (1984) Fatal Epstein–Barr-virus-associated proliferation of donor B cells after treatment of acute graft-versus-host disease with a murine monoclonal anti-T-cell antibody. *Annals of Internal Medicine* **101**: 310–315.

Martin PJ, Hansen JA, Buckner CD et al (1985) Effects of in vitro depletion of T cells in HLA-identical allogeneic marrow grafts. *Blood* **66**: 664–672.

Martin PJ, Hansen JA, Storb R & Thomas ED (1987) Human marrow transplantation: An immunological perspective. In: FJ Dixon (ed) *Advances in Immunology*, vol. 40, pp. 379–438. Orlando: Academic Press.

Martin PJ, Hansen JA, Torok-Storb B et al (1988) Graft failure in patients receiving T cell-depleted HLA-identical allogeneic marrow transplants. *Bone Marrow Transplantation* **3**: 445–456.

McDonald GB, Sharma P, Matthews DE, Shulman HM & Thomas ED (1985) The clinical curse of 53 patients with venocclusive disease of the liver after marrow transplantation. *Transplantation* **36**: 603–608.

McDonald GB, Shulman HM, Sullivan KM & Spencer GD (1986) Intestinal and hepatic complications of human bone marrow transplantation: Part I. *Gastroenterology* **90**: 460–477; 770–784.

McDonald GB, Shulman HM, Wolford JL & Spencer GD (1987) Liver disease after human marrow transplantation. *Seminars in Liver Disease* **7**: 210–229.

McGlave P, Scott E, Ramsay N et al (1987) Unrelated donor bone marrow transplantation therapy for chronic myelogenous leukemia. *Blood* **70**: 877–881.

Meyers JD (1986) Infection in bone marrow transplant recipients. *American Journal of Medicine* **81** (suppelement 1A): 27–38.

Meyers JD, Flournoy N & Thomas ED (1982) Nonbacterial pneumonia after allogeneic marrow transplantation: A review of ten years' experience. *Reviews of Infectious Diseases* **4**: 1119–1132.

Meyers JD, Flournoy N, Wade JC et al (1983) Biology of interstitial pneumonia after marrow transplantation. In RP Gale (ed.) *Recent advances in bone marrow transplantation*, pp 405–423. New York: Alan R Liss.

Meyers JD, Flournoy N & Thomas ED (1986) Risk factors for cytomegalovirus infection after human marrow transplantation. *Journal of Infectious Diseases* **153**: 478–488.

Mitsuyasu RT, Champlin RE, Gale RP et al (1986) Treatment of donor bone marrow with monoclonal anti-T-cell antibody and complement for the prevention of graft-versus-host disease: A prospective, randomized, double-blind trial. *Annals of Internal Medicine* **105**: 20–26.

Navari RM, Buckner CD, Clift RA et al (1984) Prophylaxis of infection in patients wth aplastic anemia receiving allogeneic marrow transplants. *American Journal of Medicine* **76**: 564–572.

Niederwieser D, Pepe M, Storb R et al (1988) Improvement in rejection, engraftment rate and survival without increase in graft-versus-host disease by high marrow cell dose in patients transplanted for aplastic anemia. *British Journal of Haematology* **69**: 23–28.

O'Donnell MR, Nademanee AP, Snyder DS et al (1987) Bone marrow transplantation for myelodysplastic and myeloproliferative syndromes. *Journal of Clinical Oncology* **5**: 1822–1826.

Okunewick JP & Meredith RF (1981) *Graft-versus-leukemia in man and animal models.* Boca Raton, Florida: CRC Press.

O'Reilly RJ, Dupont B, Pahwa S et al (1977) Reconstitution in severe combined immunodeficiency by transplantation of marrow from an unrelated donor. *New England Journal of Medicine* **297**: 1311–1318.

Parkman R (1986) The application of bone marrow transplantation to the treatment of genetic diseases. *Science* **232**: 1373–1378.

Peralvo J, Bacigalupo A, Pittaluga PA et al (1987) Poor graft function associated with graft-versus-host disease after allogeneic marrow transplantation. *Bone Marrow Transplantation* **2**: 279–285.

Petersen FB, Bowden RA, Thornquist M et al (1987) The effect of prophylactic intravenous immune globulin on the incidence of septicemia in marrow transplant recipients. *Bone Marrow Transplantation* **2**: 141–148.

Petz LD, Yam P, Wallace RB et al (1987) Mixed hematopoietic chimerism following bone marrow transplantation for hematologic malignancies. *Blood* **70**: 1331–1337.

Pirsch JD & Maki DG (1986) Infectious complications in adults with bone marrow transplantation and T-cell depletion of donor marrow. *Annals of Internal Medicine* **104**: 619–631.

Prentice HG, Janossy G, Skeggs D et al (1982) Use of anti-T-cell monoclonal antibody OKT3 to prevent acute graft-versus-host disease in allogeneic bone marrow transplantation for acute leukaemia. *Lancet* **i**: 700–703.

Prummer O & Fliedner TM (1986) The fetal liver as an alternative stem cell source for hemolymphopoietic reconstitution. *International Journal of Cell Cloning* **4**: 237–249.

Racadot E, Herve P, Beaujean F et al (1987) Prevention of graft-versus-host disease in HLA-matched bone marrow transplantation of malignant diseases: A multicentric study of 62 patients using 3-Pan-T monoclonal antibodies and rabbit complement. *Journal of Clinical Oncology* **5**: 426–435.

Rajantie J, Sale GE, Deeg HJ et al (1986) Adverse effect of severe marrow fibrosis on hematological recovery after chemoradiotherapy and allogeneic bone marrow transplantation. *Blood* **67**: 1693–1697.

Ramsay NKC, Kim TH, McGlave P et al (1983) Total lymphoid irradiation and cyclophosphamide conditioning prior to bone marrow transplantation for patients with severe aplastic anemia. *Blood* **62**: 622–626.

Rayfield LS & Brent L (1983) Tolerance, immunocompetence and secondary disease in fully allogeneic radiation chimeras. *Transplantation* **36**: 183–189.

Reisner Y, Kapoor N, Kirkpatrick D et al (1981) Transplantation for acute leukaemia with HLA-A and B nonidentical parental marrow cells fractionated with soybean agglutinin and sheep red blood cells. *Lancet* **i**: 327–331.

Riddell S, Appelbaum FR, Buckner CD et al (1988) High-dose cytarabine and total body irradiation with or without cyclophosphamide as a preparative regimen for marrow transplantation for acute leukemia. *Journal of Clinical Oncology* **6**: 576–582.

Sanders JE, Buckner CD, Leonard JM et al (1983) Late effects on gonadal function of cyclophosphamide, total-body irradiation,and marrow transplantation. *Transplantation* **36**: 252–255.

Sanders JE, Flournoy N, Thomas ED et al (1985) Marrow transplant experience in children with acute lymphoblastic leukemia: An analysis of factors associated with survival, relapse and graft-versus-host disease. *Medical Pediatric Oncology* **13**: 165–172.

Sanders JE, Pritchard S, Mahoney P et al (1986) Growth and development following marrow transplantation for leukemia. *Blood* **68**: 1129–1135.

Sanders JE, Buckner CD, Bensinger WI et al (1987) Experience with marrow harvesting from donors less than two years of age. *Bone Marrow Transplantation* **2** (supplement 1): 45–50.

Sanders JE, Thomas ED, Buckner CD & Doney K (1987) Marrow transplantation for children with acute lymphoblastic leukemia in second remission (Concise Report). *Blood* **70**: 324–326.

Santos GW & Colvin OM (1986) Pharmacological purging of bone marrow with reference to autografting. *Clinical Hematology* **15**: 67–83.

Santos GW, Tutschka PJ, Brookmeyer R et al (1983) Marrow transplantation for acute nonlymphocytic leukemia after treatment wih busulfan and cyclophosphamide. *New England Journal of Medicine* **309**: 1347–1353.

Schubach WH, Hackman R, Neiman PE, Miller G & Thomas ED (1982) A monoclonal immunoblastic sarcoma in donor cells bearing Epstein–Barr virus genomes following allogeneic marrow grafting for acute lymphoblastic leukemia. *Blood* **60**: 180–187.

Schubert MM, Sullivan KM, Morton TH et al (1984) Oral manifestations of chronic graft-v-host disease. *Archives of Internal Medicine* **144**: 1591–1595.

Segel GB, Simon W & Lichtman MA (1986) Variables influencing the timing of marrow transplantation in patients with chronic myelogenous leukemia. *Blood* **68**: 1055–1064.

Shulman HM, Sullivan KM, Weiden PL et al (1980) Chronic graft-versus-host syndrome in man: A long-term clinicopathological study of 20 Seattle patients. *American Journal of Medicine* **69**: 204–217.

Stiff PJ, Koester AR, Weidner MK, Dvorak K & Fisher RI (1987) Autologous bone marrow transplantation using unfractionated cells cyropreserved in demethylsulfoxide and hydroxyethyl starch without controlled-rate freezing. *Blood* **70**: 974–978.

Storb R (1987) Critical issues in bone marrow transplantation. *Transplantation Proceedings* **19**: 2774–2781.

Storb R, Doney KC, Thomas ED et al (1982) Marrow transplantation with or without donor buffy coat cells for 65 transfused aplastic anemia patients. *Blood* **59**: 236–246.

Storb R, Prentice RL, Thomas ED et al (1983) Factors associated with graft rejection after HLA-identical marrow transplantation for aplastic anaemia. *British Journal of Haematology* **55**: 573–585.

Storb R, Prentice RL, Buckner CD et al (1983) Graft-versus-host disease and survival in patients with aplastic anemia treated by marrow grafts from HLA-identical siblings: Beneficial effect of a protective environment. *New England Journal of Medicine* **308**: 302–307.

Storb R, Prentice RL, Sullivan KM et al (1983) Predictive factors in chronic graft-versus-host disease in patients with aplastic anemia treated by marrow transplantation from HLA-identical siblings. *Annals of Internal Medicine* **98**: 461–466.

Storb R, Thomas ED, Buckner CD et al (1984) Marrow transplantation for aplastic anemia. *Seminars in Hematology* **21**: 27–35.

Storb R, Deeg HJ, Whitehead J et al (1986) Methotrexate and cyclosporine compared with cyclosporine alone for prophylaxis of acute graft versus host disease after marrow transplantation for leukemia. *New England Journal of Medicine* **314**: 729–735.

Storb, R, Weiden PL, Sullivan KM et al (1987) Second marrow transplants in patients with aplastic anemia rejecting the first graft: Use of a conditioning regimen including cyclophosphamide and antithymocyte globulin. *Blood* **70**: 116–121.

Storb R, Deeg HJ, Fisher LD et al (1988) Cyclosporine versus methotrexate for graft-versus-host disease prevention in patients given marrow grafts for leukemia: Long-term follow-up of three controlled trials. *Blood* **71**: 293–298.

Sullivan KM (1986) Acute and chronic graft-versus-host disease in man. *International Journal of Cell Cloning* **4** (supplement 1): 42–93.

Sullivan KM (1987) Immunoglobulin therapy in bone marrow transplantation. *American Journal of Medicine* **83**: 34–45.

Sullivan KM & Parkman R (1983) The pathophysiology and treatment of graft-versus-host disease. *Clinical Haematology* **12**: 775–789.

Sullivan KM, Shulman HM, Storb R et al (1981) Chronic graft-versus-host disease in 52 patients: Adverse natural course and successful treatment with combination immunosuppression. *Blood* **57**: 267–276.

Sullivan KM, Storb, R, Shulman HM et al (1982) Immediate and delayed neurotoxicity after mechlorethamine preparation for bone marrow transplantation. *Annals of Internal Medicine* **97**: 182–189.

Sullivan KM, Deeg HJ, Sanders JE et al (1984) Late complications after marrow transplantation. *Seminars in Hematology* **21**: 53–63.

Sullivan KM, Appelbaum FR, Horning SJ, Rosenberg SA & Thomas ED (1986) Selection of patients with Hodgkin's disease and non-Hodgkin's lymphoma for bone marrow transplantation. *International Journal of Cell Cloning* **4** (supplement 1): 94–106.

Sullivan KM, Deeg HJ, Sanders J et al (1986) Hyperacute GVHD in patients not given immunosuppression after allogeneic marrow transplantation. *Blood* **67**: 1172–1175.

Sullivan KM, Meyers JD, Flournoy N, Storb R & Thomas ED (1986) Early and late interstitial pneumonia following human bone marrow transplantation. *International Journal of Cell Cloning* **4** (supplement 1): 107–121.

Sullivan KM, Witherspoon R, Deeg HJ et al (1987) Chronic graft-versus-host disease in man. In RP Gale & R Champlin (eds) *Progress in bone marrow transplantation*, pp 473–487. New York: Alan R Liss.

Sullivan KM, Fefer A, Witherspoon R et al (1987) Graft-versus-leukemia in man: Relationship of acute and chronic graft-versus-host disease to relapse of acute leukemia following allogeneic bone marrow transplantation. In RL Truitt, R P Gale & M M Bortin (eds) *Cellular immunotherapy of cancer*, pp 391–399. New York: Alan R Liss.

Sullivan KM, Witherspoon RP, Storb R et al (1988) Prednisone and azathioprine compared to prednisone and placebo for treatment of chronic graft-versus-host disease: Prognostic influence of prolonged thrombocytopenia after allogeneic marrow transplantation. *Blood* **72**: 546–554.

Sullivan KM, Witherspoon RP, Storb R et al (1988) Alternating-day cyclosporine and prednisone for treatment of high-risk chronic graft-versus-host disease. *Blood* **72**: 555–561.

Sullivan KM, Weiden PL, Storb R et al (1989) Influence of acute and chronic graft-versus-host disease on relapse and survival after bone marrow transplantation from HLA-identical siblings as treatment of acute and chronic leukemia. *Blood* **73**: 1720–1728.

Thomas ED (1983) Marrow transplantation for malignant diseases (Karnofsky Memorial Lecture). *Journal of Clinical Oncology* **1**: 517–531.

Thomas ED (1985) Marrow transplantation for nonmalignant disorders (Editorial retrospective). *New England Journal of Medicine* **312**: 46–47.

Thomas ED & Clift RA (1989) Indications for marrow transplantation in chronic myelogenous leukemia. *Blood* **73**: 861-864.

Thomas ED & Storb R (1970) Technique for human marrow grafting. *Blood* **36**: 507–515.

Thomas ED, Lochte HL, Cannon JH, Sahler OD & Ferrebee JW (1959) Supralethal whole body irradiation and isologous marrow transplantation in man. *Journal of Clinical Investigation* **38**: 1709–1716.

Thomas ED, Storb, R, Clift RA et al (1975) Bone-marrow transplantation. *New England Journal of Medicine* **292**: 832–843; 895–902.

Thomas ED, Buckner CD, Banaji M et al (1977) One hundred patients with acute leukemia treated by chemotherapy, total body irradiation, and allogeneic marrow transplantation. *Blood* **49**: 511–533.

Thomas ED, Buckner CD, Clift RA et al (1979) Marrow transplantation for acute nonlymphoblastic leukemia in first remission. *New England Journal of Medicine* **301**: 597–599.

Thomas ED, Clift RA & Buckner CD for the Seattle Marrow Transplant Team (1982) Marrow transplantation for patients with acute nonlymphoblastic leukemia who achieve a first remission. *Cancer Treatment Reports* **66**: 1463–1466.

Thomas ED, Clift RA, Fefer A et al (1986) Marrow transplantation for the treatment of chronic myelogenous leukemia. *Annals of Internal Medicine* **104**: 155–163.

Thompson CB, Sanders JE, Flournoy N, Buckner CD & Thomas ED (1986) The risks of central nervous system relapse and leukoencephalopathy in patients receiving marrow transplants for acute leukemia. *Blood* **67**: 195–199.

Torok-Storb BJ, Simmons P & Przepiorka D (1987) Impairment of hemopoiesis in human allografts. *Transplantation Proceedings* **19 (7)**: 33–37.

Tsoi M-S (1982) Immunologic mechanisms of graft-versus-host disease in man. *Transplantation* **33**: 459–464.

Tutschka PJ, Copelan EA & Klein JP (1987) Bone marrow transplantation for leukemia following a new busulfan and cyclophosphamide regimen. *Blood* **70**: 1382–1388.

UCLA Bone Marrow Transplant Team (1977) Bone marrow transplantation with intensive combination chemotherapy–radiation therapy (SCARI) in acute leukemia. *Annals of Internal Medicine* **86**: 155–161.

van Bekkum DW & Knaan S (1977) Role of bacterial microflora in development of intestinal lesions from graft-versus-host reaction. *Journal of the National Cancer Institute* **58**: 787–789.

Weiden PL, Sullivan KM, Flournoy N, Storb R & Thomas ED for the Seattle Marrow Transplant Team (1981) Antileukemic effect of chronic graft-versus-host disease: Contribution to improved survival after allogeneic marrow transplantation. *New England Journal of Medicine* **304**: 1529–1533.

Weiner RS, Bortin MM, Gale RP et al (1986) Interstitial penumonitis after bone marrow transplantaion. Assessment of risk factors. *Annals of Internal Medicine* **104**: 168–175.

Winston DJ, Schiffman G, Wang DC et al (1979) Pneumococcal infections after human bone-marrow transplantation. *Annals of Internal Medicine* **91**: 835–841.

Winston DJ, Ho WG, Lin C-H et al (1987) Intravenous immune globulin for prevention of cytomegalovirus infection and interstitial pneumonia after bone marrow transplantation. *Annals of Internal Medicine* **106**: 12–18.

Witherspoon RP, Lum LG & Storb R (1984) Immunologic reconstitution after human marrow grafting. *Seminars in Hematology* **21**: 2–10.

Witherspoon RP, Schubach W, Neiman P, Martin P & Thomas ED (1985) Donor cell leukemia developing six years after marrow grafting for acute leukemia. *Blood* **65**: 1172–1174.

Witherspoon RP, Sullivan KM, Lum LG et al (1988) Use of thymic grafts or thymic factors to augment immunologic recovery after bone marrow transplantation: Brief report with 2.2–12.3 (median 6.7) years follow-up. *Bone Marrow Transplantation* **3**: 425–435.

Yeager AM, Kaizer H, Santos GW et al (1986) Autologous bone marrow transplantation in patients with acute nonlymphocytic leukemia, using ex vivo marrow treatment with 4-hydroperoxycyclophosphamide. *New England Journal of Medicine* **315**: 141–147.

Yee GC, Self SG, McGuire TR et al (1988) Serum cyclosporine concentration and risk of acute graft-versus-host disease after allogeneic marrow transplantation. *New England Journal of Medicine* **319**: 65–70.

Zander AR, Culbert S, Jagannath S et al (1987) High dose cyclophosphamide, BCNU, and VP-16 (CBV) as a conditioning regimen for allogeneic bone marrow transplantation for patients with acute leukemia. *Cancer* **59**: 1083–1086.

7 Pancreas Transplantation

ROBERT A. SELLS
DAVID LESLIE

The aim of pancreas transplantation or islet implantation is to provide a source of insulin that will be sufficient to maintain normal glycaemia. As a consequence, a transplant may prevent diabetic complications, as well as improve the quality of life by releasing patients from dependence on insulin injections.

There is substantial evidence that normoglycaemic subjects do not develop diabetic nephropathy or diabetic retinopathy; also some diabetics with moderate glycaemic control may live for many years without developing significant complications. The decision to perform pancreatic transplantation in the diabetic therefore depends, first, on accurate identification of those at risk from progressive and harmful complications and, second, on the balance between the risks of transplantation and the benefits that might occur from a long-term successful transplant. In this chapter we describe the clinical and aetiological features of the complications of diabetes, the current techniques, risks and benefits of pancreas transplantation, and we discuss the considerable challenge of predicting those patients likely to devlop complications. We shall repeatedly refer to the central reality that many diabetics achieve good glycaemic control by simple insulin replacement therapy, by comparison with which the procedure of pancreas transplantation or islet implantation is undeniably invasive and potentially hazardous.

Judging which diabetics are potentially suitable for transplantation, the risks of transplantation itself, and our uncertainty about the success of a transplant ameliorating or preventing complications pose serious practical and ethical questions that pervade the debate on this subject (Pyke, 1988; Sutherland, 1988a).

RISKS OF DIABETES

Insulin-dependent diabetes occurring in young people (IDDM, type I) is currently believed to be caused by islet failure due to autoimmune injury, in patients with a genetic predisposition; it is often presaged by the appearance of insulin-binding and islet-binding antibodies and is associated with a high incidence of complications mainly attributable to progressive microangiopathy. The non-insulin-dependent (maturity onset, type II) diabetic may sometimes progress to a degree requiring insulin therapy; however, this type of diabetes is also associated with a frequency of diabetes-specific complications similar to that found in type I cases.

Before the insulin era commenced, diabetic coma was the cause of death in nearly two-thirds of type I diabetics of all ages, and the introduction of insulin therapy in 1922 in Toronto provided a means of rescuing nearly all patients from this complication, with consequent markedly improved longevity. In 1946, W. R. Campbell presented an early survivor of 25 years' insulin therapy as a person who was 'joyous, clear-eyed and vibrant' (Campbell 1946). This patient was fortunate to survive without a clinically evident retinopathy or neuropathy, but as we describe below, the increased longevity associated with successful insulin therapy has, paradoxically, created the syndrome of chronic diabetic microangiopathy with its attendant sequelae. This is graphically demonstrated in Figure 1, which demonstrates the increased mortality due to these complications and the simultaneous near-disappearance of deaths from diabetic coma in insulin-dependent diabetics.

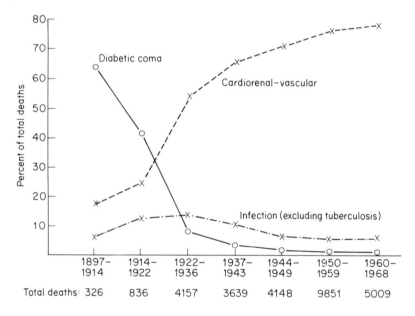

Figure 1. Causes of death in persons with diabetes, expressed as percentages of total deaths. From Marble (1972), with permission of the American Diabetes Association, Inc.

Sixty-three years after the introduction of insulin treatment, diabetics still die earlier than non-diabetics. The age- and sex-specific mortality rate in diabetics is higher at all ages than it is for normal populations. The difference in mortality rates is in part dependent on age, for between 20 and 40 years of age the risk is ten or more times greater in type I diabetics than in non-diabetics whereas in diabetics over 50 years of age it is only twice as great. The cause of death is likewise age-dependent: younger patients tend to die of nephropathy whereas in older patients the increased mortality is largely caused by cardiovascular disease. Other factors such as diabetic ketoacidosis and hypoglycaemia play a minor role in causing increased mortality.

Diabetic Retinopathy

In Britain the commonest cause of blindness during working years is diabetes. Diabetic retinopathy is to be expected in nearly all diabetics and can be detected in about 80% of diabetics with a disease duration of 20 years, and 100% after 40 years of the disease (Krolewski et al, 1986). However, only the minority of diabetics have a visual disability because of their retinopathy. In one study from Wisconsin 1.4% of type I diabetics diagnosed before the age of 30 had moderate visual impairment and 3.6% were blind. In diabetics diagnosed later, visual disability was more prevalent, though in only some 33% could the visual impairment be attributed to diabetes (Klein et al, 1984).

Diabetic Nephropathy

In type I diabetics clinical proteinuria (greater than 0.5 g/day) usually only occurs after 10 years duration of the disease. Before this time, however, low levels of proteinuria (microalbuminuria) can be found, and they may herald in some the onset of diabetic nephropathy. As the urinary concentration of albumin increases, so the body work rate under experimental conditions, corrected for standard oxygen uptake, also diminishes (Jensen et al, 1988): diabetics with micro- and macroalbuminuria were found to have an appreciably impaired aerobic work capacity that could not be explained by autonomic neuropathy and was independent of the duration of diabetes. There is a suggestion here that this generalized reduction in capacity may be due to widespread microangiopathy, possibly affecting the myocardium. The appearance of clinical proteinuria usually indicates the relentless development of renal dysfunction, and the cumulative incidence of diabetic nephropathy is 40% by 40 years duration of the disease. In a Danish study, a cohort of diabetics diagnosed under the age of 31 and before 1933 had a cumulative mortality of 50% after 35 years. A common accompaniment of the renal problem is a co-existent array of cardiovascular risk factors which include hypertension, hyperlipidaemia, and generalized atherosclerosis (Borch-Johnsen et al, 1985). In this study, 30% died from renal failure and 25% from myocardial infarction. However, in over half of the survivors in this survey no nephropathy was found. The early physiological abnormality of microalbuminuria is accompanied by minimal histological changes, which are generally thought to progress as the renal failure declines. Since the rate of progress of this complication seems to depend principally on the degree of glycaemic control, one might predict that euglycaemic diabetices of long-standing without clinical evidence of nephropathy would show a commensurately low degree of histological change at post mortem examination. This is, in fact, *not* so: in a necropsy study of 17 matched patients with and without clinical nephropathy, the prevalence and severity of glomerular and arteriolar lesions were indistinguishable in the two groups (Thomsen et al, 1984). Thus histological changes do no necessarily reflect abnormalities in renal function.

Non-insulin dependent diabetics (type II) are as a rule diagnosed at an older age than insulin-dependent diabetics. In them the date of onset of the disease is less clear as many of the diabetics are asymptomatic when they are diagnosed. The period from the clinical diagnosis to the onset of proteinuria is, not surprisingly, shorter than in insulin-dependent diabetics. Nevertheless, the death rate due to uraemia is only 1% for those patients diagnosed over the age of 60, which contrasts sharply with the younger onset patients. In these non-insulin dependent diabetics, vascular disease, and in particular ischaemic heart disease, account for much of the increase in mortality over the general population.

Diabetic Neuropathy

Approximately 15% of diabetic patients develop clinical neuropathy that may be focal, or diffuse and symmetrical. The most common clinical consequence is ulceration of the feet, a potentially disastrous complication that is commonly the cause of hospital admission in diabetic patients and for which up to 40% of patients may require amputation. Gangrene has a high mortality and a poor prognosis for social rehabilitation. Symptomatic autonomic neuropathy carries a terrible prognosis in that half of the patients may be dead within 5 years (Ewing et al, 1980). About half of these deaths are due to renal failure or cardiorespiratory arrest independent of renal failure, the precise cause of which remains unclear, but which may reflect occult progressive myocardial microangiopathy.

WHICH PATIENT IS AT RISK FROM DIABETIC COMPLICATIONS?

Diabetes is a potentially devastating disease. However, the risk of developing the complications can vary substantially between individuals. We have already discussed the age at onset and duration of disease as important risk factors. Other variables include sex (women are more at risk than men), smoking, high blood pressure, HLA or complement status and the degree of hyperglycaemia. Unfortunately it is not possible at present to determine with certainty that any one diabetic patient without complications will or will not develop complications in the future. Clearly, until we have an accurate, predictive test of the threat to life or sight in the type I diabetic population, pre-emptive pancreas grafting will remain problematical.

A pragmatic approach to this problem is to identify individuals who have minor changes in, say, renal function, and to calculate the risk of their developing diabetic nephropathy with a view to intervention therapy in those at very high risk. Such work is currently being undertaken (see below).

If pancreas transplantation could result in normoglycaemia in diabetics, diabetic complications might well be avoided. There is no clear evidence yet that normoglycaemia prevents diabetic complications, but there is substantial indirect evidence that raised glucose levels are necessary for complications to develop.

HYPERGLYCAEMIA IS ASSOCIATED WITH COMPLICATIONS

The study of identical twins with diabetes has made it possible to determine to some extent the relative role of genetic and environmental influences in at least some diabetic complications. Neither diabetic nephropathy nor retinopathy has been observed in the non-diabetic twin of the diabetic. This suggests that predisposition to one of these complications cannot be inherited or, if it is, that diabetes *per se* must play a permissive role. In addition, capillary basement membrane thickening, supposedly a histological hallmark of microangiopathy; has not been found in non-diabetic co-twins of diabetics (Steffes et al, 1985). Finally, diabetic complications occur irrespective of the aetiology of the disease: thus, haemochromatosis and pancreatitis can be accompanied by the specific complications of diabetes. This suggests that it is hyperglycaemia (and its associated metabolic derangement) that is important in causing diabetic microangiopathy.

Nevertheless, genetic factors may be important in determining the risk of developing complications, or the rate at which they occur. Type II diabetic co-twins are strikingly similar in terms of the presence and severity of retinopathy. But comparisons between non-related diabetics show that the course of microangiopathy is unpredictable, and severe hyperglycaemia in some is associated with minimal changes whereas in others mild hyperglycaemia can be associated with severe complications. There is limited evidence that certain genes may be associated with an increased risk of developing retinopathy. Genes in the Class III region of the HLA system have been implicated, particularly the complement gene C4, B3, which has a highly significant association with retinopathy, though this has yet to be confirmed (Mijovic et al, 1985). In addition a gene on chromosome 14, coding for heavy chain immunoglobulin constant region (Gm zafmbg), has been implicated as a risk factor in 47% of patients with retinopathy but in only 18% of those without the complication (Mijovic et al, 1986).

Improved Glycaemic Control Reduces Complications

Epidemiological studies clearly indicate that the degree of hyperglycaemia is a major risk factor for diabetic complications. Nevertheless, the most noted long-term studies of the quality of diabetic control and its effect on diabetic complications have been severely criticized. Particular problems with such studies include:

1. Failure to randomize patients.
2. Failure to establish a rigorous system for assessing neuropathy, retinopathy, or nephropathy.
3. Failure to determine and define levels of diabetic control.
4. Failure to account for non-glucose related factors involved in the aetiology of complications, e.g. duration of diabetes.

Current methods for obtaining diabetic control enable near-physiological blood glucose levels to be achieved. Continuous subcutaneous insulin infusion (CSII), compared with conventional insulin treatment, reduces many of the biochemical and functional abnormalities that accompany conventional insulin treatment, can maintain blood glucose and glycosolated haemoglobin concentreations at near-normal levels (Kroc Study, 1984) and can lower serum lipid values (Tamborlane et al, 1979). CSII reduces the glomerular filtration rate in patients with persistent diabetes-associated hyperfiltration and microalbuminuria. Yet only one study showed improvement after 2 years of treatment (Feldt-Rasmussen et al, 1986). Despite the convenience of this system, which allows tuning of the insulin dose according to the timing of meals, infection risk at the infusion site and a high degree of compliance required by the patient makes CSII unsuitable for the majority. Equally good control may be achieved in many patients by multiple insulin injections using a pen containing a pre-filled cartridge of insulin. Insulin delivery pumps have been implanted into a few patients (the vapour powered Infusaid device–Buchwald et al, 1985). Technical problems persist for this form of treatment, and a larger series of patients must be assembled before it can be properly assessed.

Although near-physiological blood glucose levels may be achieved using these recently developed techniques, the goal of long-term glycaemic control remains elusive. However, significant improvement occurs in many, and now that intensive long-term glycaemic control is practicable in some patients, the prevention of complications, or their reversal, can in theory be compared in groups receiving conventional versus intensive insulin regimens. It may, however, be difficult to complete such a study over a sufficiently long period in which one group of diabetics has normal or near-normal glycaemia whilst the control group suffers persistently higher blood glucose levels. So long as we lack conclusive evidence that euglycaemia or even near-normal blood sugar levels prevent or reverse diabetic complications, the most important indication for clinical pancreatic grafting is lacking. It must remain ethically dubious to submit a patient to the hazards of surgery and immunosuppression without a strong conviction that artificial euglycaemia, and therefore (by implication) homeostatically controlled euglycaemia, will be clinically beneficial in the long term.

Role of Blood Sugar Control in Preventing Specific Complications

There is no direct evidence in man that hyperglycaemia leads inevitably to diabetic complications, nor is there clear evidence that reversal of hyperglycaemia prevents complications. Nevertheless, several studies have suggested that good diabetic control may improve some, if not all complications.

Reversal of Retinopathy, Nephropathy, and Neuropathy

Retinopathy is unusual in the absence of diabetes, though some of the lesions associated with diabetic retinopathy may occur in a number of conditions including hypertension, sickle-cell disease, collagen vascular disease, and retrolental fibroplasia. A causal relationship is suggested by a number of factors, including the absence of retinopathy in non-diabetic identical twins of diabetic patients, and the frequent development of retinopathy 5 or more years after diagnosis. Randomized control trials have been reported comparing the effects of very good control (achieved by using multiple insulin injections, insulin infusion pumps or home glucose monitoring) with standard regimens involving twice daily insulin injections; in two of these studies there was a transient deterioration in retinopathy in the group with very good control; however, by 2 years, there was no difference in retinopathy between the two groups (Lawson et al, 1985; Dahl-Jorgensen, 1986).

While good glycaemic control reduces microalbuminuria it remains unclear whether improved glycaemic control slows or prevents clinically manifest diabetic nephropathy. Two important longitudinal studies (the Diabetic Control and Complications Trial, and the British Microalbuminuria Collaborative Study) are currently in progress. It is already apparent, however, that some patients with microalbuminuria do progress to diabetic nephropathy, while others do not. We cannot, therefore, at present predict diabetic nephropathy while serum creatinine levels remain normal (Mogensen, 1988).

Once diabetic nephropathy is established, diabetic control does not appear to play a major role in determining the tempo of its progression. Six patients with persistent proteinuria were treated with continuous subcutaneous insulin infusion for up to 24 months without any effect on the rate of decline of glomerular filtration rate (GFR) or the fractional clearance of albumin or IgG (Viberti et al, 1983). These studies need to be confirmed as the number of patients was small but, as with retinopathy, very good blood glucose control does not appear to have a major effect over a short period in diabetics with established renal lesions. The variation in the rate of onset and severity of the histological findings in the various groups studied, the lack of correlation of the degree of pathological change to clinical expression of the disease, and the failure of good glycaemic control to influence the decline in GFR or protein clearance confounds the idea of a simple relationship between diabetic control with exogenous insulin and renal morbidity. The progression to renal failure might depend, too, on a non-glycaemic trigger factor such as diet, smoking, and inherited susceptibility, or the development of hypertension.

The rate of flux of the blood glucose seems to play a role in the causation of neuropathy; neuropathic symptoms may be precipitated by episodes of hypo- or hyperglycaemia and they may be associated with chronic hypoglycaemia associated with insulinomas or the institution of insulin therapy (Boulton et al, 1982; Jaspan et al, 1982; Morley et al, 1984; Service et al, 1985). By the time symptoms of autonomic neuropathy have developed, autonomic nerve damage is probably irreversible and carries a poor prognosis (Ewing et al, 1980). There is as yet no evidence that modern techniques maintaining normal glycaemia have any effect on the progression of this group of complications, the most disabling symptoms of which include postural hypotension, diarrhoea, bladder dysfunction and impotence.

Somatic nerve function may, by contrast, be influenced by glucose levels. Hyperglycaemia may affect the perception of pain; in one study (Morley et al, 1984) a glucose bolus resulted in a fall in both the threshold of pain detection and the maximum tolerated pain. (The levels of maximum tolerated pain were lower in diabetics than in non-diabetic patients.) Continuous subcutaneous insulin infusions have been studied in patients with chronic painful neuropathy, with encouraging results in that the motor conduction velocity and vibration perception threshold improved (Boulton et al, 1982). These studies were open-ended, but a control study of vibration perception in insulin-treated diabetics also demonstrated a significant improvement in the intensively treated group compared with the group receiving the standard regimen (Service et al, 1985).

Summary: The Relationship of Poor Glucose Control to Complications

Blood glucose levels do appear to be related to diabetic complications, and although the nature of the relationship remains unclear, the evidence linking complications to poor glucose control provides support for the assumption that homeostatic control of blood glucose by a functioning pancreatic graft may prevent their onset. Early lesions may respond to insulin treatment that achieves near-normoglycaemia. Established lesions do not appear to improve with a controlled reduction in the blood glucose to normal levels, or to levels just above the normal range. The beneficial effect of a long period of near-normoglycaemia achieved with subcutaneous insulin injections (and therefore, by implication, the normoglycaemia that would be achieved in a functioning pancreas transplant) remains to be established.

PANCREAS PLUS KIDNEY TRANSPLANTATION

The incentives to embark on pancreas transplantation in man developed in the pre-cyclosporin era, when it became clear that the results of renal transplantation alone to correct diabetic nephropathy were substantially inferior to the results achieved by renal transplantation for other diseases. For example, the annual report of the American College of Surgeons in 1979 indicated that after cadaveric transplantation the mortality at one year in diabetics was 38%, with a graft success rate of 35%, compared with 89% patient survival and 64% graft survival following renal transplantation for other diseases (ACS/NIH Organ Transplant Registry, 1975). The results of dialysis alone in the treatment of diabetic nephropathy were also poor at that time: the European Dialysis and Transplantation Association Registry (EDTA) reported in 1981 an actuarial patient survival rate of 28% at 5 years in over 5000 diabetics accepted for all forms of treatment, compared with 56% in 20 000 non-diabetic dialysis patients. The survival of diabetics did not appear to be strongly influenced by age as it is in other patients with end-stage renal failure and 'the diabetics appear prematurely old, their survival being roughly equivalent to their non-diabetic counterparts with end-stage renal disease at a chronological age some 20–30 years older' (Jacobs et al, 1983). The cause of death in 45% of diabetics treated by dialysis or transplantation was myocardial infarction, according to one report on patients receiving steroids for immunosuppression (Okye et al, 1983); vascular disease requiring amputation or causing stroke was seen after transplantation more frequently than in non-diabetics. These complications were undoubtedly precipitated by the liberal use of prophylactic steroids and high-dose prednisolone therapy for rejection: in patients with pre-existing diabetic vascular disease, this therapy was commonly associated with severe hyperglycaemia. Infectious complications were, likewise, more common, and these factors discouraged clinicians from using immunosuppressive drugs during rejection episodes and led them to abandon the graft and return the patient to dialysis as quickly as possible. Even in those patients who survived with a graft for more than one year, the long-term prognosis would be uncertain in view of the incidence of diabetic glomerulo-sclerosis occurring in such grafts after 5 years (Mauer et al, 1983).

In some countries the poor prognosis associated with any form of therapy discouraged clinicians from accepting diabetics even for dialysis: between 1975 and 1981 only 1.3 diabetics per million population were accepted for dialysis in the United Kingdom, and these were all under the age of 40 years (Jacobs, 1983). More liberal dialysis services elsewhere, for instance Finland, allowed the acceptance of up to six new patients per million per year, although transplant rates remained low.

The decision to protect the patient and his graft from the dangers of postoperative hyperglycaemia by simultaneous pancreas and kidney grafting was taken, courageously, by Lillehei and his colleagues in 1967. After developing the appropriate model in experimental animals, they reported the first two recipients of kidney transplants with a simultaneous pancreas and duodenal transplant (Kelly et al, 1967). Despite a high failure rate in early series from these and other authors, surgeons in several centres (notably Minneapolis, Stockholm, Madison, Lyon and Cambridge) persisted in their attempts to develop a clinically successful technique.

The fundamental technical challenge was to find a successful way of draining, or preventing the secretion of, exocrine pancreatic juice. The leakage of pancreatic secretions between sutures of an anastomosis of the cut pancreas to bowel causes autodigestion of the surrounding tissue, abscess formation, and secondary thrombosis of the adjacent major blood vessels. The continual escape of enzymes into the wound results in a chronic fistula, persistent infection, and a serious risk of septicaemia until the leaking graft is removed. Yet with persistence and by the exercise of meticulous surgical technique and proper surgical principles, successful transplantation of segmental and whole (pancreatico-duodenal) human transplants were eventually achieved with acceptable clinical results (Groth et al, 1982; Sutherland et al, 1984). The endocrine secretions of the pancreas were drained into the systemic circulation via the external iliac vein, which led to an increase in the serum insulin compared with non-diabetic recipients of renal grafts only. This hyperinsulinaemia did not, however, affect glucose homeostasis, which was essentially normal. Recipients of successful grafts rapidly demonstrated normalization of their haemoglobin A1C levels; furthermore, the quality of life for pancreaticorenal transplant recipients was found to be substantially improved on psychometric assessment, compared with diabetics transplanted with kidneys alone (Voruganti et al, 1989). Striking improvements were seen in this group of pancreas recipients, e.g. improved self-image as well as better performance of work in the home and in their sexual relations. These improvements may well have been due to the release from dependence on exogenous insulin therapy rather than to any alteration in the natural history of the disease and its complications.

In an attempt to obtain a more physiological form of endocrine drainage, Calne developed the 'paratopic' technique whereby the segmental pancreatic graft is vascularized by the splenic vessels, thus allowing insulin to enter the portal circulation, and with the pancreatic duct draining into the stomach (Calne, 1984). Restoration of normal postoperative plasma insulin levels has been demonstrated in these patients, but the superiority of the technique over heterotopic grafting in the long term has not yet been demonstrated. Other workers, notably Dubernard, endeavoured to prevent leakage of exocrine secretion by abolishing it: they achieved this by injecting the exocrine duct with various polymers including neoprine, prolamine and silicone. In animal models, as well as in patients, ductal obliteration causes fibrosis, which may result in strangulation of the blood supply to the islets. However, Dubernaud and his group have reported no significant difference in results between whole pancreases transplanted with enteric diversion and those transplanted with duct obstruction (Dubernaud et al, 1988).

A major technical advance in pancreatic drainage was introduced by Sollinger and his colleagues by draining the whole pancreatic graft through the duodenum into the bladder (Cook et al, 1983). This has resulted in the near-abolition of exocrine leakage and wound sepsis, although the risk of pancreatic vessel thrombosis is still around 10%. Occasional complications of this technique have been duodenal erosions or ulceration requiring duodenal excision and reanastomosis, acidosis secondary to high bicarbonate losses in the urine during renal impairment, and cystitis. A major advantage of this form of urinary drainage is that exocrine pancreatic function can be monitored by serial urinary amylase measurement. It has been shown by Prieto et al (1987) that during early pancreatic rejection a significant decline in urinary amylase precedes hyperglycaemia by several days. This test, regularly performed after the operation, therefore allows the early treatment of rejection, and has undoubtedly contributed to the success of the procedure.

In all reported series sudden postoperative death due to myocardial infarction is still a risk. To reduce this mortality, a policy of careful cardiovascular evaluation is required, which includes isotope ventriculography and coronary arteriography for potential recipients. In one series (Corry, 1988) sudden cardiac death was abolished by preliminary screening and exclusion of all patients with evidence of significant cardiomyopathy at the time of referral. In this series, patient survival has been 100% and graft success rate at 6 months was 76%. A detailed analysis of other factors that have led to improved graft survival and patient survival are described in Appendix I by Sutherland. The short- and mid-term success of pancreas transplantation either alone or with a kidney in terms of graft and patient survival has improved commensurately with the introduction of pancreaticocystostomy, urinary amylase monitoring for rejection, preoperative cardiac screening leading to better patient selection, cyclosporin anti-rejection therapy avoiding the use of prophylactic steroids, and improvements in DR matching between the donor graft and the recipient. It remains to be seen whether the deployment of all these advances outside the major centres of expertise will bring about a general reduction in the hazards of the procedure and an improvement in long-term graft and patient survival.

PURE ISLET TRANSPLANTATION

Much has been done during the last 15 years to develop a technique of transplanting pancreatic islets alone: the great attraction of this technique is that islets could be injected intravenously to a well-vascularized site (e.g. the spleen or the liver). This would do away with the need for a surgical operation and would avoid any immunological and inflammatory consequences of exocrine tissue transplantation. Despite encouraging results in rodents, islet allografts in large animals including man have never been demonstrated to produce insulin for significant periods of time. The exhaustive work of Gray has shown that if 20–40% of the total islet tissue is transplanted in this way in cynomolgus monkeys, diabetes can be reversed for periods for more than 1 year (Gray et al, 1986). Progress has recently been made in improving the viability and yield of islets using precise density gradients for their separation (Rajotte et al, 1987).

Despite the lack of progress in the clinical application of this potentially very useful technique, the pure islet allograft has become a useful model for studying the immunobiology of graft rejection. Like cultured thyroid tissue (see Chapter 8d), the antigenic status of the tissue and its components is now well-known; it can be immunologically manipulated during culture prior to transplantation to any site in the recipient, and the endpoint of rejection is sharply defined in the recipient (rendered diabetic before transplantation) by acute hyperglycaemia. It is possible, for instance, selectively to destroy islet dendritic cells in culture; prolonged survival of islet allografts in the mouse was achieved by Faustman et al (1981) by treatment of solitary islets with complement-fixing anti-Ia antibodies and complement, as well as by treating cultured islets with specific anti-dendritic cell antibody (Faustman, 1984). Further, ultraviolet irradiation of cultured rat islets, a treatment known to destroy dendritic cells, causes increased islet survival in some strain combinations (Lau et al, 1984). Lafferty's group first suggested that the presence of passenger leukocytes (or their analogues subsequently known to be the dendritic cells) could be the initiating trigger for islet rejection, and they have shown that islets cultured at high oxygen tension or under normal conditions lost their dendritic cells and showed prolonged survival after transplantation (Bowen et al, 1980). A successful combination of techniques allowing a high yield of pure human islets, together with a uniformly successful method for reducing their immunogenicity, would provide a new method of treating diabetes with enormous clinical potential.

CAUSES OF NON-TECHNICAL FAILURE OF THE ENDOCRINE PANCREATIC GRAFT

Pancreatic allografts, in common with other vascularized grafts, are prone to rejection, the intensity of which is principally determined by the degree of HLA mismatch between donor and recipient. Preliminary clinical data from the World Pancreas Transplant Registry suggests that DR antigen matching exerts a beneficial effect on cadaveric pancreatic transplant survival. However, MHC antigens are not uniformly distributed throughout the graft: it has been noted that the islets in transplanted dog pancreas remained histologically normal despite vigorous rejection of the exocrine pancreas. It is now known from immunohistochemical studies that normal islet cells do not express class II antigens (Daar et al, 1984; Sibley et al, 1987) whereas ductal, if not acinar, epithelium is class II antigen-positive. The entire pancreatic endothelium is normally class II antigen-positive, as are dendritic cells that are present in normal human islets (Sibley et al, 1987).

One might expect that acinar damage occurring early in pancreas transplant rejection could cause the local release of injurious enzymes that would, in turn, trigger the familiar pattern of acute pancreatitis, manifested in the non-grafted pancreas by polymorphonuclear leukocyte infiltration and vasculitis. This picture complicates the histological diagnosis of rejection in the duct-obstructed graft but in drained pancreas transplants the rejection reaction is fairly typical of other vascularized organ graft, and consists of mononuclear cell infiltration in the acinar and ductal epithelium and, occasionally, the islets of Langerhans. Vasculitis, too, is common and may proceed to fibrinoid necrosis and thrombosis (Sibley, 1988). Chronic rejection is reminiscent of that condition in renal transplants and consists of a chronic, proliferative arterial sclerosis. In this condition the islets may look histologically viable, with minimal inflammatory change; it has been found that interleukin 1 (IL-1) may inhibit insulin secretion from islets (Mandrup-Poulsen et al, 1986; Comens et al, 1987). This cytokine seems a likely candidate for a functional inhibitory role in this situation, for IL-1 may well be released from neighbouring macrophages during rejection.

CLINICAL AND PATHOLOGICAL MANIFESTATIONS OF REJECTION

Pancreas transplant rejection causes fever and influenza-like symptoms, with tenderness over the graft. The accurate diagnosis of rejection is relatively simple if the clinician has access to the exocrine secretions of the graft either by 24-hour urine collections following pancreaticocystostomy or, exceptionally, when the pancreas is exteriorized or given an exterior drain for collection of juice. As stated above, a reduction in amylase secretion is an early event in transplant rejection that allows prompt anti-rejection therapy to be started at a time when damage to the graft is still only mild or moderate. Similarly, pancreatic juice cytology reveals the presence of lymphoblasts in pancreas transplants undergoing rejection, and these cells disappear promptly following successful treatment of rejection (Tyden et al, 1987a). Other tests have been unhelpful: they either take too long to perform (plasma c-peptide for serum immunoreactive insulin level), are inconclusive (serum amylase), merely confirm rejection after it has occurred (plasma blood glucose, graft angiography) or are invasive despite being valuable (pancreatic biopsy). A moderate rise in the postprandial blood glucose level is, however, an early indication of graft injury, and has been described as preceding fasting hyperglycaemia by up to 5 days (Groth et al, 1980).

IMMUNOSUPPRESSION

Cyclosporin is the lynch-pin of most successful prophylactic regimens against pancreatic transplant rejection. Its use has led to a substantial reduction in prophylactic steroids, azathioprine and high dose prednisolone having been commonly used. By 1986 Sutherland was able to report from the World Transplant Registry that the inception of cyclosporin in combination with steroids or azathioprine had resulted in a doubling of graft survival at 1 year (47%) (Sutherland et al, 1986). Patient survival at one year was likewise markedly improved (see Appendix I). Nonetheless, the benefit gained on the immunological swings may be lost on the pharmacological roundabouts. Cyclosporin turned out to be not only nephrotoxic, thereby causing the principal complication of renal injury in non-transplanted diabetics as well as in recipients of kidney and pancreas transplants, but caused hyperglycaemia in some patients (Gunnarsson et al, 1984; Bending et al, 1987; Tyden et al, 1987b). Cyclosporin-related hyperglycaemia appears to be dose-related and by reducing the dosage to a therapeutic range, islet cell damage may be reversed.

Cyclosporin is usually administered with azathioprine or prednisone, often with both, and sometimes prophylactic antithymocyte globulin or OKT3 is used to supplement double or triple therapy. The risks of quadruple therapy must not be underestimated, and high dose quadruple therapy is definitely contraindicated by the experience of Dubernard (1984, personal communication), who found that in long-term survivors of pancreatico-renal transplants, excessive immunosuppressive therapy appeared to be directly associated with a substantial increase in the incidence of lymphoma. At the other end of the spectrum, cyclosporin monotherapy may be used with acceptable results (Sells, 1987). Pancreatic transplant rejection is generally treated by pulsed steroids, antithymocyte globulin, OKT3, or Campath 1 (Brons et al, 1988).

THE RECURRENCE OF DIABETES IN THE PANCREAS GRAFT

Selective destruction of the islets of Langerhans has been described by Sibley and Sutherland in pancreatic transplants between well-matched recipients and donors. This phenomenon is distinct from typical pancreas transplant rejection found in some HLA incompatible grafts and which shows the typical histological features of widespread immunological cell-mediated injury affecting all the parenchymal components of the graft. Selective β cell loss was confined to a small group of diabetics who received transplants from HLA-identical siblings or from identical twins (Sibley and Sutherland, 1987). Eight out of the nine patients described had pancreaticojejunostomies. Clinically and biochemically patients suffering from this complication presented with progressive hyperglycaemia or sudden loss of function up to 32 months after transplantation. Although there was some evidence of exocrine infiltration with lymphocytes, and some non-specific exocrine atrophy, three out of four identical twin transplants displayed inflammation of the islets, and four out of five HLA-identical sibling transplants showed selective β cell loss. A minority of patients had improvement of islet function after antilymphocyte globulin (ALG) treatment, but in all eight enterically drained cases there was permanent partial dysfunction or non-function of the graft despite additional immunosuppressive therapy. Immunohistochemically the islet cells showed increased class I antigen expression and there was also increased class II antigen on intra-islet endothelial cells. Biopsy material taken later on indicated that the inflammation of the islets eventually resolved and β cells atrophied completely. These histological features are reminiscent of those typically found in type I diabetes. Experimental work in spontaneously diabetic BB/W rats suggests that immunological attack occurs in MHC identical normal islets transplanted to BB rats, whereas survival of MHC mismatched rat islets may be prolonged or permanent in this strain (Woehrle et al, 1986). From this work we may conclude that a minor (non-MHC) antigen is expressed on islet cells in this model, which in the presence of HLA identity stimulates an immunological response. The occurrence of such a response in MHC-identical donors and recipients appears to be an example of MHC-restricted responsiveness against a minor antigen in the graft (see Chapter 1); such an hypothesis has been put forward by Bottazzo as the mechanism of islet injury in type I diabetes in the non-grafted native pancreas (Bottazzo et al, 1985). These authors suggested that cytokine-induced upgrading of class II antigen expression in β cells or islet components permits a MHC-restricted reaction against a neo-autoantigen, possibly of viral origin, expressed on islet components. This theory remains speculative, however, and the additional injurious effect of IL-1 on islet function remains a possible additional (or alternative) mechanism of islet suppression in these immunogenetically special cases (Mandrup-Poulsen et al, 1986). Whatever the explanation, selective β cell destruction in HLA-identical recipients of pancreatic grafts may represent a re-enactment of the immunological induction of the diabetic state, and seems to be quite distinct from graft rejection: no such selective β cell loss has been described in non HLA-identical graft recipients, and the institution of additional immunosuppression may not reverse this 'recurrent disease' process. It may be that in future the prevention of such recurrent disease in MHC-identical pancreatic grafts could be achieved by giving recipients full doses of immunosuppression, or conceivably the avoidance of such a complication may paradoxically require a deliberate mismatching of donor and recipient HLA antigens.

PROGRESSION OF DIABETIC LESIONS IN PANCREAS TRANSPLANT RECIPIENTS

There is clear evidence from experimental studies conducted in rats that successful pancreatic transplantation leading to normal glycaemia in alloxan-induced diabetes is associated with the prevention of diabetic complications (Orloff et al, 1986; Federlin and Bretzel, 1984). Indeed, in long-term studies, neovascularization of the retina and cataract formation, as well as histological abnormalities of the glomerular basement membrane and mesangium, could be reversed as long as 2 years after the induction of chemical diabetes by successful pancreas transplantation (Krupin et al, 1979). These findings give cause for hope that at least a delay in the onset of microangiopathy, if not its prevention, might be achieved by pre-emptive pancreatic transplantation in man. Convincing clinical evidence to support this optimistic view is as yet lacking, for the evidence for a beneficial effect of a successful pancreas transplant can be provided only from non-uraemic or prodromally diabetic pancreas recipients, or those diabetics who receive a pancreas graft following a successful previous kidney transplant.

The bulk of the useful clinical and pathological evidence on this very important subject comes from the large series of such patients transplanted in Minneapolis and reported by Sutherland and his colleagues (Sutherland et al, 1988b). To summarize their findings: patients with established retinopathy showed no significant stabilization or improvement of retinopathy compared with controls (patients whose pancreas grafts had failed) up to 2 years after transplantation, although after that time the patients with functioning grafts appeared to have less progression of retinopathy and less deterioration in vision than those with failed grafts; mean motor nerve conduction velocity improved following successful pancreas transplantation, indicating that in the majority of cases the progression of polyneuropathy was altered if not reversed by pancreas transplantation; and in non-uraemic patients receiving a pancreas graft alone, in whom the preoperative creatinine clearance was greater than 20 ml/min (serum creatinine less than 300 μmol/l), there was a consistent reduction in glomerular mesangial volume as determined by serial biopsies up to 2 years following pancreas transplantation. This last crucial observation was confirmed by Bohman (Bohman et al, 1987), who showed that in patients who had undergone combined pancreatic and renal transplantation, renal graft biopsies taken 2–4 years after transplantation showed no histological evidence of diabetic nephropathy, and that glomerular basement membrane thickening did not occur as it did in diabetics receiving renal transplants alone.

Functional studies of the performance of renal transplants 'protected' by a pancreas graft, or in pre-uraemic patients receiving a solitary pancreas graft, are complicated by the fact that many of the long-term survivors receive cyclosporin therapy with concomitant impairment of renal function due to nephrotoxicity. Although the data from the biopsies indicates the strong possibility that a simultaneous pancreas transplant performed with a renal graft, or a pre-emptive pancreas transplant performed in a non-uraemic diabetic, may prevent microangiopathy (or may reverse mild microangiopathy) in the kidneys, a satisfactory answer to this question will remain elusive in terms of renal function until non-nephrotoxic immunosuppressive regimens can be developed.

Autonomic neuropathy has been studied in patients with established diabetic complications who received simultaneous pancreaticorenal transplants, and it has been shown that the autonomic parasympathetic nervous system is severely affected in this selected diabetic population and that no significant effect is achieved by pancreatic transplantation. However, Abendroth et al (1987) suggest that normal glycaemia following pancreas transplantation is accompanied by significant changes in skin surface temperature and transcutaneous oxygen pressure measurements, indicating that sympathetic vasomotor innervation may have improved. It should be remembered, however, that these patients also received a kidney and benefited from reversal of uraemia, a factor which may well account for their improved neurological status. The question of whether or not a pancreas transplant can significantly affect the natural history of diabetic microangiopathy remains tantalizingly uncertain. It may well be that many of the benefits reported after pancreas transplantation are due to the beneficial consequences of the concomitant reversal of uraemia caused by the simultaneous transplantation of a successful kidney transplant, a situation that obtains in most of the recipients studied so far. Nonetheless, the possible protective function of a pancreas graft in preventing diabetic nephropathy keeps alive the hope, if not the confident expectation, that pre-emptive pancreas transplantation performed at an early stage of microangiopathy might prevent the widespread progression of diabetic complications.

THE INDICATIONS FOR PANCREATIC TRANSPLANTATION

Pancreas transplantation should only be considered for type I insulin-dependent diabetics. Although the procedure itself has evolved into a relatively safe method with a high expectation of patient survival and a reasonable expectation of medium-term graft survival, the use of this technique in an attempt to cure diabetes, reverse or ameliorate its complications, or prevent them must be very carefully considered by weighing the risks of the procedure against the possible benefits. There are two major difficulties which make it inadvisable for pancreas transplantation to be done pre-emptively to prevent microangiopathy:

1. It is still impossible to identify those high-risk diabetics whose angiopathy will progress rapidly and to distinguish them from those whose complications may progress slowly or may never reach a clinically severe stage. Until those two groups can be distinguished, we must assume that widespread pre-emptive pancreatic grafting in early type I diabetics would cause unnecessary surgical risks in many patients.
2. Transplants requiring cyclosporin therapy in non-uraemic recipients of pancreatic grafts would, in the majority of patients, run the risk of renal injury caused by the immunosuppressive drug even if diabetic nephropathy were delayed or prevented. It is possible that careful control of the cyclosporin dosage by careful monitoring of blood concentrations may in the long term (i.e. more than 10 years after transplantation) produce a net beneficial effect by limiting drug nephrotoxicity. However, whilst a well-functioning pancreas transplant may be the only chance of a definitive cure of diabetes, the existing immunosuppressive regimens are too injurious and uncertain to be applicable as yet.

Simultaneous pancreas and kidney transplantation would seem a more justifiable option; the quality of life and the conservation of renal function and renal architecture appear to be preserved in those patients who receive a pancreatic graft at the same time as a renal transplant. Although there is no conclusive evidence that established diabetic complications can be reversed in such cases, in those patients who have been screened to exclude major cardiac risk factors, the benefits in the long term would be very significant. However, it remains arguable whether the benefits are attributable to the reversal of uraemia and anaemia and the freedom from dialysis engendered by a successful kidney transplant, or result from normoglycaemia produced by the pancreas graft.

There seems, therefore, to be a very strong case for conducting a prospective randomized study of pancreas plus kidney transplantation versus kidney transplantation alone in a selected group of type I diabetic patients wth end-stage renal disease, in whom significant cardiovascular contraindications to the procedure have been excluded. The lack of good data from controlled studies is the principal cause of uncertainty about the indications for this potentially very powerful therapeutic technique.

REFERENCES

Abendroth D, Illhmer VD, Landgraf R & Land W (1987) Are late diabetic complications reversible after pancreas transplantation? A new method of follow-up of microcirculatory changes. *Transplantation Proceedings* **XIX**: 23–26.

ACS/NIH Organ Transplant Registry (1975) *Journal of American Medical Association* **233**: 148–153.

Bending JJ, Ogg CS & Biberti GC (1987) Diabetogenic effect of Cyclosporin. *British Medical Journal* **294**: 401–402.

Bohman SO, Wilczek H, Tyden G et al (1987) Recurrent diabetic nephropathy in renal allografts placed in diabetic patients and protective effect of simultaneous pancreatic transplantation. *Transplantation Proceedings* **XIX**: 2290–2293.

Borch-Johnsen K, Andersen PK & Deckert T (1985) The effect of proteinuria on relative mortality in type I (insulin-dependent) diabetes mellitus. *Diabetologia* **28**: 592–596.

Bottazzo GF, Dean BM, McNally JM et al (1985) In situ characterization of autoimmune phenomena and expression of HLA molecules in the pancreas in diabetic insulitis. *New England Journal of Medicine* **313**: 353–360.

Boulton AJM, Drury J, Clark B & Ward JD (1982) Continuous subcutaneous insulin infusion in the management of painful diabetic neuropathy. *Diabetes Care* **5**: 386–390.

Bowen KN, Handras L & Lafferty K (1980) Successful allotransplantation of mouse pancreatic islets to non-immunosuppressed recipients. *Diabetes* **29** (supplement 1): 98–104.

Brons IGM & Calne R (1988) Immunosuppression in pancreatic transplantation. In Groth CG (ed.) *Pancreatic Transplantation*, p 245. London: WB Saunders.

Buchwald H, Chute FE, Rup WM et al (1985) Implantable infusion pump for insulin delivery: past present and future. *Life Support Systems* **3**: 51–53.

Calne RY (1984) Paratopic segmental pancreas grafting: a technique with portal venous drainage. *Lancet* **i**: 595–597.

Campbell WR (1946) The first clinical trials of insulin. *Proceedings of the American Diabetes Association* **6**: 95–106.

Comens PG, Woolfe BA, Unanue ER, Lacy PE & McDaniel ML (1987) Interleukin 1 is a potent modulator of insulin secretion from isolated rat islets of Langerhans. *Diabetes* **36**: 963–970.

Cook K, Sollinger HW, Warner T et al (1983) Pancreaticocystostomy. *Transplantation* **35**: 634–638.

Corry RJ (1988) Pancreaticoduodenal transplantation with urinary tract drainage. In Groth CG (ed.) *Pancreatic Transplantation*, p 151. London: WB Saunders.

Daar AS, Fuggle SV, Faber JW, Ting A & Morris PJ (1984) The detailed distribution of MHC class II antigens in normal human organs. *Transplantation* **38**: 293–298.

Dahl-Jorgensen K, Brinchmaff-Hansen O, Hanssen KF et al (1986) Effect of near-normoglycaemia for two years on progression of early diabetic retinopathy, nephropathy and neuropathy: the Oslo study. *British Medical Journal* **293**: 1195–1199.

Dubernaud JN, Martin X, Camozz IL & Nsaverino R (1988) Segmental pancreatic transplantation with ductal filling by polymer injection. In Groth CG (ed.) *Pancreatic Transplantation*, p 162. London: WB Saunders.

Ewing DJ, Campbell IW & Clarke BF (1980) The natural history of autonomic neuropathy. *Quarterly Journal of Medicine* **49**: 95–108.

Faustman DL, Hauptfeld V, Lacy P & Davie J (1981) Prolongation of murine islet allograft survival by pretreatment of islets with antibody directed to Ia determinants. *Proceedings of the National Academy of Science USA* **78**: 5159.

Faustman DL, Steinman RM, Gebel HM et al (1984) Prevention of rejection of murine islet allografts by pretreatment with antidendritic cell antibody. *Proceedings of the National Academy of Science USA* **81**: 3864–3868.

Federlin KF and Bretzel RG (1984) The effect of islet transplantation on complications in experimental diabetes in the rat. *World Journal of Surgery* **8**: 169–178.

Feldt-Rasmussen B, Mathieson ER, Hegedus L & Deckert T (1986) Kidney function during twelve months of strict metabolic control in insulin-dependent diabetic patients with incipient nephropathy. *New England Journal of Medicine* **314**: 665–670.

Gray DW, Warnock G, Sutton R et al (1986) Successful autotransplantation of isolated islets of Langerhans in a cynomolgus monkey. *British Journal of Surgery* **73**: 850–853.

Groth CG, Lundgren G, Gunnarsson R, Arner P et al (1980) Segmental pancreatic transplantation with duct ligation or drainage to a jejunal Roux-en-Y-loop in non-uraemic diabetic patients. *Diabetes* **29** (suppl. 1): 3–9.

Groth CG, Collste H, Lundgrin G, Wilczek H et al (1982) Successful outcome of segmental human pancreatic transplantation with enteric exocrine diversion after modifications in technique. *Lancet* **ii**: 522.

Gunnarsson R, Klinmalm G, Lundgren G et al (1984) Deterioration of glucose metabolism in pancreatic transplant recipients after conversion from azathioprine to Cyclosporin. *Transplantation Proceedings* **XVI** 709–712.

Jacobs C, Brunner FP & Brynger RH (1983) The first 5,000 diabetics treated by dialysis and transplantation in Europe. *Diabetic Nephropathy* **2**: 12–16.

Jaspan JA, Wollman RL, Bernstein L & Rubenstein AH (1982) Hypoglycaemic peripheral neuropathy in association with insulinoma: implication of glucopenia rather than hyperinsulinism. *Medicine* **61**: 33–44.

Jensen T, Richter CA, Feldt-Rasmussen B, Kelbaekh O & Deckert T (1988) Impaired aerobic work capacity in insulin-dependent diabetics with increased urinary albumin excretion. *British Medical Journal* **296**: 1352–1354.

Kelly WD, Lillehei RC, Mirkel FK, Idezuki Y & Goetz FC (1967) Allotransplantation of the pancreas and duodenum along with the kidney in diabetic nephropathy. *Surgery* **61**: 827.

Klein R, Klein BEK & Moss SE (1984) Visual impairment in diabetes. *Ophthalmology* **91**: 1–9.

Kroc Collaborative Study Group (1984) *New England Journal of Medicine* **311**: 365–372.

Krolewski AS, Warram JR, Rand LI et al (1986) Risk of proliferative diabetic retinopathy in type I diabetes, a 40 year follow-up study. *Diabetes Care* **9**: 443–452.

Krupin T, Waltman SR & Scharp DW (1979) Ocular Fluorophotometery in streptozotocin diabetes mellitus in the rat: Effect of pancreatic islet isografts. *Investigative Ophthalmology and Visual Science* **18**: 1185–1190.

Lau H, Reemstma K & Hardy MA (1984) Prolongation of rat allograft survival by direct ultraviolet irradiation of the graft. *Science* **223**: 607–609.

Lawson P, Holme BD & Bergenstal R (For the Kroc Collaborative Study Group) (1985) *Diabetes* **34** (supplement 1): 39A.

Mandrup-Poulsen T, Bendtzen K, Nerup J et al (1986) Affinity-purified human interleukin 1 is cytotoxic to isolated islets of Langerhans. *Diabetalogia* **6-29**: 63–67.

Marble A (1972) Insulin—clinical aspects: The first 50 years. *Diabetes* **21** (supplement 2): 632–636.

Mauer M, Steffes MW, Connett J et al (1983) The development of lesions in the glomerular basement membrane and mesangium after transplantation of normal kidneys to diabetic patients. *Diabetes* **32**: 948–952.

Mijovic C, Fletcher JA, Bradwell AR & Barnett AH (1985) Relation of gene expression (allotypes) of the fourth component of complement to insulin dependent diabetes and its microangioperative complications. *British Medical Journal* **291**: 9–10.

Mijovic C, Fletcher JA, Bradwell AR & Barnett AH (1986) Phenotypes of the heavy chains of immunoglobulins in patients with diabetic microangiopathy: evidence for an immunogenetic predisposition. *British Medical Journal* **292**: 433–435.

Mogensen CE (1988) The management of diabetic renal involvement and disease. *Lancet* **i**: 867–870.

Morley GK, Mooradian AD, Levine AL & Morlety JE (1984) Mechanisms of pain in diabetic peripheral neuropathy: effect of glucose on pain perception in humans. *American Journal of Medicine* **77**: 79–82.

Okye SE, Engen VE, Sterioff SS et al (1983) Primary and secondary renal transplantation in diabetic patients. *Journal of American Medical Association* **249**: 492–495.

Orloff M, Yamanaka N, Greenleaf G et al (1986) Reversal of mesangial enlargement in rats with longstanding diabetes by whole pancreas transplantation. *Diabetes* **35**: 347–354.

Prieto M, Sutherland DER, Fernando Cruz L, Heil J & Najarian JS (1987) Experimental and clinical experience with urine amylase monitoring for early diagnosis of rejection in pancreas transplantation. *Transplantation* **43**: 73–79.

Pyke D (1988) Pancreas Transplantation for Diabetes. *Lancet* **i**: 816–817.

Rajotte RV, Warnock GL, Evans M & Davidson I (1987) Isolation of viable islets of Langerhans from collagenase perfuse canine and human pancreata. *Transplantation Proceedings* **XIX**: 918–922.

Sells RA (1987) Experience in pancreatic/renal transplantation at Liverpool UK. *Transplantation Proceedings* **XIX** (supplement 4): 40–43.

Service FJ, Rizza RA, Dauke JR et al (1985) Near normoglycaemia improved nerve conduction and vibration sensation in diabetic neuropathy. *Diabetologia* **28**: 722–727.

Sibley K (1988) Pathology of the pancreas graft. In Groth CG (ed.) *Pancreas Transplantation*, pp 272–284. London: WB Saunders.

Sibley RK & Sutherland DER (1987) Pancreas transplantation: an immunohistologic and histopathologic examination of 100 grafts. *American Journal of Pathology* **128**: 151–170.

Steffes NW, Sutherland DER, Goetz FC, Rich SS & Mauer SM (1985) Studies of kidney and muscle biopsy specimens of identical twins, discordant for type I diabetes mellitus. *New England Journal of Medicine* **312**: 1282–1287.

Sutherland DER, Goetz FC & Najarian JS (1984) 100 pancreas transplants at a single institution. *Annals of Surgery* **200**: 414.

Sutherland DER, Goetz, FC & Najarian JS (1986) Improved pancreas graft survival rates by use of combination immunotherapy. *Transplantation Proceedings* **XVIII**: 1770–1773.

Sutherland DER, Goetz FC & Najarian JS (1988a) Pancreas Transplantation for diabetes. *Lancet* **i**: 1100.

Sutherland DER, Goetz FC & Najarian JS (1988b) Experience with single pancreas transplantation compared with pancreas transplantation after a kidney transplantation; with transplantation with pancreas graft from living related compared with cadaveric graft. In Groth CG (ed.) *Pancreatic Transplantation*, pp 175–189. London: WB Saunders.

Tamborlane WV, Genel M, Sherwin RS & Felig P (1979) *Lancet* **i**: 1250–1261.

Thomsen OF, Andersen AR, Christiansen JS & Deckert T (1984) Renal changes in long term, type II (insulin dependent) diabetic patients with and without the clinical nephropathy: a light microscopic, morphometric study of autopsy material. *Diabetalogia* **26**: 361–365.

Tyden G, Reinhellt F, Brattstrom M & Lundgren G (1987a) Diagnosis of rejection in recipients with pancreatic grafts with enteric exocrine diversion by monitoring pancreatic juice cytology and amylase secretion. *Transplantation Proceedings* **XIX**: 3892–3894.

Tyden G, Brattstrom C, Gunnarsson R et al (1987b) Metabolic control four months to four years after pancreatic transplantation with a special reference to the role of Cyclosporin. *Transplantation Proceedings* **XIX**: 2294–2296.

Viberti GC, Bilous RW, Macintosh D, Bending JJ & Keen H (1983) Long term correction of hyperglycaemia and progression of renal failure in insulin dependent diabetes. *British Medical Journal* **286**: 598–602.

Voruganti LNP & Sells RA (1989) Quality of life of diabetic patients after combined pancreaticorenal transplantation. *Clinical Transplantation* **2** (in press).

Woehrle M, Markmann JF, Silvers WK, Barker CF & Naji A (1986) Transplantation of cultured islets to BB rats. *Surgery* **100**: 334–340.

8a Current Controversies and New Horizons

Specific Immunological Unresponsiveness of Long-term Organ Transplant Recipients

BARRY D. KAHAN

The ultimate goal of transplantation immunology is to devise a strategy that induces immunological tolerance. The acceptance of donor-specific tissues without the need for immunosuppression (Billingham et al, 1953), distinct from the apparent unresponsiveness of allograft recipients under drug therapy, only rarely occurs in clinical practice (Ozaki et al, 1980; Suzuki et al, 1985). Although renal transplant recipients under combined cyclosporin and prednisone therapy generally display immunological unresponsiveness (Kahan et al, 1986), they uniformly experience severe rejection episodes and frequently graft loss if they are non-compliant and discontinue cyclosporin (Didlake et al, 1988). Despite having apparently been unresponsive for years, these patients have not developed true immunological tolerance. This natural resistance of man to the development of tolerance contrasts with findings in rats, which frequently develop this state after immunosuppression with cyclosporin for a sufficient time (Lim et al, 1988). Thus, man requires more intense or more sophisticated immunosuppressive regimens to facilitate the progression to tolerance. In one anecdotal report, three patients treated with total lymphoid irradiation (TLI) had all immunosuppressants withdrawn from them without allograft rejection (Chow et al, 1987).

Complete withdrawal of suppressive drugs nevertheless carries a high risk of graft loss, and the dosage needs to be reduced cautiously and progressively. The first step should be steroid withdrawal; this not only ameliorates toxic side-effects, but also allows one to observe immunological mechanisms concealed by the prominent non-specific effects of corticosteroids. This manoeuvre carries a high risk of rejection in patients receiving azathioprine-based immunosuppression (Naik et al, 1979) unless they carry HLA-identical grafts (First et al, 1981). Even recipients of MHC-incompatible cadaver grafts (Hillebrand et al, 1988; Maiorca, 1988) and living-related grafts (Burlingham et al, 1989) under cyclosporin–prednisone therapy display a greater than 50% risk of rejection episodes after complete steroid withdrawal. Therefore, an *a priori* index of immuno-acceptance

ORGAN TRANSPLANTATION: CURRENT CLINICAL AND
IMMUNOLOGICAL CONCEPTS   ISBN 0-7020-1393-5

prior to steroid withdrawal is urgently needed in order to avert even reversible rejection episodes, for allosensitization is associated with poor long-term graft survival, in spite of pharmacological control of the initial rejection episodes.

Whilst one approach is to seek to elucidate tolerance induction mechanisms in animal models, possibly leading to the design of tolerance-induction regimens for general clinical application, a second approach is to dissect specific anti-donor hyporesponsiveness in patients, in order to obtain indices for the reduction of immunosuppression.

IN VITRO ANALOGUES OF IN VIVO UNRESPONSIVENESS

Although in vitro assays fail to predict in vivo alloimmune responses reliably (Kahan, 1985), two types of donor-specific hyporesponsiveness broadly correlate with allograft acceptance: namely, impaired proliferative responses in one-way mixed lymphocyte reactions (MLR) and a low level of cytoaggressiveness in cell-mediated lympholysis assays (CML).

Bach et al (1972) showed that, following kidney transplantation, a cohort of MHC-incompatible recipients developed reduced responses in MLR towards their living related donors' lymphocytes. This suggested that the one-way MLR assay might predict alloacceptance. Using the stimulation index (SI; the ratio of counts per minute (cpm) of tritiated thymidine incorporated into the patient's blood lymphocytes in the presence of irradiated donor stimulator cells and the counts obtained in the presence of irradiated autologous stimulator cells), MLR hyporesponsiveness was defined as having an SI of < 6.5. Donor-specific hyporesponsiveness, apparent when the SI after stimulation by a panel of third-party cells was > 6.5, suggests that it may be possible to withdraw steroids whilst maintaining cyclosporin therapy. Unfortunately, MLR hyporesponsiveness is not an inevitable consequence of cyclosporin–prednisone therapy. Of 55 patients receiving haploidentical living-related renal grafts, only 17 (30%) displayed it (Kahan et al, 1989). Sixteen such patients, whose steroids had been withdrawn, were generally (81%) free from rejection episodes and they had an actuarial 1 year graft survival of 94%. The MLR hyporesponsive patients were, likewise, hyporesponsive in CML (Flechner et al, 1984).

A larger series of 36 recipients followed for at least 1 and up to 6 years confirmed little risk of steroid withdrawal (Kahan et al, 1989). As might be predicted, the recipients of HLA-identical grafts showed transplant survival to 4 years after withdrawal of steroids; one patient was non-compliant to the cyclosporin regimen, reducing graft survival to 95%. Among the 19 HLA-identical patients whose steroids had been withdrawn, four suffered rejection episodes requiring a return to steroids at 2, 5, 15 and 32 months. Among the patients receiving haploidentical grafts there were no losses until 2 years following steroid withdrawal, when the transplant survival rate fell to 82% because of chronic rejection. Two of this group suffered rejection episodes requiring a return to steroids at 3 and 6 months. The graft survival rate in the cohort of patients on cyclosporin only, who were steroid-withdrawn solely based on the criterion of specific MLR hyporesponsiveness, equalled the rate in persistently MLR-responsive patients maintained on cyclosporin plus prednisone.

Other workers have failed to document significant differences in MLR responsiveness before and after transplantation in patients on azathioprine–prednisone therapy (Thaysen and Lokkegaard, 1977; Pfeffer et al, 1983). Goulmy et al (1981) found that CML, but not

MLR, hyporesponsiveness predicted a benign post-transplant course in 20 recipients of HLA-mismatched, azathioprine–prednisone immunosuppressed cadaver kidney grafts, an observation supported by Wonigeit et al (1979) and Harmon et al (1982). Donor-specific CML hyporesponsiveness, defined as $\leqslant 10\%$ lysis of specific kidney donor splenocytes, correlated with both a reduced frequency of rejection episodes and better renal allograft function. In living-related donor transplantation, CML but not MLR hyporesponsiveness was observed in recipients bearing successful allografts under azathioprine–prednisone (Thomas et al, 1977; Liburd et al, 1978) and under cyclosporin–azathioprine–prednisone immunosuppressive regimens (Burlingham et al, 1989). As CML hyporesponsiveness was not a prerequisite of graft survival after withdrawal of steroids from a cyclosporin–azathioprine–prednisone regimen, it is unclear whether those in vitro assays truly reflect the clinical status of patient unresponsiveness or merely represent incidental findings.

IMMUNOLOGICAL MECHANISMS

The in vivo mechanisms that lead to in vitro findings of hyporesponsiveness are not clear. Although Pfeffer et al (1983) described depletion of alloreactive antidonor lymphocytes, Goulmy et al (1985) documented the presence of cells able to become cytotoxic following the addition in vitro of exogenous interleukin 2. These observations reinforce the widely held hypothesis that hyporesponsiveness is due to cellular or humoral immunoregulatory elements. Suppressor cells have been demonstrated using 'three-cell assays': lightly-irradiated, post-transplant patient peripheral blood lymphocytes (PBL), which are themselves incapable of proliferation but which retain any in vitro suppressor function, are added to mixtures of cryopreserved, pre-transplant patient PBL responding to heavily-irradiated donor stimulators.These mixtures are analysed either at 5 days for incorporation of ^{3}H-thymidine in proliferative MLR assays, or at 10 days for lysis of added ^{51}Cr-labelled, concanavalin A-stimulated donor lymphoblasts. One cohort of MLR hyporesponsive recipients under cyclosporin–prednisone therapy had peripheral blood mononuclear leukocytes (PMBL) that inhibited autologous pre-transplant recipient PBL proliferation toward the donor 4–10 times more potently than toward third-party stimulators. By contrast, PBML from persistently MLR-responsive recipients failed to inhibit proliferation (Flechner et al, 1985). The suppressive activity was not caused by cytotoxicity toward the MLR responders.

Suppressor elements have been documented in two cellular compartments: a lymphocyte-mediated, specific component which is non-adherent to plastic was present in 35% of 255 cadaver kidney transplant patients who were immunosuppressed with cyclosporin–prednisone (Kerman et al, 1987). A greater (46%) fraction of this patient cohort displayed a non-specific suppressive effect mediated by plastic adherent cells. HLA-DR matching of donor and recipient appeared to facilitate the induction of suppressive cells. The presence of suppressive activity correlated with OKT4–OKT8 ratios $\leqslant 1.0$, and a decreased incidence of allograft rejection episodes (Kerman et al, 1987). These findings parallel work in total lymphoid irradiation (TLI)-treated patients. Strober (1984) described the initial activation of non-specific suppressor cells. In vitro analysis of the three patients in whom tolerance had been induced by TLI revealed specific MLR hyporesponsiveness toward stimulator cells sharing HLA antigens with the allograft donor (Chow et al, 1987). Furthermore, suppressor cells have been documented that mediate unresponsiveness in animals treated with antilymphocyte serum and bone marrow (Kilshaw et al, 1975; Kilshaw and Brent, 1977; Wood and Monaco, 1980) or with CsA and extracted histocompatibility antigen (Yasumura and Kahan, 1984) tolerance models. It is unclear whether the specific and non-specific suppressive elements are independent effectors, or whether the adherent non-specific elements are actually triggered by humoral factors produced by non-adherent, specific suppressor lymphocytes (Waltenbaugh, 1979).

The emergence of suppressor cells in patients under long-term cyclosporin therapy is consistent with the drug's selective sparing of this cellular element. Suppressor cells appear and mature despite the presence of potent cyclosporin immunosuppression during the induction of alloimmune reactions. In vitro addition of CsA does not affect the appearance of cellular suppressors in MLR and CML reactions (Hess and Tutschka, 1980). Suppressor cells that appear in human renal transplant recipients during in vivo cyclosporin adminstration may be detected either in vitro by inhibition of MLR (Agostino et al, 1982) or pokeweed mitogen-stimulated B cell activation (Van Buren et al, 1982) or, in vivo, by adoptive transfer tests in normal or irradiated rat hosts (Yasumura and Kahan, 1984). Clarification of the cellular mechanism of cyclosporin-sparing of suppressor cells has been impeded by controversy concerning not only the three-cell assay system but also the identity of the cells as discrete elements of CD4 (Dorsch and Roser, 1977) or CD8 (Yoshimura and Kahan, 1985) lineages. Although only one of seven CML hyporesponsive patients under azathioprine–prednisone therapy displayed suppressor cell activity in three-cell assays in the study of Goulmy et al (1981), such activity has been documented in similar studies by Seki et al (1983) and by Pfeffer et al (1983). Thus, suppressor cells may mediate many but not all forms of allo-unresponsiveness and tolerance.

Tolerance induction under azathioprine therapy may depend on humoral mechanisms. Goulmy et al (1985) correlated the pattern of CML unresponsiveness with the presence of donor HLA-B (or HLA-B/HLA-C region), but not HLA-A, determinants, a finding that paralleled the apparent HLA-B genetic specificity of anti-idiotypic antibodies. Humoral substances are believed to affect in vivo cellular maturation (Miyajima et al, 1980; Suzuki et al, 1985), particularly in patients rendered allo-unresponsive by pre-transplant, donor-specific blood transfusions (Singal and Joseph, 1982). Thus, HLA-DR gene restriction of suppressor cell induction may be complemented by an HLA-specificity of CML hyporesponsiveness.

LIMITATIONS OF PRESENT ASSAYS OF HYPORESPONSIVENESS

Because present techniques assess alloreactivity based on PBL responses toward donor cells, they represent late reflections of the immunoadaptive events that presumably occur in the central lymphoid compartment and determine the progression from unresponsiveness to tolerance under the cover of immunosuppression. Thus, blood cells may only poorly reflect primary events in the tolerance process that occur elsewhere. In addition to the lymph nodes and spleen, the thymus and the allograft itself act as two major sites in this process. Autoreactive anti-MHC cells are normally eliminated in the course of fetal development in the thymic medulla as part of the acquisition of self/non-self discrimination. This thymic site (or its analogue in adult hosts) imprints H-2-restricted T-cell specificity (Lo and Sprent, 1986). Tolerance may thus be induced by extending the auto-

MHC restriction to a narrow range of donor-specific alloantigens via cellular or possibly humoral mechanisms. Functional blockade of the H-2 IE molecule with monoclonal antibody prevented thymic organ cultures from developing specifically reactive elements towards allogeneic MHC class I determinants (McDuffie et al, 1988). The transplant itself provides unique conditions for the maturation of allo-unresponsiveness. Tolerance models using either anti-lymphocyte serum and bone marrow (Kilshaw et al, 1975; Kilshaw and Brent, 1977; Wood and Monaco, 1977) or cyclosporin and extracted histocompatibility antigen (Yoshimura and Kahan, 1986) require the presence of alloantigens for the maintenance of the unresponsive state. Indeed in the latter system, intragraft lymphoid cells transfer allo-unresponsiveness more potently than those harvested from peripheral blood or spleen. Presumably this potent effect of the allotransplant is connected wth the unique environment it provides for immunocompetent cells of the host, possibly by a special tolerogenic form, or high concentration of foreign histocompatibility antigens in the transplant, or by unique biochemical or physiological factors in the graft environment.

Further, in vitro essays of PBL reactivity suffer the limitations of (i) at least a temporal delay between the induction of central allo-unresponsiveness and its peripheral manifestations; (ii) the probability that in vitro separation, culture and activation conditions are sufficiently artificial to induce spurious allo-aggressiveness or unresponsiveness (Kilshaw et al, 1975); (iii) the presence of either the immunosuppressive agents or their metabolites or their residual effects inhibiting the responses of isolated cells; and (iv) the possibility that isolated cells acting in vitro in the absence of co-existent humoral factors present in vivo do not reflect allo-acceptance conditions in the patient.

THE FUTURE

Dissection of the in vitro, anti-donor, immunological responses of successfully engrafted transplant recipients represents the only available avenue for the assessment of mechanisms of in vivo allo-unresponsiveness in man. Under azathioprine–prednisone therapy for CML, and under cyclosporin–prednisone therapy for MLR and CML, hyporesponsiveness is associated with a benign clinical course and, in the latter, with a good prognosis for withdrawal of steroids. However, the correlations are not exact – some patients who display uninhibited MLR and/or CML responses in vitro likewise tolerate steroid withdrawal without rejection episodes. Thus, advances in the analysis of clinical events must depend on the development of direct assays for humoral and/or cellular vectors mediating allo-unresponsiveness to replace tests measuring proliferative and cytotoxic reactivity resulting from such vectors. Further, not only rational steroid withdrawal, but also clinical evaluation of numerous tolerance induction strategies that have already been developed in rodents and verified in canine and the baboon transplant models, depends on the definition of valid in vitro correlates of in vivo allo-acceptance.

REFERENCES

Agostino GJ, Kahan BD & Kerman RH (1982) Suppression of mixed lymphocyte culture using leukocytes from normal individuals, uremic patients and allograft recipients. *Transplantation* **34**: 367–371.

Bach ML, Engstrom MA, Bach FH, Etheredge EE & Najarian JS (1972) Specific tolerance in human kidney allograft recipients. *Cellular Immunology* **3**: 161–166.

Billingham RE, Brent L & Medawar PB (1953) Actively acquired tolerance to foreign cells. *Nature (London)* **172**: 603–606.

Burlingham WJ, Grailer A & Sollinger HW (1989) Changes in donor-specific cell-mediated lympholysis response associated with success of early steroid withdrawal in DST-azathioprine-treated renal transplant recipients. *Transplantation Proceedings* **21**: 1818–1819.

Chow D, Soper V & Strober S (1987) Renal transplant patients treated with total lymphoid irradiation show specific unresponsiveness to donor antigens in the mixed leukocyte reaction. *Journal of Immunology* **138**: 3446–3750.

Didlake R, Dreyfus K, Kerman RH, Van Buren CT & Kahan BD (1988) Patient noncompliance: a major cause of late graft failure in cyclosporine-treated renal transplants. *Transplantation Proceedings* **20** (supplement 3): 63–69.

Dorsch S & Roser B (1977) Recirculating suppressor T cells in transplantation tolerance. *Journal of Experimental Medicine* **145**: 1144–1149.

First, MR, Munda R, Kant KS, Fidler JP & Alexander JW (1981) Steroid withdrawal following HLA-identical related donor transplantation. *Transplantation Proceedings* **13**: 319–322.

Flechner SM, Kerman RH, Van Buren CT, Epps L & Kahan BD (1984) The use of cyclosporine in living related renal transplantation: donor specific hyporesponsiveness and steroid withdrawal. *Transplantation* **38**: 685–691.

Flechner SM, Kerman RH, Van Buren CT & Kahan BD (1985) Mixed lymphocyte culture hyporesponsiveness as a marker for steroid withdrawal in cyclosporine-treated living related renal recipients. *Transplantation Proceedings* **17**: 1260–1264.

Goulmy E, Persijn G, Blokland E, D'Amaro J & van Rood JJ (1981) Cell-mediated lympholysis studies in renal allograft recipients. *Transplantation* **31**: 210–217.

Goulmy E, Blokland E, Persijn G et al (1985) HLA regulates postrenal transplant CML nonreactivity. *The Journal of Immunology* **135**: 3082–3086.

Harmon WE, Parkman R, Lavin PT et al (1982) Comparison of cell-mediated lympholysis and mixed lymphocyte culture in the immunologic evaluation for renal transplantation. *The Journal of Immunology* **129**: 1573–1577.

Hess AD & Tutschka PJ (1980) Effect of CsA on human lymphocyte responses in vitro: I. CsA allows for the expression of alloantigen activated suppressor cells while preferentially inhibiting the induction of cytolytic effector lymphocytes in MLR. *The Journal of Immunology* **124**: 2601–2608.

Hillebrand DG, Krumme D, Schleibner S, Land W & Gurland HJ (1988) Is withdrawal of steroids hazardous to cadaveric renal transplants under treatment with cyclosporine? *Transplantation Proceedings* **20** (supplement 3): 126–129.

Kahan BD (1985) Immunologic monitoring: utility and limitations. *Transplantation Proceedings* **17**: 1537–1545.

Kahan BD, Van Buren CT, Flechner SM, Wideman CA & Kerman RH (1986) Allograft rejection in renal allograft recipients under cyclosporine-prednisone immunosuppressive therapy. In GM Williams, JF Burdick & K Solez (eds) *Kidney Transplant Rejection: Diagnosis and Treatment*, pp 411–422. New York: Marcel Dekker.

Kahan BD, Kerman RH, Van Buren CT et al (1989) Clinical outcome in 36 patients after at least one and up to 5 years of steroid withdrawal based upon specific mixed lymphocyte reaction hyporesponsiveness toward the living related donor. *Transplantation Proceedings* **21**: 1579–1580.

Kerman RH, Flechner SM, Van Buren CT, Lorber MI & Kahan BD (1987) Immunoregulatory mechanisms in cyclosporine-treated renal allograft recipients. *Transplantation* **43**: 205–210.

Kilshaw PJ & Brent L (1977) Further studies on suppressor T cells in mice made unresponsive to H-2 incompatible with skin grafts. *Transplantation Proceedings* **9**: 717–719.

Kilshaw PJ, Brent L & Pinto M (1975) Suppressor T cells in mice made unresponsive to skin allografts. *Nature* **255**: 489–491.

Liburd EM, Pazderka V, Kovithavongs T & Dossetor JB (1978) Evidence for suppressor cells and reduced CML induction by the donor in transplant recipients. *Transplantation Proceedings* **10**: 557–561.

Lim SML, White DJG & Calne RY (1988) Cyclosporine coverage during the risk period leads to 100% long-term graft acceptance in the rat. *Transplantation Proceedings* **20** (supplement 3): 1013–1015.

Lo D & Sprent J (1986) Identity of cells that imprint H-2-restricted T cell specificity in the thymus. *Nature* **319**: 672–673.

McDuffie M, Roehm N, Kappler JW & Marrack P (1988) Involvement of major histocompatibility complex products in tolerance induction in the thymus. *The Journal of Immunology* **141**: 1840–1847.

Maiorca R, Cristinelli L, Brunori G et al (1988) Prospective controlled trial of steroid withdrawal after 6 months in renal transplant patients treated with cyclosporine. *Transplantation Proceedings* **20** (supplement 3): 121–125.

Miyajima T, Higuchi H, Kashiwabara H, Yokoyama T & Fujimoto S (1980) Antiidiotypic antibodies in a patient with a functioning renal graft. *Nature* **283**: 306–308.

Naik RB, Abdeen H, English J et al (1979) Prednisolone withdrawal after 2 years in renal transplant patients receiving only this form of immunosuppression. *Transplantation Proceedings* **11**: 39–44.

Ozaki A, Iwasaki Y & Miyajima T (1980) Withdrawal of azathioprine after renal transplantation. *Transplantation Proceedings* **12**: 513–514.

Pfeffer PF, Thorsby E & Hirschberg H (1983) Donor specific decreased cell-mediated cytotoxicity in recipients of well functioning, one HLA haplotype-mismatched kidney allografts. *Transplantation* **35**: 156–160.

Seki Y, Sakagami K, Takeuchi H et al (1983) Evidence for donor-specific cell-mediated lympholysis unresponsiveness and suppressor cells in well-functioning kidney transplants. *Transplantation Proceedings* **15**: 2131–2133.

Singal DP & Joseph S (1982) Role of blood transfusions on the induction of antibodies against recognition sites on T-lymphocytes in renal transplant patients. *Human Immunology* **4**: 93–98.

Strober S (1984) Natural suppressor cells, neonatal tolerance, and total lymphoid irradiation: exploring obscure relationships. *Annual Reviews of Immunology* **2**: 219–237.

Suzuki S, Mizuochi I, Sada M & Amemiya H (1985) Transplantation tolerance mediated by suppressor T cells and suppressive antibody in a recipient of a renal transplant. *Transplantation* **40**: 357–362.

Thaysen JH & Lokkegaard H (1977) Permanent withdrawal of prednisone in necro-kidney transplantation. *Scandinavian Journal of Urology and Nephrology* **42**: 198–199.

Thomas J, Thomas F, Mendez-Picon G & Lee H (1977) Immunological monitoring of long-surviving renal transplant recipients. *Surgery* **81**: 125–131.

Van Buren C, Kerman R, Agostino G et al (1982) The cellular target of cyclosporin A action in humans. *Surgery* **92**: 167–174.

Waltenbaugh C (1979) Specific and nonspecific suppressor T cell factors. In S Cohen, E Pick & J Oppenheim (eds) *Biology of the Lymphokines*, pp 421–431.

Wonigeit K, Boekhorn H & Pichlmayr R (1979) Posttransplant changes in specific precursor T-cell reactivity: comparison between liver and kidney allograft recipients. *Transplantation Proceedings* **15**: 1250–1252.

Wood ML & Monaco AP (1977) The effect of timing of skin grafts on subsequent survival in ALS-treated, marrow-infused mice. *Transplantation* **23**: 78–85.

Wood ML & Monaco AP (1980) Suppressor cells in specific unresponsiveness to skin allografts in ALS-treated, marrow-injected mice. *Transplantation* **29**: 196–201.

Yasumura T & Kahan BD (1984) Prolongation of allograft survival by repeated cycles of donor antigen and cyclosporine in rat kidney transplantation. *Transplantation* **38**: 418–423.

Yoshimura N & Kahan BD (1985) Nature of the suppressor cells mediating prolonged graft survival after administration of extracted histocompatibility antigen and cyclosporine. *Transplantation* **39**: 162–168.

8b   Current Controversies and New Horizons

Induction of MHC Antigens in Organ Transplants: Cause or Effect?

JOHN W. FABRE

The parenchymal cells of the body have been regarded traditionally as passive 'spectators' of the immune system's battles against micro-organisms and, in the context of the transplanted organ, as passive targets of the recipient's rejection response. However, it is now emerging that parenchymal cells might play an active role in the body's defences, by secreting lymphokines (cytokines) such as interleukin-1 (Kupper et al, 1986; Coleman et al, 1987; Chodakewitz et al, 1988) and by greatly increasing their expression of MHC molecules, the physiological function of which is now known to be the presentation of peptide fragments of foreign antigens to the T lymphocyte system. When these 'immune' functions of parenchymal cells are triggered by physiological inflammation, for example, in viral infections, it seems highly likely that the immune response against the pathogen is enhanced and the prospects of survival for the host thereby improved. It is presumably the survival value of these traits which has established them during the course of evolution. However, when the parenchymal cell happens to find itself in a foreign environment as a result of the work of transplant surgeons, what are the consequences of switching on these 'immune' functions? The release of lymphokines by some parenchymal cells has potentially very interesting consequences in transplantation and has been discussed in detail previously (Fabre, 1988). Here the role of MHC induction in the rejection response is discussed. My own view is that by over-expressing its MHC molecules in response to the inflammatory component of rejection, the parenchymal cell almost certainly plays an active and essential role in its own destruction. If this is true, it puts the rejection process in a rather more interesting perspective and has potentially important diagnostic and therapeutic applications in clinical transplantation.

THE NORMAL DISTRIBUTION OF MHC ANTIGENS

The advent of monoclonal xenoantibodies to MHC antigens made possible detailed immunohistological studies on the distribution of class I and class II MHC antigens in the

ORGAN TRANSPLANTATION: CURRENT CLINICAL AND
IMMUNOLOGICAL CONCEPTS   ISBN 0-7020-1393-5

commonly transplanted organs (e.g. Hart and Fabre, 1981a,b; Hart et al, 1983; Daar et al, 1984a,b). Until the 1980s, there was no clear view of how MHC antigens are expressed in the body. It is interesting and relevant to the present discussion to note that the parenchymal cells of the commonly transplanted organs express little, and sometimes no, MHC antigen. The widely accepted dictum that all nucleated cells express class I MHC antigens is simply not true. For example, the exocrine cells of the pancreas do not express class I antigens. The myocardial cell has no detectable class I except at the intercalated discs. The hepatocyte appears to show species and individual or strain variation with respect to class I expression and has been reported as expressing class I either weakly or not at all (reviewed in Settaf et al, 1988) or strongly (Brent et al, 1981). Renal tubular cells are all weakly positive for class I, with the proximal tubular cells additionally showing weak expression of class II. However, it is important to note that the vascular endothelial cells of all organs strongly express class I antigens at the time of transplantation, a point to which I shall return later.

THE PHENOMENON OF MHC INDUCTION

In experimental models using inbred rat strains, it is possible to perform grafts between genetically identical individuals, and thereby to note any effects on MHC expression of the transplantation procedure itself, in the absence of rejection (Milton and Fabre, 1985; Milton et al, 1986a; Settaf et al, 1988). The general rule that emerges is that transplantation of itself gives rise to very weak class I induction which begins at day 3 and persists for at least 2 weeks, but that class II induction does not occur.

During rejection episodes, the overall level of expression of MHC antigens within a grafted organ can increase very dramatically, increases of ten- to thirty-fold being common. The phenomenon has been studied in experimental (Milton and Fabre, 1985; Steiniger et al, 1985a) and clinical (Rose et al, 1986; Ahmed-Ansari et al, 1988) heart transplantation; experimental (Benson et al, 1985; Milton et al, 1986a) and clinical (Hall et al, 1984; Fuggle et al, 1986; Barrett et al, 1987) kidney transplantation; experimental (Settaf et al, 1988) and clinical (Tacacs et al, 1983; Demetris et al, 1985; So et al, 1987; Steinhoff et al, 1987) liver transplantation; and in experimental pancreas transplantation (Steiniger et al, 1985b).

The overall picture for class I antigens is relatively straightforward: class I is readily induced on all cell types (except possibly the smooth muscle of small vessels). At the height of rejection episodes, all cells in the commonly transplanted organs (except vascular smooth muscle) strongly express class I MHC antigens. This is illustrated in Figure 1a and b for heart allografts in rats. The normally class I negative myocardial cells (Figure 1a) are seen to develop very strong membrane expression of class I by the fifth day after grafting (Figure 1b).

The situation with regard to class II antigens is more complicated. The various cell types within the commonly transplanted organs show markedly different propensities for class II induction, a fact of potentially great importance. Epithelial cells of the renal tubules, the exocrine pancreas and the pancreatic and hepatic ducts show marked induction, as illustrated in Figures 1c and d. A biopsy taken from a kidney graft at the time of transplantation showed no staining for class II antigens on the epithelial cells of the tubules (Figure 1c). However, during a rejection episode, the same kidney had strongly class II positive tubular cells (Figure 1d). Myocardial cells are able to express class II, but this is not as readily induced as in the tissues just mentioned, and probably occurs only during the more violent rejection episodes. Hepatocytes are the cells most resistant to class II induction. At the height of even very fierce rejection episodes most hepatocytes remain resolutely class II negative.

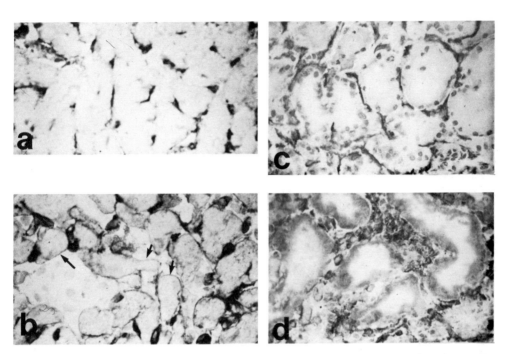

Figure 1.   Immunohistological studies on MHC induction. Frozen sections of (a) normal DA rat heart and (b) DA heart 5 days after grafting to a PVG rat were stained for class I MHC antigens using the indirect immunoperoxidase technique. Note the absence of class I on the myocardial membranes of the normal heart but strong class I expression on the myocardial membranes (arrowed) in the rejecting heart. Frozen sections from a human kidney transplant were stained for class II MHC antigens (c) before grafting and (d) during a rejection episode. Note that the renal tubular epithelial cells were class II-negative at the time of grafting but became class II-positive during rejection. (All original magnifications × 400 reduced to 60%).

There is little doubt that the MHC induction seen in rejecting grafts is a consequence of lymphokine release by the invading host leucocytes. Gamma interferon (IFNγ) is probably the major lymphokine involved in class II and probably also in class I induction (Wong et al, 1984), but it is now clear that other lymphokines are likewise involved. The α and β interferons can induce class I but not class II antigens (Vignaux and Gresser, 1977). Tumour necrosis factor α can augment both class I and class II antigen induction produced by IFNγ (Pfizenmaier, 1987; Weetman and Rees, 1988) and interleukin 4 induces class I and class II antigens on macrophages (Stuart et al, 1988).

Lymphokine release within the rejecting graft could conceivably increase systemic levels of lymphokines to a level where MHC induction might occur in recipient tissues. This was investigated by removing recipient heart and kidney at the height of rejection of heart and kidney grafts in the rat, for immunohistological studies. No MHC induction could be seen in the recipient organs (Milton et al, 1986a). However, at the International Congress in Sydney, it was reported that, in the dog, MHC induction does occur in the recipient's own kidneys during kidney allograft rejection (Miller et al, 1989). There does therefore appear to be an interesting species difference.

CAUSE OR EFFECT?

Is MHC induction an incidental byproduct of lymphokine release from infiltrating host leucocytes within the transplanted organ or does it play a vital role in the rejection process? There is at the moment no definitive answer to this question. However, the circumstantial evidence implicating induction as an important process is strong.

It is important to note that the class I and class II antigens evoke different types of rejection responses. The cytotoxic T cell response of the host is effected primarily by CD8-positive T cells directed against class I antigens. Although CD4-positive cytotoxic T cells directed at class II antigens occur, the class II antigens act primarily by stimulating CD4-positive T cells to delayed-type hypersensitivity (DTH) responses. Whereas the cytotoxic T cell response involves direct cell-to-cell contact between the effector and target cells, the DTH response involves the release of damaging lymphokines into the connective tissues. These lymphokines are either directly toxic, or cause oedema and the recruitment and activation of macrophages and other leucocytes. (For a detailed analysis of the rejection process, see Chapter 2.)

Class I MHC Antigens

One would guess, *a priori*, that the myocardial cells illustrated in Figure 1a are not susceptible to cytotoxic T cells: there is simply no target antigen on the myocardial cell membrane with which the cytotoxic cell can interact. However, there can be little doubt that the myocardial cells in the rejecting heart illustrated in Figure 1b are susceptible to class I specific cytotoxic T cells. Cells which are weakly class I-positive, such as renal tubular cells, might well be poor targets for cytotoxic T cells. Recently, Niederwieser and coworkers (1988) have demonstrated that keratinocytes (which normally express low levels of class I antigens) are not susceptible to cytotoxic T cells unless MHC antigens have been induced by IFNγ.

Given the low level of class I expression on the parenchymal cells of the commonly transplanted organs, it seems likely that organ grafts are initially relatively invulnerable to the host's cytotoxic effector responses. The induction of class I MHC antigens, however, renders the graft highly susceptible to these important effectors.

It was, however, mentioned above that the vascular endothelial cells of all the commonly transplanted organs are strongly class I-positive at the time of grafting. It is likely that these cells are susceptible to cytotoxic T cells from the beginning and might therefore represent the grafted organ's Achilles' heel with respect to cytotoxic T cells. The importance of the vascular endothelial cell as a target for the cytotoxic T cell response remains, nevertheless, uncertain. Moreover, it is possible that, even in the presence of susceptible vascular endothelial cells, shielding of the parenchymal cells from the cytotoxic T cell response (by prevention of class I MHC induction – see below) would reduce the overall 'strength' of the rejection response and make it more easy to control.

Class II MHC Antigens

At the time of grafting there is very little class II antigen in most organs. In the rat, the only class II-positive structures in heart, pancreas and liver are isolated leucocytes scattered in the connective tissues. These are the interstitial dendritic cells (Hart and Fabre, 1981b) and almost certainly represent the immunogenic passenger leucocytes. In man (but not in the rat) the vascular endothelial cells, and the Kupffer cells of the liver, are likewise class II-positive. Despite this sparse distribution of class II antigens, experiments with congenic rat strains have demonstrated that class II incompatibilities alone evoke very strong rejection responses, usually stronger than isolated class I incompatibilities (Klempnauer et al, 1985; Tsuchimoto et al, 1985).

How the anti-class II rejection response is generated has not been precisely defined. However, it is possible that foci of activated cells develop, perhaps around the interstitial dendritic cells, and that lymphokine release within these foci causes the expression of class II antigens on the local parenchymal cells. CD4-positive cells can then respond to these class II positive parenchymal cells by further lymphokine release, thereby causing further class II induction, and so on, in a self-regenerating ('vicious') circle.

It should be borne in mind that there is more to T cell stimulation than the simple expression of class II antigens. Thus, whereas dendritic cells can stimulate resting T cells to proliferate, class II-positive fibroblasts cannot do so although they can stimulate primed T cells (Geppert and Lipsky, 1985). This implies that T cells, primed by the interstitial dendritic cells either within the graft or in the draining lymphoid tissues, will be responsive to the class II-positive parenchymal cells. However, the essential difference between the dendritic cell and the class II-positive fibroblast in T cell stimulators might be connected with the capacity of dendritic cells to secrete lymphokines. If this is so, it should be remembered that the interstitial tissues of a rejecting graft are bathed in high concentrations of a variety of lymphokines. In this milieu, the class II-positive parenchymal cells could conceivably stimulate even non-primed T cells.

It has not been proven that the above sequence of events occurs. However, the strength of the anti-class II rejection response, combined with the sparsity of class II expression at the time of grafting, would suggest that class II induction is likely to make a major contribution to the stimulation of the host CD4 T cells and therefore to the overall development of the rejection response. If so, the resistance to class II induction seen in hepatocytes might contribute to the relative immunological privilege of liver grafts in transplantation (Settaf et al, 1988).

The Role of γ-Interferon

We have been investigating the role of IFNγ in graft rejection and MHC induction in rats by treating recipients with IFNγ or antibodies to it. Contrary to our expectations, antibodies to IFNγ *shortened* graft survival in otherwise untreated recipients. Gamma interferon itself, although it had no effect on otherwise untreated recipients, unexpectedly potentiated the prolongation of graft survival induced by pre-transplant blood transfusion (Paineau et al, 1989). Similarly, antibodies to IFNγ have been reported to exacerbate, and IFNγ itself to suppress, experimental allergic encephalomyelitis in mice (Billiau et al, 1988). This suggests that IFNγ might have suppressor effects on immune responses, in addition to its well known MHC-inducing capacity – a somewhat paradoxical situation. However, the effects of IFNγ appear to be multiple and complex. Thus, although it usually augments in vitro effector responses by T cells (Spiegel, 1988) and macrophages (Okutoni and Yamazaki, 1988) and augments lymphocyte recruitment in vivo (Issekutz et al, 1988) it appears also to augment suppressor activity (Holda et al, 1988) and to suppress IL-1 secretion (Ghezi and Dinarello, 1988). Although it suppresses experimental allergic encephalomyelitis (EAE) in mice and can prolong graft survival in certain situations (see preceding paragraph), it has been reported to exacerbate multiple sclerosis (Panitch et al, 1987) and also to shorten graft survival (see Chapter 2). The overall effects of IFNγ appear to depend on the precise details of individual situations in a manner that is as yet unpredictable.

These data might be relevant to some recent interesting observations in rats treated with donor-strain blood prior to kidney transplantation (Armstrong et al, 1987; Wood et al, 1988). The transfusion resulted in long-term survival of the graft but, contrary to expectations, the infiltration of host leucocytes and the induction of class I and class II antigens was actually more marked than in untreated controls rejecting their grafts. Although unexpected, this result does not mean that MHC induction is not important for rejection. The situation after sensitization by blood transfusion is likely to be complex, with the operation of both positive and negative factors. For example, sensitized cells secrete more IFNγ (Sanders et al, 1988) and this might favour suppressor responses in this situation as well as causing more marked MHC induction.

CLINICAL IMPLICATIONS

Therapeutics

If the induction of donor MHC antigens within the graft makes an important contribution to the development of the rejection response, its prevention would be a novel and interesting approach to immunosuppression. A rational evaluation of this approach requires detailed knowledge of the molecular mechanisms involved in normal MHC expression and during MHC induction, a field in which we remain profoundly ignorant.

As IFNγ is likely to be the major MHC-inducing lymphokine, we have used a monoclonal antibody to it, which gave the unexpected result of shortening graft survival times, with no diminution in MHC induction (Paineau et al, 1989; see also above). Prostaglandins of the E series have been reported to suppress lymphokine-mediated MHC induction (Snyder et al, 1982), and we are currently evaluating these compounds. However, even if they were to prove useful in this respect, it would be difficult to pinpoint the precise mechanism of action, for they have many other suppressor effects on the immune system. Additionally, they are vasodilators and interfere with platelet aggregation.

Diagnostics

It is in this area that the phenomenon of MHC induction (irrespective of its importance to the rejection process) might prove of immediate value. There are two clinical situations where the diagnosis of rejection can be particularly difficult: in pancreatic transplantation and in kidney graft recipients treated with cyclosporin A.

In kidney transplant patients it is important, but sometimes difficult, to distinguish cyclosporin toxicity from rejection as potential causes of graft dysfunction. In preliminary experiments in the rat, we have established that the cellular infiltrate often seen in grafts from cyclosporin A-treated recipients did not cause MHC induction (Milton et al, 1986b). We went on to perform a clinical trial which evaluated MHC induction using immunohistological techniques on frozen sections of biopsies taken during periods of graft dysfunction. In nine out of ten biopsies taken during periods of dysfunction attributed retrospectively (on clinical and laboratory criteria) to rejection, there was easily-recognized class II induction in the tubular epithelial cells. Conversely, eight of nine biopsies taken during periods of drug toxicity failed to show class II induction (Barrett et al, 1987). It must be borne in mind that class II induction is not pathognomonic of rejection. Any infiltrate of activated leucocytes (e.g. in response to viral infections) will cause MHC induction. Moreover, following an episode of rejection, class II levels can remain elevated for several weeks, depending on how effectively the rejection crisis is treated. Nevertheless, given that immunohistological results can be available within 2 hours of biopsy, the evaluation of MHC induction might well be of value in distinguishing cyclosporin nephrotoxicity from kidney graft rejection. The use of fine needle aspirates instead of biopsies would simplify matters and could be a better approach.

In pancreatic transplantation, the diagnosis of rejection sufficiently early to allow treatment before the graft is destroyed can be difficult. In this context, the fact that the epithelial cells of the pancreatic ducts show class II induction very readily during rejection might be of value. It is now common practice to drain the exocrine pancreas to the bladder and monitor the secretions for the diagnosis of rejection; epithelial cells from the pancreatic ducts could be recovered and examined for class II expression.

REFERENCES

Ahmed-Ansari A, Tadros TS, Knopf WD et al (1988) Major histocompatibility complex class I and class II expression by myocytes in cardiac biopsies post-transplantation. *Transplantation* **45**: 972–978.

Armstrong HE, Bolton EM, McMillan I, Spencer SC & Bradley JA (1987) Prolonged survival of actively enhanced rat renal allografts despite accelerated cellular infiltration and rapid induction of both class I and class II MHC antigens. *Journal of Experimental Medicine* **165**: 891–907.

Barret M, Milton AD, Barrett J et al (1987). Needle biopsy evaluation of class II MHC expression for the differential diagnosis of cyclosporin nephrotoxicity from kidney graft rejection. *Transplantation* **44**: 223–227.

Benson EM, Colvin RB & Russell PS (1985) Induction of Ia antigens in murine renal transplants. *Journal of Immunology* **134**: 7–9.

Billiau A, Heremans H, Vandekerckhove F et al (1988) Enhancement of experimental allergic encephalomyelitis by antibodies against IFN gamma. *Journal of Immunology* **140**: 1506–1510.

Brent L, Bain AG, Butler R et al (1981) The antigenicity of pure liver parenchyma cells. *Transplantation Proceedings* **13**: 860–862.

Chodakewitz JA, Kupper TS & Coleman DL (1988) Keratinocyte-derived granulocyte/macrophage colony-stimulating factor induces DNA synthesis by peritoneal macrophages. *Journal of Immunology* **140**: 832–836.

Coleman DL, Kupper TS, Flood PM, Fultz CC & Horowitz MC (1987) Characterisation of a keratinocyte-derived T cell growth factor distinct from interleukin 2 and B cell stimulatory factor 1. *Journal of Immunology* **138**: 3314–3318.

Daar AS, Fuggle SV, Fabre JW, Ting A & Morris PJ (1984a) The detailed distribution of HLA-ABC antigens in normal human organs. *Transplantation* **38**: 287–292.

Daar AS, Fuggle SV, Fabre JW, Ting A & Morris PJ (1984b) The detailed distribution of MHC class II antigens in normal human organs. *Transplantation* **38**: 293–298.

Demetris AJ, Lasky S, Thiel DHV, Starzl TE & Whiteside T (1985) Induction of DR/IA antigens in human liver allografts. *Transplantation* **40**: 504–509.

Fabre JW (1988) 'Immune' functions of parenchymal cells might contribute to their susceptibility to rejection. *Transplantation International* **1**: 165–167.

Fuggle SV, McWhinnie DL, Chapman JR, Taylor HM & Morris PJ (1986) Sequential analysis of HLA-Class II antigen expression in human renal allografts. *Transplantation* **42**: 144–150.

Geppert TD & Lipsky PE (1985) Antigen presentation by interferon gamma treated endothelial cells and fibroblasts: differential ability to function as antigen-presenting cells despite comparable Ia expression. *Journal of Immunology* **135**: 3750–3762.

Ghezzi P & Dinarello CA (1988) IL-1 induces IL-1. III Specific inhibition of IL-1 production by interferon gamma. *Journal of Immunology* **140**: 4238–4244.

Hall BM, Duggin CG, Philips J et al (1984) Increased expression of HLA-DR antigens on renal tubular cells in renal transplants: relevance to the rejection response. *Lancet* **ii**: 247–251.

Hart DNJ & Fabre JW (1981a) Endogenously produced Ia antigens within cells of convoluted tubules of rat kidney. *Journal of Immunology* **126**: 2109–2113.

Hart DNJ & Fabre JW (1981b) Demonstration and characterisation of Ia positive dendritic cells in the interstitial connective tissues of rat heart and other tissues, but not brain. *Journal of Experimental Medicine* **154**: 347–361.

Hart DNJ, Newton MR, Reece-Smith H, Fabre JW & Morris PJ (1983) Major histocompatibility complex antigens in the rat pancreas, isolated pancreatic islets, thyroid and adrenal. Localisation with monoclonal antibodies and demonstration of interstitial dendritic cells. *Transplantation* **36**: 431–435.

Holda JH, Maier T & Claman HN (1988) Evidence that interferon gamma is responsible for natural suppressor activity in GVHD spleen and normal bone marrow. *Transplantation* **45**: 772–777.

Issekutz TB, Staltz JM & van der Meide P (1988) The recruitment of lymphocytes into the skin by T cell lymphokines: role of interferon gamma. *Clinical and Experimental Immunology* **73**: 70–75.

Klempnauer J, Steiniger B, Wonigeit K & Gunther E (1985) Genetics of heart allograft rejection in the rat. *Transplantation Proceedings* **17**: 1897–1899.

Kupper TS, Ballard DW, Chua AO et al (1986) Human keratinocytes contain mRNA indistinguishable from monocyte interleukin 1α and β mRNA. *Journal of Experimental Medicine* **164**: 2095–2100.

Miller SM, Gupta R, Lee SH & Belitsky P (1989) Renal allograft rejection induces MHC class II upregulation in autologous kidney and liver of the recipient. *Transplantation Proceedings* **21**: 328.

Milton AD & Fabre JW (1985) Massive induction of donor type class I and class II MHC antigens in rejecting cardiac allografts in the rat. *Journal of Experimental Medicine* **161**: 98–112.

Milton AD, Spencer SC & Fabre JW (1986a) Detailed analysis and demonstration of differences in the kinetics of induction of class I and class II MHC antigens in rejecting cardiac and kidney allografts in the rat. *Transplantation* **41**: 499–508.

Milton AD, Spencer SC & Fabre JW (1986b) The effects of cyclosporin A on the induction of donor class I and class II MHC antigens in heart and kidney allografts in the rat. *Transplantation* **42**: 337–347.

Niederwieser D, Aubock J, Troppmair J et al (1988) IFN-mediated induction of MHC antigen expression on human keratinocytes and its influence on in vitro alloimmune responses. *Journal of Immunology* **140**: 2556–2564.

Okutoni T & Yamazaki M (1988) Augmentation of release of cytotoxin from murine bone marrow macrophages by gamma interferon. *Cancer Research* **48**: 1808–1811.

Paineau J, Priestley C, Fabre JW et al (1989) Effects of gamma interferon and interleukin 2 and of gamma interferon antibodies on the rat immune response against allografts. *Transplantation Proceedings* **21**: 99–1001.

Panitch H, Hirsch RL, Haley AS & Johnson KP (1987) Enocerbations of multiple sclerosis in patients treated with gamma interferon. *Lancet* **i**: 893–895.

Pfizenmaier K, Scheurich P, Schluter C & Kronke M (1987) Tumor necrosis factor enhances HLA-A,B,C and HLA-DR gene expression in human tumor cells. *Journal of Immunology* **138**: 975–980.

Rose ML, Coles MI, Griffin RJ, Pomereance A & Yacoub M (1986) Expression of class I and class II major histocompatibility antigens in normal and transplanted human heart. *Transplantation* **41**: 776–782.

Sanders ME, Makgoba MW, Sharrow SO et al (1988) Human memory T lymphocytes express increased levels of three cell adhesion molecules (LFA-3, CD2, and LFA-1) and three other molecules (UCHL1, CDw29, and Pgp-1) and have enhanced interferon gamma production. *Journal of Immunology* **140**: 1401–1407.

Settaf A, Milton AD, Spencer SC, Houssin D & Fabre JW (1988) Donor class I and class II MHC antigen expression following liver allografting in rejecting and non-rejecting rat strain combinations. *Transplantation* **46**: 32–40.

Snyder DS, Beller DI & Unanue ER (1982) Prostaglandins modulate macrophage Ia expression. *Nature* **299**: 163–165.

So SKS, Platt JL, Ascher NL & Snover DC (1987) Increased expression of class I major histocompatibility complex antigens on hepatocytes in rejecting human liver allografts. *Transplantation* **43**: 79–85.

Spiegel JP (1988) Effects of interferon gamma on the activation of human T lymphocytes. *Cellular Immunology* **111**: 461–472.

Steinhoff G, Wonigeit K, Ringe B et al (1987) Modified patterns of major histocompatibility complex antigen expression in human liver allografts during rejection. *Transplantation Proceedings* **19**: 2466–2469.

Steiniger B, Klempnauer J & Wonigeit K (1985a) Expression of class I and class II major histocompatibility complex antigens during heart allograft rejection in the rat. *Transplantation Proceedings* **17**: 1907–1910.

Steiniger B, Klempnauer J & Wonigeit K (1985b) Effect of the rejection process on class I and class II major histocompatibility complex antigen expression in the rat pancreas. *Transplantation Proceedings* **17**: 407–411.

Stuart PM, Zlotnik A & Woodward JG (1988) Induction of class I and class II MHC antigen expression on murine bone marrow-derived macrophages by IL-4 (B cell stimulatory factor 1). *Journal of Immunology* **140**: 1542–1547.

Tacacs L, Szende B, Monostori E et al (1983) Expression of HLA-DR antigens on bile duct cells of rejected liver transplants. *Lancet* **ii**: 1500.

Tsuchimoto S, Mizuno K, Matsuno Y et al (1985) The effect of RT1 subregion differences on liver allograft survival in the rat. *Transplantation Proceedings* **17**: 1900–1901.

Vignaux F & Gresser I (1977) Differential effects on the expression of H-2K, H-2D and Ia antigens on mouse lymphocytes. *Journal of Immunology* **118**: 721–723.

Weetman AP & Rees AJ (1988) Synergistic effects of recombinant tumour necrosis factor and interferon-gamma on rat thyroid cell growth Ia antigen expression. *Immunology* **63**: 285–289.

Wong GH, Clark-Lewis WI, Harris AW & Schrader JW (1984) Effect of cloned interferon gamma on expression of H-2 and Ia antigens on cell lines of haemopoietic, lymphoid, epithelial, fibroblastic and neuronal origin. *European Journal of Immunology* **14**: 52–56.

Wood KJ, Hopley A, Dallman MJ & Morris PJ (1988) Lack of correlation between the induction of donor class I and class II major histocompatibility complex antigens and graft rejection. *Transplantation* **45**: 759–767.

8c Current Controversies and New Horizons

Gene Therapy

D. J. WEATHERALL

The development of methods for cloning and sequencing genes from patients with single gene disorders has led to the characterization of the molecular pathology of a number of these conditions (Caskey, 1987; Davies and Robson, 1987). It turns out that most of them result from simple point mutations, deletions or rearrangements of structural genes: so-called distant regulatory mutations seem to be quite unusual. These observations have raised the possibility of treating at least some of these conditions by replacing the defective gene.

One of the major difficulties in developing gene therapy is our present lack of understanding about how genes are regulated. It is now apparent that most mammalian genes have upstream promotor sequences that are involved in regulating their rates of transcription, and elements called enhancer sequences that are probably involved in the specificity of transcription in particular tissues. The actions of many genes are modified by external regulatory signals such as growth factors or hormones. This involves a complex series of interactions in which these molecules bind to and activate specific receptors that generate second messengers, including cyclic adenosine monophosphate. The latter triggers off a chain of intracellular reactions that involve the phosphorylation of effector enzymes by protein kinase. These changes may, in turn, activate a battery of genes that work as an orchestrated whole to promote normal cellular function. There is increasing evidence that co-ordination of this type is mediated through the activity of interactions of regulatory transcription factors which work in *trans*, that is on both pairs of homologous structural genes. It is against this complex regulatory background that human gene therapy will have to be developed.

Over the last few years some progress has been made in gene transfer although we are still very far from even contemplating its widespread use for correcting genetic disease. Here I shall review briefly the current state of this complex field and attempt to define some of the hurdles that will have to be overcome before gene therapy becomes a part of clinical practice.

ORGAN TRANSPLANTATION: CURRENT CLINICAL AND IMMUNOLOGICAL CONCEPTS   ISBN 0-7020-1393-5

PREREQUISITES FOR HUMAN GENE THERAPY

Clinicians will want to ensure that several prerequisites are fulfilled before patients are subjected to somatic gene therapy, that is the transfer of genes into cells other than those of the germ line in order to cure an inherited disease (Table 1).

Table 1.   Requirements for gene therapy.

Full understanding of genotype/phenotype
Gene and regulatory regions isolated
Target cell defined and accessible
Efficient and safe transfer vector
Proliferative advantage and long survival
of treated cell population

First, to be able to counsel a prospective patient or their family it must be possible to give an accurate account of the clinical course of the illness and its response to more conventional therapy: genetic diseases vary enormously in their severity and even when the underlying molecular lesions are known the reasons for their clinical heterogeneity still remain largely unexplained. Second, we must be able to isolate the appropriate gene and define, at least in outline, its major regulatory regions. Third, we have to identify and harvest the appropriate target cells and develop efficient and safe vectors with which to introduce the new gene. Finally, there must be clear evidence from animal experiments that the inserted gene will function adequately, that the recipient cell population will have a reasonably long lifespan, and that the gene that we have inserted will produce no deleterious effects in its new environment. Recently published accounts emphasize just how far we are from meeting these requirements (Williams and Orkin, 1986; Nichols, 1988; Friedmann, 1989).

SOMATIC VERSUS GERM CELL GENE TRANSFER

There are two main approaches to gene transfer therapy. First, genes may be inserted into somatic cells, that is any body cell other than a germ cell. This approach raises no new ethical issues and is, essentially, no different from organ transplantation therapy in that any changes in the genotype of a cell population will die with the individual. Germ line therapy, on the other hand, involves the introduction of genes into fertilized eggs. In this case the genes will become distributed in both somatic cells and germ cells and be passed on to future generations. This approach raises all sorts of new ethical issues and is not being contemplated for human gene therapy.

METHODS FOR GENE TRANSFER

The transfer of genes into foreign cells may be achieved either directly or using a form of delivery system.

Direct Insertion

There are a variety of ways in which DNA can be inserted into another cell (Anderson, 1984). One of the simplest methods is based on the principle of the uptake of calcium microprecipitates of DNA which can be used to insert cloned genes. Although selective it is very inefficient and the rate of stable transfection is probably only about one cell in 10^5. A number of variations on this theme have been attempted including transfection of cells in suspension or following their treatment with dimethylsulphoxide (DMSO), glycerol, chloroquine, or sodium butyrate. Unfortunately the efficiency of transfection by these techniques varies widely between different cell lines and is often unacceptably low. Furthermore, even when a better level of efficiency is achieved it is often confined to a specific cell line and hence is not generally applicable. By and large these techniques seem unlikely to be suitable for use in human gene therapy.

Another direct approach is to microinject DNA directly into the nucleus of cells. This requires considerable expertise, and because it involves treating one cell at a time is unlikely to have any practical application in gene therapy. Automated methods for injection may improve matters, however.

A more recent method for direct insertion of genes involves the exposure of cells to a pulsed electric field, a technique called electroporation. It is believed that cells treated in this way open up pores in their plasma membranes. Although when it was first developed this approach likewise gave a low efficiency of transfection, there have been some recent improvements. For example, a modification has been described that has resulted in more than 1% of the viable cells showing stable expression of a selectable marker gene (Chu et al, 1987). To date there is no information about the long-term viability of cells that have been treated in this way or about the possibility of genetic damage caused by exposure to a strong electrical field.

Finally, Tao et al (1987) have described a relatively efficient method of DNA transfer using laser micropuncture of cell membranes.

RNA Viruses (Retroviruses)

Retroviruses are adapted by evolution for the efficient delivery of their genome into cells, with integration into the host genome and a high level of expression of their internal sequences. At present the use of retroviral vectors seems to be the most promising approach to gene therapy (Anderson, 1984; Anderson et al, 1986; Miller et al, 1986; Williams and Orkin, 1986; Yee et al, 1986; Nichols, 1988).

Retroviruses have a complicated structure and lifestyle (Varmus, 1988). The virion particle consists of a dimer of viral RNA within a protein coat surrounded by a lipid bilayer that contains viral-specific glycoproteins that attach themselves to cells during infection. The virion contains the virus-coded enzyme, reverse transcriptase. After entering cells the coat is shed and the RNA genome is copied into DNA by reverse transcriptase. A double-stranded DNA circle is formed and specific retroviral sequences direct the integration of viral DNA into the host genome. After integration viral sequences transcribe full-length and spliced RNAs. The spliced RNAs are translated to generate glycoproteins while the full length RNA is either translated into internal structural proteins of the virion core and reverse transcriptase or packaged into virion particles as new genomic RNA. The subsequent assembly and budding of virion particles from infected cells is non-lytic.

The main features of the genome of a typical retrovirus are shown in Figure 1. A variety of recombinant retrovirus vectors have been constructed. The viral genome needed for the infection, integration and transcriptional control of the genome, which is all contained in the long terminal repeat sequences (LTRs), is preserved together with the packaging sequence (*Psi*), but viral sequences whose function can be supplied in *trans* are taken out. Thus the *gag* sequences which encode internal structural proteins of the virion core, *pol* genes which encode reverse transciptase, and *env* genes which encode the envelope glycoproteins are all deleted and are replaced by a dominant selectable marker and a restriction enzyme site into which the sequence that is to be transferred (that is the gene we wish to insert) can be cloned (Figure 1).

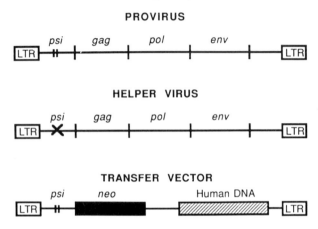

Figure 1. Retroviral constructs for gene transfer. The main genes of the provirus are described in the text. The helper virus has had its packaging sequence (*psi*) removed. The transfer vector has had the *gag*, *pol*, and *env* genes removed and replaced by a selectable marker (*neo*) and a human DNA sequence carrying a gene for transfer.

The recombinant and now defective retroviral genome in the form of plasmid DNA is then introduced by transfection into murine fibroblasts to generate cell lines that produce the recombinant retrovirus. Simultaneous infection with wild-type helper viruses that have had their packaging sequences removed (Figure 1) can provide the required packaging proteins although it is now possible to achieve the same result by the use of specialized packaging cell lines that contain helper virus sequences within their genomes. In essence, the engineered vector retrovirus uses its packaging sequences to package proteins produced by the helper virus which, because it lacks these sequences, remains trapped in the cells (see Figure 1). Vector virus particles are shed into the surrounding medium, which can then be harvested and used to infect the recipient cells, or the latter can be incubated directly with the cells that are budding off the viral particles.

Experiments using recombinant retroviruses of this type have demonstrated that gene transfer can be achieved. For example, murine bone marrow has been cultivated with packaging cell lines that produce recombinant retrovirus and injected into lethally irradiated recipient mice (Williams et al, 1986; Dzierzak et al, 1988). Because injected stem cells colonize the spleen it is possible to follow the fate of the transfected genes by analysis of the DNA of colonies formed in the spleen of the mice or in the blood of the animal. Studies of this kind have shown that genes have been transferred into pluripotential haemopoietic stem cells and that the transfected cells appear to be long-lived, at least up to 4 months after transplantation. Furthermore, they are totipotential, i.e. they give rise to both lymphoid and myeloid progeny.

A variety of genes have been transferred into intact mice using retroviral vectors, including G418 (a neomycin resistance gene), hypoxanthine phosphoribosyl transferase (HPRT), dihydrofolate reductase (DHFR) and human adenosine deaminase (ADA) (see Nichols, 1988). In addition to murine stem cells, retrovirus-mediated transfer and expression of drug resistance genes has also been achieved using human haemopoietic progenitors in culture (Miller et al, 1986); and the human ADA gene has been transferred into, and expressed in, diploid skin fibroblasts obtained from an ADA-deficient human (Willis et al, 1984).

While these results are encouraging, the level of expression of many of these transferred genes has been extremely variable. Retrovirus mediated transfer of genes into cultured haemopoietic cells has often resulted in their expression at levels similar to or even higher than that of the endogenous genes. For example, a homozygous Lesch–Nyhan lymphoblast line, deficient in HPRT, was used to determine whether the defect could be corrected by a retroviral vector containing a functional HPRT gene. This turned out to be the case and the metabolic derangements associated with HPRT deficiency were almost completely corrected (Willis et al, 1984). On the other hand, transplantation of transfected haemopoietic cells into mice has often resulted in low or almost undetectable expression of the inserted genes although encouraging improvements have been reported recently (Dzierzak et al, 1988). Similarly, although expression of human ADA or neomycin-resistant genes has been demonstrated in monkeys after transfection of their bone marrow the expression was confined to a very small proportion of peripheral blood white cells (Anderson et al, 1986).

It is not yet clear why the expression of transferred genes is so low in these in vivo experiments. One problem is that retroviruses only infect cells in cycle, and most haemopoietic stem cells are out of cycle in the adult marrow. Furthermore, it is possible that the genes may be inactivated or rearranged during haemopoietic differentiation. In this context it has been possible to obtain expression of the genes for factor VIII and HPRT in human or mouse skin fibroblasts. It will be interesting to see whether these cells can maintain more persistent expression of transferred genes, particularly as they undergo very little differentiation after engraftment (Anson et al, 1987; St Louis and Verma, 1988). Retrovirus-mediated gene transfer has also been achieved using primary cultures of mouse or rat hepatocytes (Ledley et al, 1987; Wilson et al, 1988).

Many problems remain, in particular the efficiency of transfection and level of expression using retroviral vectors for gene transfer. A number of ingenious attempts have been made to improve the level of expression (reviewed by Anderson, 1984 and Nichols, 1988). For example, some encouraging results have been obtained by inserting the sequence for rat growth hormone together with 237 bases of genomic 5' flanking sequence into a retroviral vector. The growth hormone genes were regulated in fibroblasts by their own promotor and regulatory sequences, as evidenced by stimulation by glucocorticoid and thyroid hormones. But there are still enormous problems concerning the level and stability of expression to be overcome using retroviral vector systems. Whether it will be possible to improve the situation by the incorporation of internal enhancer sequences into these vectors remains to be seen (Yee et al, 1987).

Retroviruses have their own enhancers immediately upstream from their promotors in the LTR. But the species and tissue specificity of enhancers, as mentioned earlier, may be of particular importance in determining the appropriate expression of inserted genes. In this context the recent discovery of sequences upstream from the human β-globin-like gene cluster that have strong enhancer-like properties is very encouraging (Grosveld et al, 1987).

Finally, as mentioned earlier, it should be emphasized that very little is known about the safety of retroviral delivery systems. There is no doubt that they can rearrange their own structure as well as exchange sequences with other retroviruses including helper viruses. There is still a distinct possibility that a retroviral vector might recombine with an endogenous viral sequence to produce an infectious recombinant virus. Although the properties of a virus of this type are difficult to anticipate a distant possibility remains that they might be oncogenic. Recently, self-destructing retroviruses have been engineered to try to solve this problem.

Targeted Modification of Human Genes

Targeted modification of genes by exogenous DNA has been possible in yeast for many years. However, it is only recently that preliminary studies of this approach to the alteration of the human genome have been attempted (Gregg and Smithies, 1986; Thomas and Capecchi, 1986).

In principle, this approach to the replacement of defective genes has many attractions. In particular, it is site-directed and hence should not cause the problems of random integration. The idea is that the exogenous DNA should contain a region with the same nucleotide sequence as the target gene so that homologous recombination can occur between the regions of sequence identity. In other words, the method uses nature's way of gene mixing. Depending on the arrangement of the incoming sequences relative to the target the recombination event could either introduce new sequences into the recipient chromosome by a single crossover or substitute sequences by gene conversion or double crossover events.

Several ingenious attempts at targeted gene modification have been made recently (Nandi et al, 1988). Plasmids have been linearized with restriction enzymes to produce a double strand break within the region homologous to the gene target. These have tended to be much more efficient than closed circular molecules which are also capable of generating recombination. It is presumed that the ends of the DNA molecules are more active in recombination. Although there have been some spectacular successes with this approach many problems remain. In particular the efficiency is low and there is a worrying tendency to induce new mutations afer recombination with the 'foreign' DNA. However, because of its potential specificity it is very important that work continues in this promising area.

Specific Correction of Genetic Defects with Suppressor tRNA Genes

Many single gene disorders result from so-called nonsense mutations. These are single base changes that produce premature stop codons in the middle of exons and which therefore make it impossible for the affected genes to produce full-length protein products. It is possible to correct these defects by the use of so-called suppressor transfer

RNAs, i.e. transfer RNAs that can insert amino acids into the altered codons (see Ho et al, 1986).

Recent work has suggested that functional suppressor genes of this type can be constructed by site-specific mutagenesis. Unfortunately these molecules mediate only low levels of suppression. Thus a major problem is whether it would be possible to achieve a level of suppression at which the appropriate genes could function in such a way as to produce adequate amounts of gene product. Current work in this field is directed towards constructing retrovirus vectors that contain the suppressor transfer RNA genes so that they can be inserted with high efficiency into bone marrow sells.

Transgenic Approaches

The introduction of DNA into fertilized eggs and subsequent integration into both somatic cells and germ cells has been achieved successfully in a variety of species. These experiments have been carried out with the object of developing the transgenic animal system as a model for studying gene regulation. DNA has been injected directly into fertilized eggs and genes have also been transferred using retroviral vectors.

There is no doubt that foreign DNA introduced either by microinjection or retroviral transfection integrates into chromosomal DNA and is carried in germ cells and is then transmitted to subsequent generations (Palmiter and Brinster, 1985). Some remarkable results have been obtained. For example, the introduction of metallothionein–growth hormone fusion genes into mice stimulates the production of growth hormone in tissues that normally synthesize metallothionein. Suitable induction of the metallothionein genes with metals has caused treated mice to grow to about twice their normal size. Tissue specific expression of a variety of genes has been obtained and a number of genetic diseases of mice, including thalassaemia, have been corrected (Nichols, 1988). This model is also extremely useful for studying the effects of oncogene expression and for analysing defective embryonic development by insertional mutagenesis and the expression of genes for histocompatibility antigens and related cell surface molecules (see below).

DISEASES SUITABLE FOR EARLY CONSIDERATION FOR GENE THERAPY (Table 2)

Table 2.   Candidate disorders for gene therapy.

Disorder	Enzyme or protein
SCID*	Adenine deaminase
Lesch–Nyhan	Hypoxanthine-guanine phosphoribosyl transferase
α or β Thalassaemia	α or β globin
PNP deficiency	Purine nucleoside phosphorylase
Phenylketonuria	Phenylalanine hydroxylase
Gaucher disease	Lysomal glucocerebrosidase
α_1-Antitrypsin deficiency	α_1-Antitrypsin

* Severe combined immunodeficiency

It seems likely that the best candidates for gene therapy for the immediate future are disorders like Lesch–Nyhan disease, purine nucleoside phosphorylase deficiency, or ADA deficiency. These diseases are due to deficiencies of enzymes produced by so-called housekeeping genes, genes that are 'on' in most cells and which do not require very precise regulation. All three conditions are severely disabling and it is hoped that a low level expression of inserted genes into deficient cells will correct at least some of their functional abnormalities. The limited in vitro experience with hypoxanthine-guanine phosphoribosyl transferase (HGPRT) deficiency suggests that this is the case. However, even in these disorders there are enormous difficulties to be overcome. In particular, although the defect in each of these conditions is expressed in cells of bone marrow origin, at least in the case of the Lesch–Nyhan syndrome there is deficiency of HGPRT in brain cells which could probably not be corrected by current technology. If it proves possible to obtain prolonged and relatively high levels of production of factor IX in skin fibroblasts, Christmas disease might be another condition for early consideration for gene therapy of this type (see Anson et al, 1987).

Other single gene disorders will be even more difficult to correct. For example, although a great deal is known about the molecular defects in thalassaemia and some of the structural haemoglobin disorders, it seems unlikely that it will be possible to insert normal globin genes in the immediate future. These genes have to be under extremely tight regulation; for example it would be no good inserting a β gene into the haemopoietic stem cells of a patient with β thalassaemia only to see it over-expressed in their progeny, with the production of the clinical phenotype of α thalassaemia!

One encouraging fact for the future of gene therapy is that ADA deficiency can be corrected by bone marrow transplantation, as can a number of other single gene disorders that affect haemopoietic stem cells, β thalassaemia for example (see Thomas, 1986; Nichols, 1988) (Table 3). Hence there is no reason why these conditions should not be cured by somatic gene therapy once the difficulties of transfection and expression are overcome. But until it becomes possible to transfect a sufficient number of stem cells it may still be necessary to attempt to provide the treated population with some form of selective advantage; cells must be in cycle to be infected with retroviruses and since the majority of haemopoietic stem cells are out of cycle the efficiency of transfection will remain a serious problem. However, it is conceivable that, by the use of the recently purified haemopoietic growth factors, it may be possible to encourage a greater number of stem cells into cycle.

A recent study (Madsen et al, 1988) is an example of how gene transfer is beginning to play an important role in transplantation. In an attempt to determine the mechanism whereby immunological unresponsiveness to allografts can be achieved by pre-treating recipients with cells expressing donor-specific histocompatibility antigens, murine class I or II major histocompatibility genes of the donor strain were introduced into cells of the recipient strain. This allowed murine recipients of cardiac allografts to be pre-treated with syngeneic cells sharing only an isolated class I or class II MHC locus product with the donor organ. Pre-treatment with either donor class I or class II antigens was shown significantly to prolong graft survival. Furthermore, the capacity of a particular donor MHC antigen to induce unresponsiveness appeared to be the product of its intrinsic immunogenicity and the antigen load delivered during pre-treatment. As well as explaining certain discrepancies in earlier studies of antigen-induced unresponsiveness these experiments suggest a novel approach to specific immunosuppression in clinical transplantation.

Table 3. Transplantation for genetic disease.

Bone marrow
    SCID* and related disorders
    Storage disorders
    Haemoglobinopathy

Liver
    α_1-Antitrypsin deficiency
    Haemophilia A
    Tyrosinaemia
    Wilson's disease

Kidney
    Cystinosis
    Alport syndrome

Heart
    Cardiomyopathy

---

* Severe combined immunodeficiency

THE FUTURE: ETHICAL ISSUES

In considering the clinical applications of this new technology it is very important to make a clear distinction between somatic and germline gene therapy. The replacement of a gene into somatic cells raises no fundamentally new ethical issues. In a sense it is no different from organ transplantation or, for that matter, blood transfusion. On the other hand, germline therapy, that is injecting genes into fertilized eggs so that they become incorporated into both somatic and germline genes, is quite a different matter. These genes would be handed on to the progeny and this would open up a completely new area of human genetics. Nobody is contemplating transgenic therapy in man and there is no reason why they ever should. As techniques for the identification of genetic disorders improve, it should be possible to diagnose single gene disorders in tissue obtained from fertilized ova. Using in vitro fertilization it would then be possible to sort through a number of fertilized ova and to discard those that carried a single gene defect and implant those that were normal in this respect.

It is very important to develop guidelines for early attempts at somatic gene therapy (Anderson and Fletcher, 1980). Efforts to develop a sensible code of practice for this field have been made recently in both Europe and the USA (Nichols, 1988; Recommendations of the European Research Councils, 1988). These include careful measures to ensure the safety of the procedure and strict criteria for selection of cases.

Thus although somatic gene therapy is no different in principle to organ transplantation, it remains a highly emotive topic. Many clinicians are still concerned that, in their haste to be first, workers in this field will cut corners, both scientific and ethical. However, provided the guidlines set out in Europe and the United States are adhered to, and the prerequisites set out earlier in this chapter are fulfilled, there seems no reason why gene therapy should not be developed within the next few years for at least a limited number of single gene disorders. It is important that this work goes ahead because although improved methods for prenatal diagnosis will have some impact on the frequency of single gene disorders, many cases will go unrecognized. Indeed, many genetic diseases are due to new mutations. Current treatment is largely unsatisfactory and correction by gene therapy offers the best hope for the management of these distressing conditions in the future. Meanwhile, the transplantation of bone marrow and organ allografts (see Table 3) as an alternative therapy should certainly continue.

REFERENCES

Anderson WF (1984) Prospects for human gene therapy. *Science* **226**: 401–409.

Anderson WF & Fletcher JC (1980) Gene therapy in human beings: when is it ethical to begin? *New England Journal of Medicine* **303**: 1293–1297.

Anderson WF, Kantoff P, Eglitis M et al (1986) Gene transfer and expression in nonhuman primates using retroviral vectors. *Cold Spring Harbor Symposium on Quantitative Biology* **51**: 1065–1072.

Anson DS, Hock RA, Austen D et al (1987) Towards gene therapy for hemophilia B. *Molecular Biology and Medicine* **4**: 11–20.

Caskey CT (1987) Disease diagnosis by recombinant DNA methods. *Science* **236**: 1223–1227.

Chu G, Hayakawa H & Berg P (1987) Electroporation for the efficient transfection of mammalian cells with DNA. *Nucleic Acids Research* **15**: 1311–1326.

Davies KE & Robson KJH (1987) Molecular analysis of human monogenic disease. *Bioessays* **6**: 247–253.

Dzierzak EA, Papayannopoulou T & Mulligan RC (1988) Lineage-specific expression of a human β-globin gene in murine bone marrow transplant recipients reconstituted with retrovirus-transduced stem cells. *Nature* **331**: 35–41.

Friedmann T (1989) Progress towards human gene therapy. *Science* **244**: 1275–1281.

Gregg RG & Smithies O (1986) Targeted modification of human chromosomal genes. *Cold Spring Harbor Symposium on Quantitative Biology* **51**: 1093–1100.

Grosveld F, van Assendelft GB, Greaves DK & Kollias G (1987) Position-independent, high-level expression of the human β-globin gene in transgenic mice. *Cell* **51**: 975–985.

Ho T-S, Norton GP, Palese P, Dozy AM & Ka YW (1986) Expression and function of suppressor tRNA genes in mammalian cells. *Cold Sring Harbor Symposium on Quantitative Biology* **151**: 1033–1040.

Ledley FD, Darlington GJ , Hahn T & Woo SLC (1987) Retroviral gene transfer into primary hepatocytes: Implications for genetic therapy of liver-specific functions. *Proceedings of the National Academy of Sciences, USA* **84**: 5335–5339.

Madsen JC, Superina RA, Wood KJ & Morris PJ (1988) Immunological unresponsiveness induced by recipient cells transfected with donor MHC genes. *Nature* **332**: 161–164.

Miller AD, Palmer TD & Hock RA (1986) Transfer of genes into human somatic cells using retrovirus vectors. *Cold Spring Harbor Symposium on Quantitative Biology* **51**: 1013–1020.

Nandi AK, Roginski RA, Gregg RG, Smithies O & Skoultchi AI (1988) Regulated expression of genes inserted at the human chromosomal β-globin locus by homologous recombination. *Proceedings of the National Academy of Sciences, USA* **85**: 3845–3849.

Nichols EK (1988) *Human Gene Therapy*. Cambridge, Massachusetts: Harvard University Press.

Nicholls RD, Fischel-Ghodsian N & Higgs DR (1987) Recombination at the human α-globin gene cluster: sequence features and topological constraints. *Cell* **49**: 369–378.

Palmiter RD & Brinster RL (1985) Transgenic mice. *Cell* **41**: 343–345.

Recommendation of European Medical Research Councils (1988) Gene Therapy in Man. *Lancet* **i**: 1271–1272.

St. Louis A & Verma IM (1988) An alternative approach to somatic cell gene therapy. *Proceedings of the National Academy of Sciences, USA* **85**: 3150–3154.

Tao W, Wilkinson J, Stanbridge EJ & Berns MW (1987) Direct gene transfer into human cultured cells facilitated by laser micropuncture of the cell membrane. *Proceedings of the National Academy of Sciences, USA* **84**: 4180–4184.

Thomas ED (1986) Marrow transplantation and gene transfer as therapy for hematopoietic diseases. *Cold Spring Harbor Symposium on Quantitative Biology,* **51**: 1009–1012.

Thomas KR & Capecci MR (1986) Targeting of genes to specific sites in the mammalian genome. *Cold Spring Harbor Symposium on Quantitative Biology* **51**: 1101–1114.

Varmus H (1988) Retroviruses. *Science* **240**: 1427–1435.

Williams DA & Orkin SH (1986) Somatic gene therapy. Current status and future prospects. *Journal of Clinical Investigation* **77**: 1053–1056.

Williams DA, Orkin SH & Mulligan RC (1986) Retrovirus-mediated transfer of human adenosine deaminase gene sequences into cells in culture and into murine hematopoietic cells in vivo. *Proceedings of the National Academy of Sciences, USA* **83**: 2566–2570.

Willis RC, Jolly DJ, Miller AD et al (1984) Partial phenotypic correction of human Lesch–Nyhan (hypoxanthine-guanine phosphoribosyltransferase-deficient) lymphoblasts with a transmissible retroviral vector. *Journal of Biological Chemistry* **259**: 7842–7849.

Wilson JM, Jefferson DM, Chowdhury JR et al (1988) Retrovirus-mediated transduction of adult hepatocytes. *Proceedings of the National Academy of Sciences, USA* **85**: 3014–3018.

Yee J-K, Jolly DJ, Moores JC, Respess JD & Friedman T (1986) Gene expression from a transcriptionally disabled retroviral vector. *Cold Spring Harbor Symposium on Quantitative Biology* **51**: 1021–1026.

Yee J-K, Moores JC, Jolly DJ et al (1987) Gene expression from transcriptionally disabled retroviral vectors. *Proceedings of the National Academy of Sciences, USA* **84**: 5197–5201.

8d Current Controversies and New Horizons

Is There a Clinical Future for the Modulation of Donor Organ Immunogenicity?

KEVIN J. LAFFERTY
RONALD G. GILL

The classical rules governing allograft rejection were laid down by Medawar and his colleagues (Medawar 1957, 1963). The rejection process is immunologically mediated and requires the recognition of transplantation antigen carried on cells of the grafted tissue. Because these antigens are genetically regulated, there seems little hope that the antigenic composition of a graft could be altered by treatment of the tissue prior to grafting. Facilitation of graft acceptance would therefore require immunosuppression of the host. This procedure has been outstandingly successful and with the development of new immunosuppressive agents has led to a great expansion of clinical allografting. Morbidity and mortality associated with organ grafting is primarily the result of immune suppression of the recipient. Better immunosuppressants may improve this situation. However, there is now a hope that we can reduce tissue immunogenicity prior to grafting. In some animal models successful allografting can be carried out with little or no recourse to immune suppression. Here we discuss this approach and speculate on its potential for clinical application.

TISSUE IMMUNOGENICITY

Although allograft rejection clearly represents a response to transplantation (predominantly major histocompatibility complex, MHC) antigens, this classic view of allograft immunity is not entirely straightforward. Early attempts to isolate and characterize transplantation antigens found them to be quite weak immunogens (Snell, 1957) and some early experiments even produced the unexpected result that immunization with extracts of transplantation antigen led to the enhancement of allogeneic tumour growth (Flexner and Jobling, 1907). More recent work from Batchelor's group has shown that

ORGAN TRANSPLANTATION: CURRENT CLINICAL AND
IMMUNOLOGICAL CONCEPTS   ISBN 0-7020-1393-5

purified forms of class I or class II MHC antigens are relatively weak immunogens (Batchelor et al, 1978). This leads us to the 'transplantation paradox', composed of three propositions:

1. Graft rejection is an immune process characterized by the recognition of and a response to transplantation antigens.
2. The allograft response is among the most violent of immune reactions.
3. Isolated transplantation antigens, whether they be class I or class II MHC antigens, are weak immunogens.

The solution to this paradox comes from understanding antigen presentation and its role in immune induction. This solution forms the foundation of a theory of tissue immunogenicity that leads us back to an early concept, namely, that graft immunogenicity can be reduced by appropriate treatment of the tissue prior to grafting (Snell, 1957).

THE TWO-SIGNAL HYPOTHESIS IN THE IMMUNE SYSTEM

Resolution of the transplantation paradox has come from understanding signal transmission in the immune system. To early theorists such as Burnet, Talmage and Medawar, antigen recognition and immune induction were seen as part of the same process. One signal, provided by antigen, was seen as sufficient to drive the differentiation process through engagement of the lymphocyte receptor (Medawar, 1963). Later, more complex notions of immune induction had to be considered. With the recognition that lymphocytes were composed of two major classes, T and B cells, and that B cell activity was T cell dependent, Bretscher and Cohn developed the idea that two signals were required for B cell induction (Bretscher and Cohn, 1970). Signal one was provided, as in the classical sense, by antigen engagement with the B cell receptor. However, induction only occurred when signal one was delivered in conjunction with a second signal that Bretscher and Cohn postulated was provided by the helper T cell. This model provided a simple explanation for self-tolerance, that is, that signal one alone was tolerogenic.

Perplexed by the species specificity of alloreactivity, Lafferty and Cunningham later used this two-signal concept to explain species-specific T cell activation (Lafferty and Cunningham, 1975). These investigators and others found that a strong graft-versus-host reaction (GVHR) occurred when adult chicken leukocytes were placed on the chorioallantoic membrane (CAM) of immunologically-incompetent allogeneic chicken embryos (Simonsen, 1962; Lafferty et al, 1969). The surprising finding was that the intensity of this reaction actually *decreased* as the phylogenetic separation between donor and recipient increased, despite the fact that the donor lymphocytes could survive and function on the xenogeneic CAM (Lafferty et al, 1969). The mixed leukocyte reaction (MLR), the in vitro analogue of the allograft reaction, was likewise shown to express a degree of species specificity (Woolnough et al, 1979). Further, the capacity to stimulate in the MLR was shown to be a function of metabolically active stimulator cells (Lafferty et al, 1980). Taken together, these findings challenged the traditional view of T cell activation by demonstrating that antigen recognition alone could not account for T cell activation by alloantigen, either in vitro or in vivo.

The solution to these problems was provided by the proposition that two signals are required for T cell activation (Lafferty and Cunningham, 1975), a model analogous to Bretscher and Cohn's idea for B cell activation. Signal one was provided by engagement of the T cell receptor complex and signal two was provided by an inductive molecule (co-stimulator) produced by the metabolically active 'stimulator' cell (antigen presenting cell, Figure 1). Release of the co-stimulator (CoS) is regulated by a control structure (c) on the surface of the stimulator cell; that is, CoS release is triggered by an interaction with c (Figure 1). The species specificity of alloreactivity would result from the species specificity of the second signal, or CoS (Lafferty and Cunningham, 1975). This proposition has since been shown to be consistent with experimental observation (Woolnough et al, 1979).

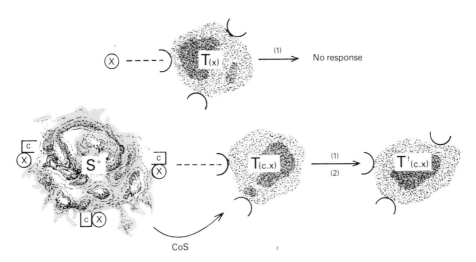

Figure 1. Stimulator cell model. Two signals are required for T cell activation. Binding of the antigen (x) alone provides only the first signal and so does not cause T cell activation (activated T cell = T'). However, T cell activation occurs when two signals are provided for the responsive T cell. Antigen binding by the T cell provides the first signal (1), and a stimulator cell (S$^+$) provides an inductive molecule, a co-stimulator (CoS), that serves as the second signal (2). A control structure (solid squares) on the surface of the S$^+$ cell (which may well be an MHC molecule) regulates the release of the CoS. Therefore, CoS is released when the responsive T cell interacts with the control structure on the S$^+$ cell.

Experimental support for the two-signal model for T cell activation comes from a study of the immunogenicity of cloned tumour cell lines for allogeneic T cells in vitro (Table 1). Talmage et al demonstrated the existence of stimulating (S$^+$) and non-stimulating (S$^-$) tumour lines expressing the same MHC antigens (Talmage et al, 1977). The gamma-irradiated P815 tumour presents H-2^d class I MHC antigen and expresses the S$^+$ phenotype by stimulating a strong cytotoxic lymphocyte (CTL) response in vitro. The epithelial cell, carcinoma D2, presents the same antigens but expresses the S$^-$ phenotype and does not elicit a CTL response. Further, the S$^+$ phenotype of the P815 tumour is inhibited by ultraviolet (UV) irradiation of the cell. This treatment inhibits the metabolic activity of the P815 cell; the uptake of both amino acids and RNA precursors is totally blocked following UV irradiation. The clear demonstration that the non-stimulatory UV-irradiated P815 and gamma-irradiated carcinoma D2 cell lines express recognizable antigen comes from the finding that specific CTL activity is restored when a source of CoS activity is added to the cultures in the form of supernatants from concanavalin A-activated spleen cells. CoS activity alone does not induce a significant CTL response (Talmage et al, 1977). These results have been confirmed using purified CD8 T cells as the responding population (Sprent and Schaefer, 1986), and emphasize the distinction between the antigenicity and the immunogenicity of MHC antigens. Similar studies using congenic mouse strains have shown the same requirement for activation of the allogeneic response to class II MHC antigen (Lafferty et al, 1980). The significant contribution of this two-signal hypothesis to transplantation biology is the notion that alloantigen alone is *not* the barrier to allografting (Lafferty et al, 1983).

Table 1.   Activation of T cells by S^+ versus S^- cells.

	Cytotoxic activity[†] ($\log_{10}$ CU/culture)	
Stimulator cell*	No co-stimulator added	Co-stimulator[‡] added
Irradiated P815 (S^+)	5.4	6.0
UV-P815 (S^-)	< 2.5	6.1
Irradiated CaD2 (S^-)	< 3.7	6.0
None	< 3.7	< 3.7

* One ml cultures contained 10^6 C57B1/6 responding lymph node cells and, where indicated, 2×10^5 P815 or 2×10^4 carcinoma D2 (CaD2) tumour cells (Talmage et al, 1977).
[†] Cytotoxic activity expressed as cytotoxic units (CU) per culture (Woolnough et al, 1979).
[‡] 0.1 ml of supernate from concanavalin A-stimulated mouse spleen cells was added to 1 ml cultures.

THEORY OF ALLOGRAFT IMMUNITY – PASSENGER LEUKOCYTE CONCEPT

The above two-signal model for immune induction has a profound influence on the way we view allogeneic interactions. Cells expressing the S^+ phenotype have the capacity to produce CoS activity, and thus can present antigen directly to allogeneic T cells (Figure 2). Other cells, such as tissue parenchymal cells, which carry the same antigen but are unable to produce CoS activity, express the S^- phenotype, and do not lead to direct T cell activation. Thus, in an allograft made up of both S^+ and S^- cells, only the antigen-bearing S^+ cells will have the capacity to stimulate allogeneic T cells. It is only in this situation that the two signals required for T cell activation are provided co-ordinately. Because the S^+ phenotype is expressed only by cells of lymphoreticular origin, we can see why leukocytes are strong stimulators of allogeneic T cells in vitro, and why these cells provide the major source of tissue immunogenicity. The key role of MHC in this process is that of a control molecule on the surface of the S^+ cell; that is, production and/ or release of the CoS requires some form of interaction of the responsive T cell with MHC on the surface of the S^+ cell (Figures 1 and 2) (Lafferty et al, 1983).

This theory provides a solution to the transplantation paradox. The immunogenicity of MHC antigen is not due to its inherent structural properties but rather to its *functional* role as a control structure. This means that MHC antigens will be highly immunogenic when presented on the surface of metabolically active S^+ cells; isolated MHC antigens or MHC antigens on the surface of S^- cells will not be immunogenic in the sense of inducing a graft-specific T cell response. This model predicts that depletion of S^+ cells from the graft prior to transplantation will reduce tissue immunogenicity. Any antigens shed from S^- cells of the graft and presented by host antigen-presenting cells will generate activated T cells specific for graft antigen in association with the host class II MHC antigen. That is, such cells will not be graft-specific. They would, however, be specific for host B cells that have a specificity for graft antigens and thus could act as helper cells for a graft-specific antibody response. Such a phenomenon would account for the immunological enhancement observed by Flexner in 1907 when he immunized animals with antigenic preparations of allogeneic tumours (Flexner and Jobling, 1907).

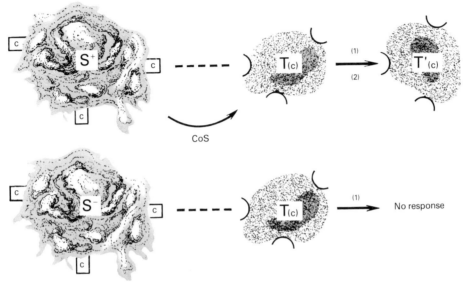

Figure 2.   Theory of alloreactivity. Alloantigen presentation by an S^+ cell will provide a source of both signals (antigen and CoS) required for T cell activation (active antigen presentation). Alloantigen presented on the surface of an S^- cell will not be directly immunogenic because these cells cannot provide a source of the second signal (passive antigen presentation).

EXPERIMENTAL MODIFICATION OF TISSUE IMMUNOGENICITY

Vascularized Organ Grafts

Snell was the first to propose that passenger lymphocytes were a major source of tissue immunogenicity (Snell, 1957). He argued that these cells, being mobile, were able to transport antigen to the regional lymph node and there initiate the rejection process. Initial attempts to remove passenger leukocytes from vascularized organs prior to transplantation were not successful. These attempts involved the induction of leukopenia in the tissue donor by procedures such as whole body irradiation, cyclophosphamide pre-treatment, or treatment with antilymphocyte serum (Guttman et al, 1967; Stuart et al 1971). At best, only marginal effects were observed with tissues transplanted across major barriers, or with rat heart allografts transplanted across multiple minor differences (Freeman et al, 1971). Stuart et al (1971) attempted to remove passenger leukocytes by first allografting rat kidneys to passively enhanced intermediate hosts. At 60–300 days post-transplantation the kidney grafts were retransplanted to naive recipient rats syngeneic with the intermediate host. Only a delay in the onset of rejection was achieved in these studies. These marginal effects led to some confusion over the extent to which passenger leukocytes contribute to tissue immunogenicity (Billingham, 1971).

Later studies from Batchelor's laboratory clarified the role passenger leukocytes play in renal allografting (Batchelor, 1978; Batchelor et al, 1979; Lechler and Batchelor, 1982). This group demonstrated that long-surviving, immunologically-enhanced, MHC-incompatible rat kidney grafts, when transplanted from a primary to a secondary recipient of the same genotype, did not elicit T cell alloimmunity in the secondary host. In contrast, normal primary kidney allografts in the relevant donor–recipient combination were rejected in 12 days. The failure of long-surviving kidney grafts to activate a T cell response could not be attributed to a lack of either class I or class II MHC antigens (Lechler and Batchelor, 1982), leading Batchelor's group to conclude that the effect resulted from a loss of passenger leukocytes. They later showed that donor strain dendritic cells in very low numbers would trigger rejection of kidneys taken from an intermediate, enhanced recipient (Lechler and Batchelor, 1982). The earlier failure of Stuart et al (1971) to see such a dramatic effect probably resulted from the strain combinations used in those studies.

Tissue Pre-treatment by Organ Culture

Unlike studies with vascularized organ grafts, tissue pre-treatment has proved spectacularly successful with cultured endocrine grafts. As early as the 1930s, Stone et al (1934) reported the clinical benefit of culturing parathyroid tissue prior to transplantation to patients with hypoparathyroidism. However, these studies were not genetically controlled and, without the support of an adequate theoretical base, enthusiasm for these experiments quickly waned. Spurred by the report of Summerlin et al (1973) of skin allograft acceptance through culture pre-treatment and by the theoretical implications of the passenger leukocyte concept, the 1970s saw a resurgence of investigation into the effect of organ culture on the immunogenicity of endocrine organs (Lafferty et al, 1983).

Allotransplantation of thyroid grafts provided a useful model for studying tissue pre-treatment. Mouse thyroid can be transplanted under the kidney capsule of syngeneic, thyroidectomized recipients, where the graft can survive and concentrate radioactive iodine as an indicator of graft function (Lafferty et al, 1976). Organ culture of thyroid tissue in an atmosphere of 95% O_2 and 5% CO_2 for 14 days extended allograft survival (Lafferty et al, 1975), while culture for 3–4 weeks resulted in indefinite survival and function of thyroid allografts (Lafferty et al, 1976). Donor pre-treatment with cyclophosphamide reduced the period of organ culture required to eliminate thyroid immunogenicity to 2 weeks (Lafferty and Woolnough, 1977). Under these conditions, both thyroid and parathyroid show indefinite survival in allogeneic, immunocompetent recipients (Lafferty and Woolnough, 1977). Similar results were reported with other species (Naji et al, 1979) as well as for xenotransplantation of thyroid and islet tissue from rat to mouse (Sollinger et al, 1976; Lacy et al, 1982). The first clinical application of this technology was reported by Sollinger et al (1983), who used the passage of donor parathyroid tissue through an athymic mouse (interim host) as a means of eliminating passenger leukocytes. This technique allowed successful allotransplantation of parathyroid tissue without recipient immunosuppression.

What accounts for the survival of cultured tissues in immunocompetent allogeneic recipients? Is the antigenicity of the graft reduced through antigen modulation in culture as proposed by Jacobs and Huseby (1967), or does the effect result from the postulated loss of passenger leukocytes? During organ culture, a rapid degeneration of the vascular bed and blood elements occurs but the tissue retains MHC antigens detectable by immunoferritin labelling (Parr et al, 1980a,b). Further, rejection of established cultured thyroid allografts is triggered by challenging the host with as few as 10^3 viable donor-type peritoneal (S^+) cells (Talmage et al, 1976). Established cultured thyroid allografts also are rejected when a second, donor-type uncultured thyroid is transplanted to the recipient (Lafferty and Woolnough, 1977). Clearly, the cultured allograft expresses recognizable alloantigens in vitro and in vivo, supporting the view that organ culture acts by depleting tissues of passenger leukocytes. The success of organ culture again illustrates the distinction between antigenicity and immunogenicity; the cultured graft cannot trigger allograft immunity but can serve as a target for immune destruction.

Similar results from high oxygen culture have been reported in the case of islet allografting (Bowen et al, 1980; Lafferty et al, 1983). In the case of this particular tissue, differing results have been reported by groups using different techniques to eliminate S^+ cells from the tissue prior to grafting (Faustman et al, 1981; Lacy et al, 1983; Hardy et al, 1984; Hegre et al, 1984). If this purging of S^+ cells from the tissue is sufficiently effective, islet allografting can be carried out without immunosuppression. Experiments in Hardy's laboratory have been successful in reducing the immunogenicity of islet allografts by UV-irradiation of the tissue prior to grafting (Hardy et al, 1984; Lau et al, 1984a,b). UV-irradiation inactivates S^+ cells in the graft (see Table 1). Other studies from Hegre and coworkers show that purified perinatal rat islets isolated by in vitro cultivation are accepted in non-immunosuppressed, allogeneic recipients (Hegre et al, 1984; Serie and Hegre, 1987). Faustman et al demonstrated a dependence of islet immunogenicity on the presence of Ia^+ cells in the transplanted tissue by achieving allograft survival with anti-Ia serum and complement pre-treatment of donor tissue (Faustman et al, 1981). However, Ia antigen allorecognition is not required for islet allograft rejection; transplantation studies using congenic strains show that islet allograft rejection can occur when there is I-region compatibility between donor and recipient (Morrow et al, 1980). The fact that rejection is dependent on the presence of an Ia^+ cell in the tissues is consistent with the notion that the S^+ stimulator cell carries Ia antigen on its surface (Yamashita and Shevach, 1977; Silberg-Sinakin et al, 1980). In other cases, brief and transient immune suppression has been shown to facilitate indefinite allograft acceptance. Taken together, this evidence shows that the obstacle of islet allograft immunity can be overcome without the requirement for chronic immunosuppression of the recipient.

THE FUTURE – CLINICAL APPLICATION

The removal of active antigen-presenting cells from a graft prior to transplantation can reduce or eliminate graft immunogenicity. However, such treatments do not eliminate antigen from the graft. Transplants of tissue modified in this way are in a metastable state during the early post-transplantation period; the metastable graft is acutely rejected if the host is immunized against graft antigens (Bowen et al, 1981). With the passage of time the graft establishes a stable relationship with the host, which is maintained by a state of suppressive tolerance (Bowen et al, 1981; Donohoe et al, 1983; Hao et al, 1987; Shizuru et al, 1987; Gotoh et al, 1988). Clinical application of technologies that eliminate active APC's from the graft must await a more complete understanding of this tolerant condition. Animal studies in which tolerance is achieved indicate that tolerance may not be obtained in 100% of trials, and currently there is no reliable test for the expression of the tolerant state that may not also pose a threat to the graft. The hope is that the future will see allografting carried out after graft pre-treatment to reduce tissue immunogenicity, and under the cover of short-term immunosuppression. Once procedures have been developed that indicate when a state of tolerance is obtained it will be possible gradually to reduce the immune suppression required to maintain the graft.

REFERENCES

Batchelor JR (1978) The riddle of kidney graft enhancement. *Transplantation* **26**: 139–141.

Batchelor JR, Welsh KI & Burgess H (1978) Transplantation antigens per se are poor immunogens within a species. *Nature* **273**: 54–56.

Batchelor JR, Welsh KI, Maynard A et al (1979) Failure of long surviving passively enhanced allografts to provoke T dependent alloimmunity I. Retransplantation of (AS × AUG)F1 kidneys into secondary AS recipients. *Journal of Experimental Medicine* **150**: 455–464.

Billingham RE (1971) The passenger cell concept in transplantation immunology. *Cellular Immunology* **2**: 13–17.

Bretscher P & Cohn M (1970) A theory of self–nonself discrimination. *Science* **169**: 1042–1048.

Bowen KM, Andrus L & Lafferty KJ (1980) Successful allotransplantation of mouse pancreatic islets to non-immunosuppressed recipients. *Diabetes* **29**: 98–104.

Bowen KM, Prowse SJ & Lafferty KJ (1981) Reversal of diabetes by islet transplantation: vulnerability of the established allograft. *Science* **213**: 1261–1262.

Donohoe JA, Andrus L, Bowen KM et al (1983) Cultured thyroid allografts induce a state of partial tolerance in adult recipient mice. *Transplantation* **35**: 62–67.

Faustman D, Hauptfeld V, Lacy P et al (1981) Prolongation of murine islet allograft survival by pretreatment of islets with antibody directed to Ia determinants. *Proceedings of the National Academy of Science, USA* **78**: 5156–5159.

Flexner S & Jobling JW (1907) On the promoting influence of heated tumor emulsions on tumor growth. *Proceedings of the Society for Experimental Biology and Medicine* **4**: 156–157.

Freeman JS, Chamberlain EC, Reemtsma K et al (1971) Prolongation of rat heart allografts by donor pretreatment with immunosuppressive agents. *Transplantation Proceedings* **3**: 580–582.

Gotoh M, Porter J, Monaco AP et al (1988) Induction of antigen-specific unresponsiveness to pancreatic islet allografts by antilymphocyte serum. *Transplantation* **45**: 429–433.

Guttman TD, Carpenter CB, Lindquist RR et al (1967) An immunosuppressive site of action of heterologous antilymphocyte serum. *Lancet* **i**: 248–249.

Hao L, Wang Y, Gill RG & Lafferty KJ (1987) Role of the L3T4[+] T cell in allograft rejection. *Journal of Immunology* **139**: 4022–4026.

Hardy M, Lau H, Weber C et al (1984) Induction of graft acceptance by ultraviolet irradiation of donor tissue. *Annals of Surgery* **200**: 441–450.

Hegre OD, Hickey GE & Marshall S (1984) Modification of allograft immunogenicity in perinatal islets isolated and purified in vitro. *Transplantation* **37**: 227–233.

Jacobs BB & Huseby RA (1967) Growth of tumors in allogeneic hosts following organ culture explantation. *Transplantation* **5**: 410–419.

Lacy PE, Davie JM & Finke EH (1979) Prolongation of islet allograft survival following in vitro culture (24°C) and a single injection of ALS. *Science* **204**: 312–313.

Lacy PE, Finke EH, Janney G et al (1982) Prolongation of islet xenograft survival by in vitro culture of rat megaislets in 95% O$_2$. Transplantation 33: 588–592.

Lafferty KJ & Cunningham AJ (1975) A new analysis of allogeneic interactions. Australian Journal for Experimental Biology and Medical Science 53: 27–42.

Lafferty KJ & Jones MAS (1969) Reactions of the graft versus host (GVH) type. Australian Journal of Experimental Biology and Medical Science 47: 17–54.

Lafferty KJ & Woolnough JA (1977) The origin and mechanism of the allograft reaction. Immunological Reviews 35: 231–262.

Lafferty KJ, Cooley MA, Woolnough S et al (1975) Thyroid allograft immunogenicity is reduced after a period in organ culture. Science 188: 259–261.

Lafferty KJ, Bootes A, Kilby VA et al (1976) Mechanism of thyroid allograft rejection. Australian Journal of Experimental Biology and Medical Science 54: 573–586.

Lafferty KJ, Andrus L & Prowse SJ (1980) Role of lymphokine and antigen in the control of specific T cell responses. Immunological Reviews 51: 279–314.

Lafferty KJ, Prowse SJ & Simeonovic CJ (1983) Immunobiology of tissue transplantation: a return to the passenger leukocyte concept. Annual Reviews of Immunology 1: 143–173.

Lau J, Reemtsma K & Hardy MA (1984a) Prolongation of rat islet allograft survival by direct ultraviolet irradiation of the graft. Science 223: 607–609.

Lau H, Reemtsma K & Hardy MA (1984b) The use of direct ultraviolet irradiation and cyclosporin in facilitating indefinite pancreatic islet allograft acceptance. Transplantation 36: 566–569.

Lechler RI & Batchelor JR (1982) Restoration of immunogenicity to passenger cell-depleted kidney allografts by the addition of donor strain dendritic cells. Journal of Experimental Medicine 155: 31–41.

Medawar PB (1957) The Uniqueness of the Individual, pp 143–185. New York: Basic Books.

Medawar PB (1963) The immunologically competent cell: Its nature and origin. In Wolstenholme GEW and Knight J (eds) CIBA Foundation Study Group, 16th edn. Boston and London: Little Brown.

Morrow CE, Sutherland DER, Steffes MW et al (1980) The effect of isolated H-2 K,D, and I region encoded histocompatibility antigen differences on mouse pancreatic islet allograft rejection. Transplantation 30: 135–141.

Naji A, Silvers WK & Barker CF (1979) Effect of culture in 95% O$_2$ on the survival of parathyroid allografts. Surgical Forum 30: 109–111.

Parr EL, Bowen KM & Lafferty KJ (1980a) Cellular changes in cultured mouse thyroid glands and islets of Langerhans. Transplantation 30: 135–141.

Parr EL, Lafferty KJ, Bowen KM & McKenzie IFC (1980b) H-2 complex and Ia antigens on cells dissociated from mouse thyroid and islets of Langerhans. Transplantation 30: 142–148.

Serie JR & Hegre OD (1987) Allotransplantation of neonatal islets in nonimmunosuppressed normal and diabetic rats. Transplantation Proceedings 19: 962–964.

Shizuru JA, Gregory AK, Chao CTB et al (1987) Islet allograft survival after a single course of treatment of recipient with antibody to L3T4. Science 237: 278–280.

Silberg-Sinakin I, Gigli I, Baer R et al (1980) Langerhans cells: role in contact hypersensitivity and relationship to lymphoid dendritic cells and to macrophages. Immunological Reviews 53: 203–223.

Simonsen M (1962) Graft versus host reactions. Their natural history and applicability as tools of research. Progress in Allergy 6: 349–467.

Snell GD (1957) The homograft reaction. Annual Reviews of Microbiology 11: 339–341.

Sollinger HW, Burkholder PM, Rasmus WR et al (1976) Prolonged survival of xenografts after organ culture. Transplantation Proceedings 96: 359–362.

Sollinger HW, Mack E, Cook K et al (1983) Allotransplantation of human parathyroid tissue without immunosuppression. Transplantation 36: 599–602.

Sprent J & Schaefer M (1986) Capacity of purified Lyt-2$^+$ T cells to mount primary proliferative and cytotoxic responses to Ia$^-$ tumour cells. Nature 322: 541–544.

Stone HB, Owings JC & Grey C (1934) Transplantation of living grafts of thyroid and parathyroid glands. Annals of Surgery 100: 613–626.

Stuart FP, Bastien E, Holter A et al (1971) Role of passenger leukocytes in the rejection of renal allografts. Transplantation Proceedings 3: 461–464.

Summerlin WT, Broutbar C & Foanes RB (1973) Acceptance of phenotypically differing cultured skin in man and mice. Transplantation Proceedings 5: 707–710.

Talmage SW, Dart G, Radovich J et al (1976) Activation of transplant immunity: Effect of donor leukocytes on thyroid allograft rejection. *Science* **191**: 385–388.

Talmage DW, Wollnough JA, Hemmingsen H et al (1977) Activation of cytotoxic T cells by nonstimulating tumor cells and spleen cell factor(s). *Proceedings of the National Academy of Sciences, USA* **74**: 4610–4613.

Woolnough JA, Misko IS & Lafferty KJ (1979) Cytotoxic and proliferative lymphocyte responses to allogeneic and xenogeneic antigens in vitro. *Australian Journal of Experimental Biology and Medical Science* **57**: 467–477.

Yamashita U & Shevach E (1977) The expression of Ia antigens on immunocompetent cells in the guinea pig. II. Ia antigens on macrophages. *Journal of Immunology* **119**: 1584–1588.

8e Current Controversies and New Horizons

Transplantation of Neural Tissue to the Brain: A New Treatment for Parkinson's Disease?

ROBERT Y. MOORE

Transplantation of neural tissue has been used for many years as an experimental method in the analysis of neural development. Recent work has attempted to apply it to the restoration of functional deficits produced by experimental lesions of the nervous system. The success of these studies (for reviews see Azmitia and Björklund, 1987; Björklund et al, 1987; Hoffer et al, 1988; Sladek and Gash, 1988) has led to the application of neural transplantation as an experimental tool for the treatment of a common neurological disorder. Parkinson's disease, first described by James Parkinson in 1817, is one of the best known of all neurological diseases. Its onset is usually late in life and sufferers typically show a progressive loss of motor function with relatively stereotyped features. These include a poverty of voluntary movement, increased muscle tone, loss of postural reflexes, and tremor. The aetiology of the disorder is unknown but the major pathophysiology has been well characterized. The studies of Hornykiewicz and his associates (see Hornykiewicz, 1982) demonstrated the now well known loss of the dopamine-producing neurones of the substantia nigra, with a concomitant denervation of the neostriatal nuclei that receive nigral dopamine neurone projections. This led to the view of Parkinson's disease as a 'deficiency' state and the introduction of a replacement therapy. The administration of the dopamine precursor, L-DOPA. L-DOPA is an effective treatment for the symptoms of Parkinson's disease, particularly early in the course, but the disease usually progresses relentlessly to a state in which the response to medical treatment is unsatisfactory. Further, many individuals are either refractory to medical treatment or unable to tolerate it. This has led to the search for other modalities of treatment. In this context, I shall review briefly the experimental background for neural transplantation, the status of current work on transplantation in Parkinson's disease and the prospects for future advances in this area.

ORGAN TRANSPLANTATION: CURRENT CLINICAL AND
IMMUNOLOGICAL CONCEPTS   ISBN 0-7020-1393-5

EXPERIMENTAL BACKGROUND

Although studies early in this century demonstrated that fetal tissue transplanted to adult brain could survive and establish connections, this approach was not systematically explored and applied to functional studies until the late 1970s (Hoffer et al, 1988). Transplantation of fetal tissue has now been used in a variety of experimental situations and the application to a model of parkinsonism is exemplary of the field. The signs of Parkinson's disease can be simulated in animals using two methods for the selective destruction of the substantia nigra dopamine neurones or their projections. The most extensive analysis has been in a rodent model with the neurotoxin, 6-hydroxydopamine. When injected into the ascending nigrostriatal bundle, 6-hydroxydopamine brings about a massive, widespread loss of the dopaminergic innervation of the neostriatum (Björklund et al, 1987). The animals become akinetic with increased tone and exhibit sensory neglect. Transplantation of fetal substantia nigra to the neostriatum, either as a solid transplant or injections of dissociated cells, results in reinnervation by dopaminergic axons in a pattern that approximates the normal pattern of innervation (Björklund et al, 1979). The area innervated depends upon the size of the transplant. Fetal tissue provides the most extensive reinnervation, presumably because it has the greatest intrinsic growth potential. Postnatal donor tissue does not survive well and does not provide an extensive reinnervation. The fetal nigral transplants restore much of the functional deficits produced by the 6-hydroxydopamine lesions (see Björklund et al, 1987; Hoffer et al, 1988).

The second experimental method for producing selective lesions is injection of the neurotoxin, 1-methyl-4-phenyl-1,2,3,6-4-tetrahydropyridine (MPTP), into monkeys to elicit an experimental parkinsonism. MPTP, first identified as a neurotoxin because it produces parkinsonism in man, can be used to produce a unilateral or bilateral syndrome with akinesia, rigidity, flexed posture and, occasionally, tremors in the monkey. Like 6-hydroxydopamine, MPTP produces a striking destruction of the nigrostriatal dopamine system with marked loss of neostriatal innervation (Sladek et al, 1987). As in humans, administration of L-DOPA is effective in ameliorating symptoms for a period of time (Bakay et al, 1987) but the restorative effects of transplantation of fetal substantia nigra are dramatic and appear long-lasting in monkeys (Bakay et al, 1987; Sladek et al, 1987).

One further point should be noted. Because of the difficulty of obtaining fetal material, attempts have been made to use other sources of neural cells for transplants (Hoffer et al, 1988; Sladek and Gash, 1988). The most commonly used source is the adrenal medulla, the cells of which originate from the neural crest and produce catecholamine. When transplanted to denervated neostriatum, they can survive and produce a functional recovery (Freed et al, 1986a). The mechanism of this recovery is unknown but there are data which suggest that the transplanted adrenal medullary cells exert a trophic action, inducing growth of surviving nigrostriatal projections (Bohn et al, 1987). The second approach, which is only at an early developmental stage, is to employ cultured cells (Freed et al, 1986b; Gash et al, 1986). Ideally, a cell line would be developed for each potential application that would have all of the required transmitter systems and that could be induced to stop dividing and growing and, yet, differentiate after transplantation.

Regardless of the source of tissue, the mechanism of neural transplant effects on function is an important issue. This has been reviewed recently in detail by Björklund and his collaborators (1987) (Table 1). A transplant could affect function in four major ways.

1. It could have a non-specific action that might improve or, more likely, increase the functional deficit produced by the initial process.
2. It could improve function by the release of a neuroactive substance. In Parkinson's disease, for example, a continuous release of dopamine to the neostriatum should improve the symptoms even though the release is diffuse and non-specific. Alternatively, the release of a trophic substance modifying the host brain to restore a functional deficit would represent another possible activity of a neuroactive substance.
3. The innervation of the host brain by the graft, with the formation of specific synaptic contacts, represents a higher level of graft–host interaction. This appears to be the mechanism of action of fetal nigral transplants. They innervate the host neostriatum in a homotypic pattern but are not themselves integrated into the host circuitry.
4. The transplant could exert a direct functional effect by being incorporated into the host circuitry with reciprocal connnections (Sotelo and Alvarado-Mallart, 1986).

These alternative mechanisms are not mutually exclusive and any combination of them might occur in a particular situation.

Table 1. Mechanisms of neural graft–host interaction. Modified from Björklund et al (1987).

Non-specific effects, either positive or negative
Production and release of neuroactive substances
Innervation of host brain by grafted neurons
Establishment of circuitry with reciprocal graft–host connections

PARKINSON'S DISEASE

Parkinson's disease has, typically, a course characterized by the inexorable progression of symptoms and signs and a failure of response to medical therapy. In addition, medical therapy may provide its own problems. As the disease progresses, those treated with L-DOPA not only exhibit a failure of response but may show a striking variability in response, the 'on–off' phenomenon, and drug-induced involuntary movements. It is therefore not surprising that the success of experimental transplantation studies has led to human trials. In order to avoid problems of graft rejection and immunosuppression, the initial studies have utilized autografts of adrenal medulla (Figure 1). This tissue contains modified nerve cells that produce catecholamines, noradrenaline and adrenaline, and peptides. The hope is that grafted adrenal medullary cells will differentiate in the neostriatum, make connections and release dopamine. It seems unlikely, however, that this would happen.

Two studies have been reported in the refereed literature. A Swedish group (Backlund et al, 1985; Lindvall et al, 1987) has transplanted fragments of autologous adrenal medullary tissue into the substance of the neostriatum. In these very carefully studied patients there was an initial, brief improvement, which then receded. There were no evident adverse effects of the operation. In contrast, a Mexican group (Madrazo et al, 1987) has reported dramatic, sustained improvement in two individuals. The two studies differed primarily in surgical technique. The Mexican group placed the adrenal medullary

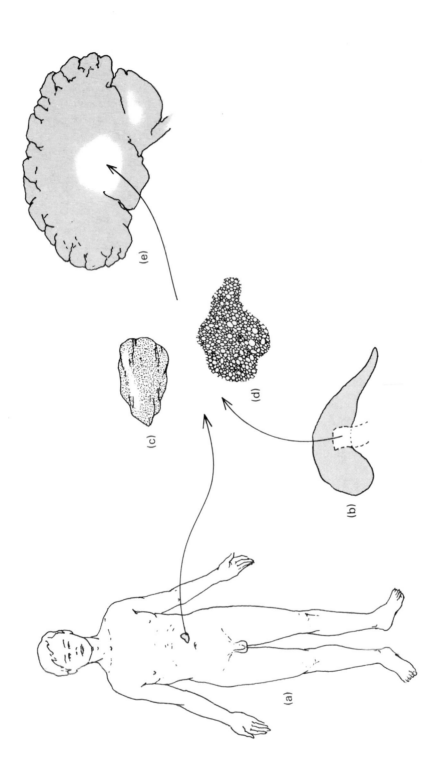

Figure 1. Transplantation of neural tissue in Parkinson's disease. Tissue is obtained as an adrenal medullary autograft (a) or from fetal mesencephalon (b). It is transplanted either as solid pieces (c) or as dissociated cells (d) into the neostriatal nuclei (e).

tissue in a site on the ventricular surface of one neostriatum. As they report bilateral improvements, the effects can only be interpreted as reflecting release of a neuroactive substance into the ventricular fluid. Since these original reports were published, a relatively large number of patients have been given adrenal medullary autografts. Preliminary reports of these more recent studies have been presented at medical meetings and in the popular press but details of their results are not yet available for scientific appraisal. In addition, trials are under way using human fetal tissue, but no reports from these have so far been presented. Nevertheless, the experimental studies do raise the hope that neural transplantation will be beneficial in Parkinson's disease and this is, at least in part, borne out by the early clinical trials. Much remains to be learned before this methodology is accepted or rejected, either in Parkinson's disease or in other chronic neurological illness for which effective treatment does not exist.

SUMMARY

Transplantation of neural tissue is now a well-established technique for the experimental study of the development and function of the nervous system. Animal studies establish that the transplantation of embryonic brain tissue to adult hosts can be used to restore functional impairments produced by focal lesions of the adult brain. The mechanisms underlying functional recovery are complex and range from apparent restitution of neural circuitry to provision of a trophic substance that induces neural reorganization in the host brain. The success of experimental neural grafts in animals reflects in large part the fact that the brain is to some degree an immunologically privileged site.

These studies have now been extended to the use of neural transplants in clinical trials as a treatment for Parkinson's disease. Autografts of adrenal medullary tissue placed in the head of the caudate nucleus appear to improve some patients. Additional studies are in progress using fetal brain tissue. Further application of neural transplantation in Parkinson's disease, and extension to other neurological disorders, requires additional animal experimentation and a careful assessment of the clinical trials in progress.

REFERENCES

Azmitia CC & Björklund A (1987) *Cell and Tissue Transplantation into the Adult Brain.* New York: New York Academy of Sciences.

Backlund E-D, Gramberg P-O, Hamberger B et al (1985) Transplantation of adrenal medullary tissue to striatum in parkinsonism. First clinical trials. *Journal of Neurosurgery* **62**: 169–173.

Bakay RAE, Barrow DL, Fiandaca MS et al (1987) Biochemical and behavioral correction of MPTP Parkinson-like syndrome by fetal cell transplantation. *Annals of the New York Academy of Sciences* **495**: 623–640.

Björklund A & Stenevi U (1979) Reconstruction of the nigrostriatal dopamine pathway by intracerebral nigral transplants. *Brain Research* **177**: 555–560.

Björklund A, Linkvall O, Isacson O et al (1987) Mechanisms of action of intracerebral neural implants: studies on nigral and striatal grafts to the lesioned striatum. *Trends in Neurosciences* **10**: 509–513.

Bohn MC, Cupit L, Marciano F & Gash DM (1987) Adrenal medulla grafts enhance recovery of striatal dopaminergic fiber. *Science* **237**: 913–916.

Freed WJ, Cannon-Spoor HE & Krauthammer E (1986a) Intrastriatal adrenal medulla grafts in rats: Long term survival and behavioral effects. *Journal of Neurosurgery* **65**: 664–670.

Freed WJ, Patel-Vaidya U & Geller HM (1986b) Properties of PC12 pheochromocytoma cells transplanted to the adult rat brain. *Experimental Brain Research* **63**: 557–566.

Gash DM, Notter MFD, Okawara SH, Kraus AL & Joynt RJ (1986) Amitotic neuroblastoma cells used for neural implants in monkeys. *Science* **233**: 1420–1422.

Hoffer BJ, Granholm AC, Stevens JO & Olsen L (1988) Catecholamine-containing grafts in parkinsonism: past and present. *Clinical Research* **36**: 189–195.

Hornykiewicz O (1982) Neurotransmitter changes in Parkinson's disease. In Marsden CD & Fahn S (eds), *Movement Disorders*, pp 41–58. London: Butterworths.

Lindvall O, Backlund E-O, Farde L et al (1987) Transplantation in Parkinson's disease. Two cases of adrenal medullary grafts to pitamen. *Annals of Neurology* **22**: 457–468.

Madrazo I, Drucker-Cokin R, Diaz V et al (1987) Open microsurgical autograft of adrenal medulla to the right caudal nucleus in two patients with intractable Parkinson's disease. *New England Journal of Medicine* **316**: 831–834.

Sladek JR Jr & Gash DM (1988) Nerve-cell grafting in Parkinson's disease. *Journal of Neurosurgery* **68**: 337–351.

Sladek JR Jr, Redmond DE Jr, Collier TJ et al (1987) Transplantation of fetal dopamine neurons in primate brain reverses MPTP induced parkinsonism. In Seil FJ, Herbert E & Carlson MB (eds), *Progress in Brain Research*, pp 309–323. Amsterdam: Elsevier.

Sotelo S & Alvarado-Mallart RM (1986) Growth and differentiation of cerebellar suspensions transplanted into the adult cerebellum of mice with heredodegenerative ataxia. *Proceedings of the National Academy of Sciences, USA* **83**: 1135–1139.

Appendices

Ia (i) Renal Transplantation in Europe

GERHARD OPELZ (for the Collaborative Transplant Study)

This report is based on data provided by centres participating in the Collaborative Transplant Study, a co-operative effort with strictly scientific aims. It is estimated that approximately 80% of European transplants are reported to the Transplant Study. Data from transplant units in the following cities were included in this analysis: Aachen, Amsterdam, Angers, Baracaldo, Barcelona, Basel, Belfast, Berlin-East, Berlin-West, Bern, Bicetre-Paris, Brimingham, Bologna, Bonn, Brussels, Budapest, Cambridge, Cardiff, Cologne, Dublin, Düsseldorf, Edinburgh, Erlangen-Nürnberg, Essen, Frankfurt, Freiburg, Geneva, Gent, Glasgow, Göttingen, Gothenburg, Groningen, Hamburg, Hann.-Münden, Hannover, Heidelberg, Helsinki, Homburg-Saar, Innsbruck, Kaiserslautern, Kiel, Lausanne, Leicester, Leuven, Liverpool, Lisbon, Ljubljana, London, Lübeck, Lund-Malmö, Lyon, Maastricht, Madrid, Malaga, Manchester, Marburg, Milan (Northern-Italy-Transplant), Montpellier, Münster, München, Nancy, Nantes, Nice, Nijmegen, Novi Sad, Oviedo, Oxford, Pamplona, Paris, Prague, Reims, Rennes, Rijeka, Rome, Santander, St Etienne, St Gallen, Stoke-on-Trent, Szeged, Thessaloniki, Toulouse, Tübingen, Turin, Ulm, Uppsala, Valencia, Vienna, Warsaw, Zagreb, and Zürich. Graft survival rates were computed by actuarial methods and no exclusions were made. Patients who died were regarded as graft failures.

Figure 1 shows graft survival rates for the three main categories of histocompatibility. Patients whose baseline immunosuppressive protocol included cyclosporin are compared to patients on 'conventional' immunosuppression. Importantly, both with and without cyclosporin treatment, HLA-identical sibling transplants have the highest graft survival rate followed by HLA 1-haplotype matched related transplants and then by transplants from (HLA 2-haplotype mismatched) cadaver donor transplants. The advantage of immunosuppression with cyclosporin is most evident in transplants from cadaver donors.

Figure 2 shows the corresponding patient survival rates. Because transplant recipients who reject their graft usually return to dialysis, patient survival rates are higher than graft survival rates. Histocompatibility can be seen to correlate with patient survival, too, although the differences are smaller than for graft survival.

An analysis of first cadaver transplants performed during each consecutive year since 1982 shows a small but steady improvement in graft outcome among patients treated without cyclosporin (Figure 3). Cyclosporin was widely prescribed in European centres from 1982 onwards. In cyclosporin treated recipients, the results of transplants done in 1982 (during the learning phase of cyclosporin management) were inferior compared

ORGAN TRANSPLANTATION: CURRENT CLINICAL AND
IMMUNOLOGICAL CONCEPTS   ISBN 0-7020-1393-5

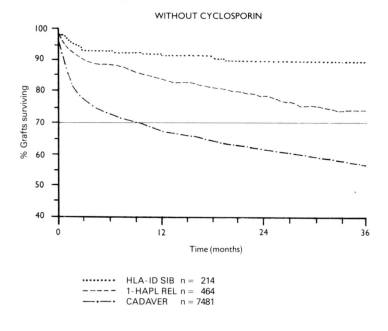

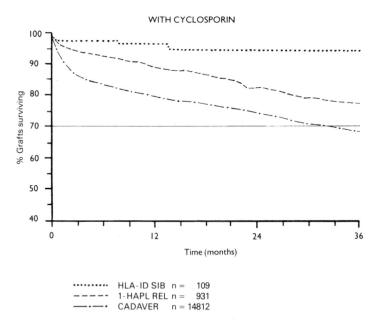

Figure 1.   Graft survival rates of first kidney transplants in patients treated with or without cyclosporin for immunosuppression. HLA-identical sibling transplants (HLA-ID SIB), HLA 1-haplotype matched related transplants (1-HAPL REL), and cadaver transplants were analysed separately. The correlation of graft survival with compatibility for the HLA phenotypes is highly significant with both types of immunosuppression ($p < 0.0001$).

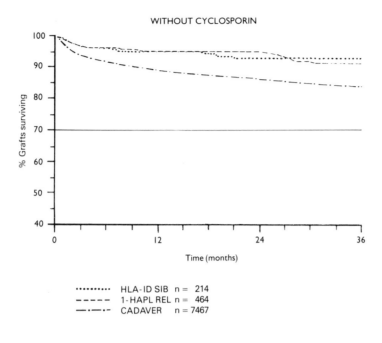

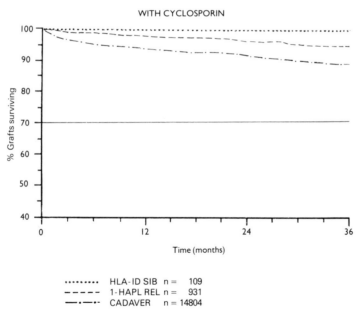

Figure 2.   Patient survival rates for first kidney transplants. The main three types of HLA compatibility were analysed: HLA-identical siblings, HLA 1-haplotype matched related transplants, and cadaver transplants. Patients with or without cyclosporin treatment were analysed separately.

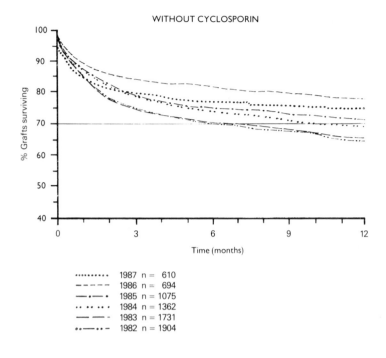

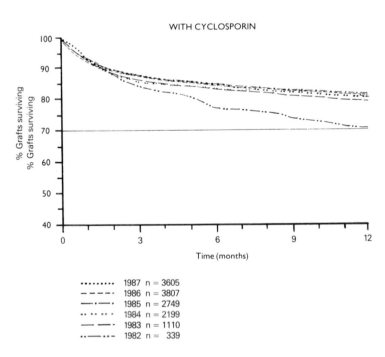

Figure 3. Graft survival rates in recipients of first cadaver kidney transplants treated with or without cyclosporin for immunosuppression. Transplants performed in each of the calendar years 1982–1987 were analysed separately.

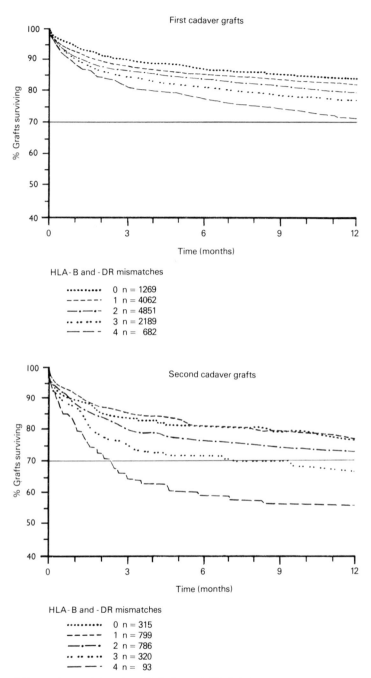

Figure 4. Effect of matching for HLA-B and HLA-DR antigens in cyclosporin-treated recipients of cadaver transplants. Graft survival rates are plotted for first cadaver transplants on the left and for second cadaver transplants on the right. The numbers of mismatched HLA antigens and the numbers of patients studied are indicated for each curve. Statistically, the correlation of matching with graft survival was highly significant both in first and second grafts ($p < 0.0001$, weighted regression analysis).

with subsequent years. The numbers of patients in Figure 3 indicate the shift towards treatment with cyclosporin in recent years. Because relatively few recently transplanted patients were immunosuppressed without cyclosporin it must be suspected that selection of 'good risk recipients' may have played a role in the improvement of results for these patients. Most patients are currently on immunosuppressive protocols including cyclosporin; therefore, we selected only cyclosporin-treated recipients for the following analyses.

In previous studies we found that matching for the HLA-B and -DR antigens correlated better with graft survival than matching for HLA-A and -B or for HLA-DR alone (Opelz, 1985). A comparison of matching for HLA-B and -DR in first and second cadaver transplants is shown in Figure 4. The correlation of matching with graft outcome is statistically highly significant for both first and second grafts; however, the impact of the beneficial matching effect is greater in second transplants.

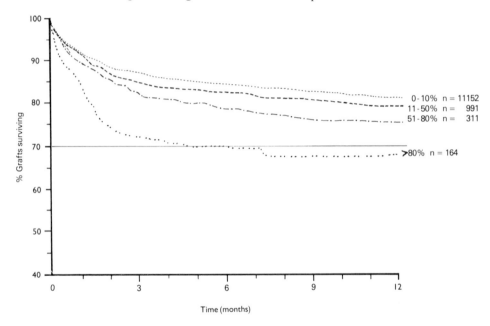

Figure 5.   Effect of preformed lymphocytotoxic antibodies on graft survival in cyclosporin-treated recipients of first cadaver kidney transplants. The antibody reactivity of the latest pre-transplant serum sample was analysed.

Figure 5 depicts the influence of preformed lymphocytotoxic antibodies on graft survival. Patients with highly reactive antibodies in their latest pre-transplant serum (> 80% reactivity against the random test panel) have an inferior graft outcome in spite of immunosuppression with cyclosporin. That the differentiation of patients with or without significant lymphocytotoxic antibody levels is important for the assessment of HLA matching is shown in Figure 6. In patients with > 50% antibody reactivity, grafts with 3 or 4 mismatches for HLA-B and -DR showed extremely poor success rates. Thus, it would appear prudent to avoid poorly matched grafts especially in patients with high antibody reactivity.

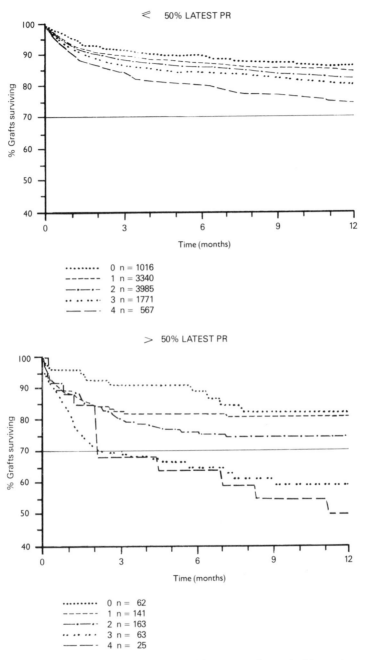

Figure 6. Effect of HLA-B and HLA-DR matching on graft survival in cyclosporin-treated recipients of first cadaver transplants. Patients with ≤50% lymphocytotoxic antibody reactivity in their latest pre-transplant serum were compared with patients with >50% reactivity. The correlation of matching with outcome was significant both in recipients with ≤50% ($p < 0.0001$) or >50% ($p < 0.001$) antibody reactivity; however, the impact of poor matching was greater with highly reactive antibodies. PR, Panel reactivity, i.e. percentage reactivity of recipient serums against a random test panel.

Figure 7 demonstrates the dramatic improvement in the graft survival rate of non-transfused recipients since 1982. Among first cadaver transplants performed from 1984–1987, the European results show a difference between transfused and non-transfused cyclosporin-treated patients of only 1 percentage point at one year (81 ± 1% v. 82 ± 1%).

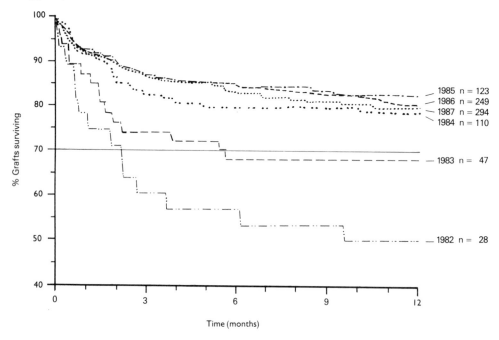

Figure 7. Graft survival rates in non-transfused recipients of first cadaver transplants. All patients were treated with cyclosporin. The results are shown for transplants done during each of the calendar years from 1982 to 1987.

Immunosuppressive regimens vary between centres in Europe and the USA, but more than 90% of recipients receive cyclosporin therapy, alone, or in combination with azathioprine and prednisolone. The rationale for adding azathioprine or prednisolone, or both to cyclosporin is that the dosage of cyclosporin may be reduced and thus the nephrotoxic effects might be minimized. Figure 8 addresses this question: patients treated between 1984 and 1987 are categorized into different immunosuppressive regimens, and within each of these groups into three categories of renal function according to the serum creatinine level at 1 year post-transplant. (Serum creatinine less than 130 μmol/l – good; 130–260 μ/l – moderate; > 260 μmol/l – poor). There seems little evidence from this preliminary analysis that the addition of azathioprine and prednisolone to cyclosporin reduces nephrotoxicity, since patients receiving cyclosporin monotherapy prophylaxis have as good, or better renal function at 1 year as all the other groups.

Approximately 55% of all transplants reported to the Collaborative Transplant Study are reported by European centres, the remainder by centres on other continents. It has been a remarkable observation that, at least with respect to the variables analysed thus far, there have been no striking differences in the results of transplants done in Europe or on other continents. Of course, there are factors that cannot be analysed in the European data, such as the influence of recipient or donor race other than Caucasian, or the effect of HLA matching in non-Caucasian recipients. The results analysed in this report are remarkably similar to the overall results derived from the complete Collaborative Transplant Study data file (Opelz, 1985, 1987).

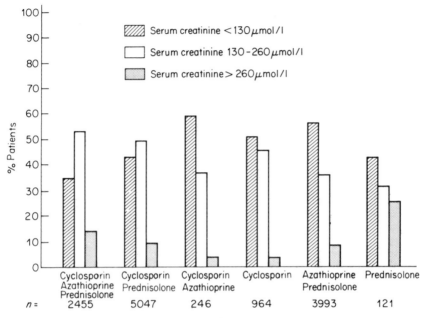

Figure 8. Creatinine values and drug protocols at 1 year, first cadaver transplants, 1984–1987, Collaborative Transplant Study.

Acknowledgement

The generous cooperation of transplant centres participating in the Collaborative Transplant Study is gratefully acknowledged.

REFERENCES

Opelz G, for the Collaborative Transplant Study (1985) Correlation of HLA matching with kidney graft survival in patients with or without cyclosporine treatment. *Transplantation* **40**: 240–243.
Opelz G, for the Collaborative Transplant Study (1987) Effect of HLA matching in 10,000 cyclosporine-treated cadaver kidney transplants. *Transplantation Proceedings* **19**: 641–646.

Ia (ii) Renal Transplantation on the American Continent

DANIEL J. COOK
PAUL I. TERASAKI

In contrast to most other organs, renal transplantation may involve either cadaver donors or living, usually related, donors as a source of the allograft. Figure 1 examines trends relating to the source of transplanted kidneys in transplants reported to the UCLA International Kidney Transplant Registry from 1968 to 1986. The bars represent the proportions of cadaver and living donor grafts for each year. Over the years, the percentage of transplants involving living donors has decreased from nearly 50% in 1968 to 20% in 1986. The lines represent the 1-year graft survival rate for transplants in each group.

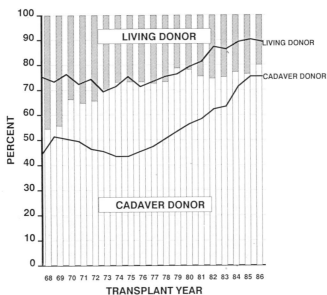

Figure 1. Donor source of kidney transplants performed in the period 1968–1986: graft survival at 1 year (UCLA International Kidney Registry). The lightly and heavily shaded bars indicate the proportion of cadaveric and living related donors, respectively.

ORGAN TRANSPLANTATION: CURRENT CLINICAL AND
IMMUNOLOGICAL CONCEPTS   ISBN 0-7020-1393-5

This figure illustrates a number of points concerning the development of kidney transplantation. Foremost among the reasons for the decreasing use of living donors is the steady improvement in graft survival rates of cadaver donor transplants seen since the mid-1970s – a strong argument for avoiding the removal of a kidney from a healthy donor and the risks of such a procedure. However, the survival of living donor transplants has likewise risen over the years, and is now averaging 90% at 1 year. While improvements in the results of cadaver donor transplants have been impressive, transplanting living related donor grafts continues to provide the best opportunity for success in both 1-year and long-term (see below) survival rates.

In contrast to the source of the transplanted organs, the proportion of second ('regraft') cadaveric kidneys has remained constant over the years, at about 20% (Figure 2). Since the mid-1970s their survival rates have been consistently lower than those of primary grafts, but there has been a steady improvement. The effect of cyclosporin, which first became a factor in these data in 1983–1984, appears to be somewhat stronger for first transplants than for second kidneys.

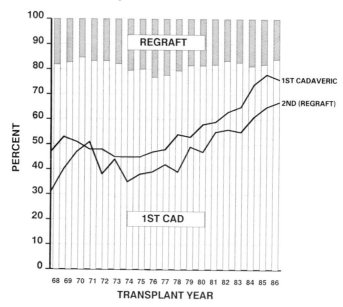

Figure 2. Primary and subsequently transplanted ('regrafted') cadaveric kidneys transplanted in the period 1968–1986: graft survival at 1 year. The lightly and heavily shaded bars indicate the proportion of primary (first) and second (regraft) cadaveric kidneys, respectively.

The problem of the regrafted patient is only partially revealed by graft survival. The fact that second transplants are not given more frequently is disturbing, considering that this group represents an increasingly greater proportion on most transplant waiting lists. Essentially this is due to a failure to overcome the problem of sensitization in patients who have lost their first kidney allograft.

Perhaps one of the more confusing observations concerning kidney transplantation has been the effect of pre-transplant blood transfusions. The lines in Figure 3 represent 1-year graft survival rates for transplants involving transfused and non-transfused recipients of primary cadaveric grafts. The beneficial effect of pre-transplant transfusions that was first described by Opelz in the 1970s is clearly seen in this figure. What is not so clear is the reason for the lessening of this effect in the 1980s. The explanation probably lies in the improvement of graft survival rates in non-transfused recipients, which began in the late 1970s. This preceded the widespread use of cyclosporin, and followed a dramatic rise in the percentage of patients who did receive transfusions, as shown by the shaded area. It is possible that the apparent disappearance of the transfusion effect is due to reporting errors, as centres have changed from a policy of avoiding pre-transplant transfusions, for fear of sensitizing the patient, to a regimen of deliberate transfusion in the hope of improving graft survival. Factors such as the fear of infection and the introduction of recombinant erythropoietin will now probably decrease the number of patients receiving pre-transplant transfusions, and the existence of a larger pool of non-transfused patients should allow the problem of the transfusion effect to be resolved.

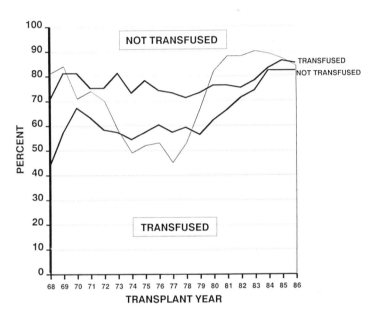

Figure 3.   Primary cadaveric kidney transplants, with or without blood transfusion, in the period 1968–1986: graft survival at 1 year. The shaded and non-shaded areas denote the proportion of patients who were transfused and those given no blood, respectively.

The introduction of cyclosporin has unquestionably brought about the greatest change that has occurred in kidney transplantation in recent years. The use of this immuno-suppressant has resulted in an overall 10–15% increase in 1-year graft survival for first cadaveric transplants. Figure 4 illustrates that while cyclosporin has increased graft survival, it has not entirely overcome the effects of histoincompatibility. Virtually no improvement in graft survival is seen for HLA-identical sibling transplants (whose survival is already very good), and very little effect is observed with one-haplotype matched living donor grafts. Cyclosporin has certainly improved the graft survival rates of both well-matched (0–1 HLA-A,-B,-DR mismatch) and poorly matched (5–6 HLA-A,-B,-DR mismatch) primary cadaveric grafts as well as that of second kidney allografts.

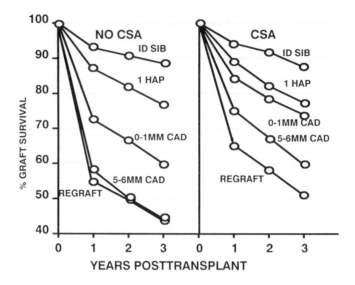

Figure 4.   The effect of cyclosporin A (CSA) on kidney allograft survival since 1980: a 3-year follow-up period. ID SIB, HLA-identical sibling; I HAP, one haplotype mismatched living related donor; 0–1 MM CAD, not more than 1 HLA mismatched cadaveric donor; 5–6 MM CAD, 5 or 6 HLA antigen mismatched cadaveric donor; regraft, second kidney transplanted after rejection of the first.

The use of cyclosporin has clearly had a beneficial effect on kidney transplantation, particularly for those transplants involving cadaveric donors. Figure 4 suggests that efforts should continue to be made to avoid HLA mismatching. With cyclosporin, well matched cadaver donor transplants survive nearly as well as haploidentical living donor grafts; poorly matched grafts fare considerably worse. It seems that even in the cyclosporin era of kidney transplantation, tissue matching will have to be a priority for primary transplants in order to both optimize graft survival and avoid the problems that tend to be encountered by second grafts (i.e. sensitization).

After the first year or two of kidney transplantation, graft losses tend to be quite regular, and Figure 5 takes advantage of this fact to extrapolate graft survival rates beyond 10 years without taking into account HLA matching. Projections of survival rates of 3-year cohorts are given for cadaver and living donor primary transplants, dividing the 1983–1985 transplants according to whether cyclosporin was used. It is clear that relatively few of the cadaveric donor kidneys transplanted up to 1985 can be expected to survive to the year 2000. Even with the use of cyclosporin, only about 15% of first grafts are likely to be functioning at that time. The situation is more promising for the living related donor transplants. Cyclosporin-treated grafts in this group appear to have a greater loss rate than grafts in patients who did not receive this drug, but this is due to a larger proportion of HLA non-identical grafts in this treated group.

The effects of histocompatibility in kidney transplantation are strongest when long-term results are examined. Thus, while 1-year graft survival rates of cyclosporin-treated primary transplants are relatively high, the late graft loss rates appear to be similar to those seen prior to the introduction of this drug. Transplants involving living donors offer much improved long-term results. However, by additionally matching for HLA in cadaveric grafts, results approaching those obtained with living related donor transplants can be obtained (see Figure 4).

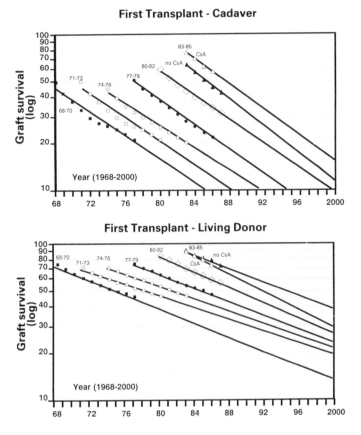

Figure 5. Long-term survival of cadaveric and living related kidney allografts without regard to HLA matching: retrospective and extrapolated survival curves covering the period 1968–2000. CSA, cylosporin A.

SUMMARY

In the two decades of its existence, the UCLA International Kidney Transplant Registry has accumulated data on more that 70 000 transplants. The data presented here examine some of the changes that have occurred over the years in the field of renal transplantation. It is clear that graft survival rates have improved quite dramatically over the last 10–15 years. This improvement is not the result of a single factor, but most likely represents the accumulation of numerous advances in the field. Even the influence of cyclosporin, which is seen in Figure 2 as an increase in primary cadaveric graft survival following its widespread use in 1984, does not seem so remarkable in view of the steady improvements that had preceded the introduction of the drug. It is, indeed, only recently that cadaveric donor transplants have reached the level of success that living related donor transplants enjoyed 20 years ago.

With the 1-year survival rates of cyclosporin-treated primary cadaveric donor grafts at about 80%, it would seem that there remains little room for improvement. If, however, kidney transplantation is meant to provide long-term remission of end-stage renal disease, then the emphasis should be placed on success rates 5, 10 or even 20 years following the transplant. Few patients would be interested in a short-term resolution of the condition, but that is all that has been offered to the recipients of cadaveric donor kidneys up to now. Most of these patients will not have a functioning graft 10 years after transplantation. Grafts from living related donors fare much better in the long-term, but this approach is not possible for the majority of the patients.

From the data now available, the approach most likely to improve the long-term results of cadaveric donor transplants would involve efforts to increase the degree of matching for HLA antigens. Well-matched grafts not only have higher 1-year survival rates but, perhaps more importantly, have lower rates of graft loss in the long-term. As the numbers of transplants performed increases, it becomes even more important to optimize the use of the kidneys that are available. Those patients who have lost their first graft usually become sensitized and therefore have to wait for a long time to obtain another transplant; the chances of success of the subsequent transplant are also reduced. The difficulties involved with the establishment of histocompatibility-based organ sharing are not insignificant, and would require co-ordinated efforts at the national or international level. Yet, until approaches are developed that can overcome the effects of histoincompatibility, minimizing disparities by means of tissue matching is a solution within our reach.

Ib   Summary of Clinical Data: Liver Transplantation

KEITH ROLLES

Clinical liver transplantation is now in its 26th year following the first case reported by Starzl in 1963. In 1983, the National Institutes of Health held a consensus meeting in Bethesda, Maryland, hearing the experiences from the four major centres actively engaged in liver transplantation at that time (Pittsburgh, USA; Cambridge/Kings, UK; Hanover, West Germany; Groningen, The Netherlands). The consensus panel concluded that liver transplantation could henceforth be considered a 'therapeutic modality'. Subsequently, enormous expansion has occurred within this field. More than 50 liver transplant programmes are currently active in the USA and Canada, with a further 40 in western Europe. Two centres are currently active in Australia. The current estimate of the numbers of liver transplants worldwide is around 5000. The longest surviving recipient of a liver graft is now more than 16 years post-transplant.

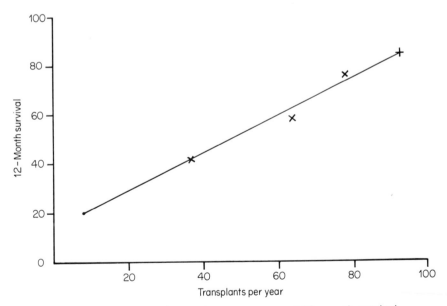

Figure 1.   Number of transplants per year and 12-month survival.

ORGAN TRANSPLANTATION: CURRENT CLINICAL AND
IMMUNOLOGICAL CONCEPTS   ISBN 0-7020-1393-5

OVERALL RESULTS

Most centres have seen improving results over the last 3–4 years. Such improvements have frequently correlated directly with increased numbers of transplants (Figure 1). The biggest single series in the world, by era, remains that of Dr Starzl. Of 172 patients immunosuppressed with azathioprine and prednisone between 1963 and 1981, actuarial 5-year survival was 20%. Between 1981 and mid 1988, 1000 patients treated with cyclosporin and prednisone yield a 65% 5-year survival (Figure 2).

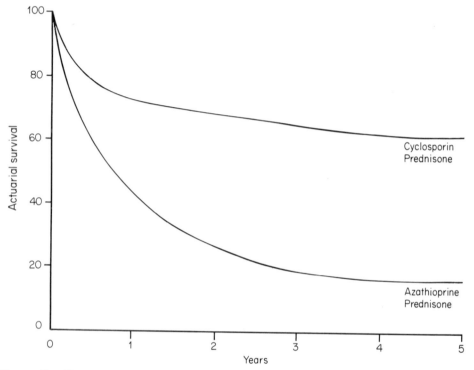

Figure 2.   Five-year survival of 1000 patients treated with cyclosporin and prednisone. 1981–1988.

The European liver transplant registry currently analysing data from over 2000 liver transplants began accumulating data in 1985 and showed marked improvement in 1-year actuarial survival in 1986 and again in 1987 (Figure 3).

Some of the more recently established, smaller centres pursuing a policy of careful case selection are achieving 1-year survival figures of more than 80%.

OVERALL RESULTS/PAEDIATRIC (less than 15 years old)

The European liver transplant registry has shown an overall 61% survival of children undergoing liver transplantation at 3 years, 4 years and 5 years of age. Results according to age are presented in Figure 4. In contrast to the reports of the Pittsburgh group, the European registry does not, at present, show consistently better survival of children when compared with adults.

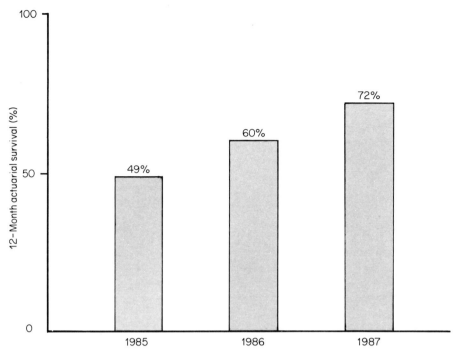

Figure 3. European liver transplant registry data for 12-month actuarial survival.

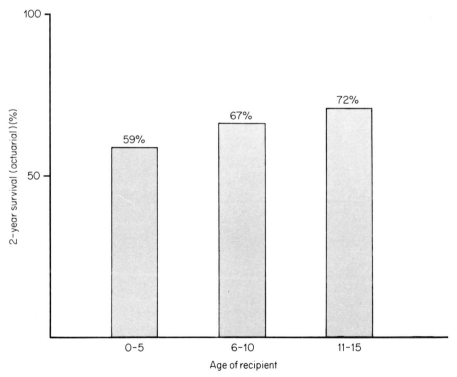

Figure 4. Survival of children undergoing liver transplantation, by age.

SPECIFIC INDICATIONS AND RESULTS (see Tables 1 and 2)

The indications for liver transplantation are currently widening, but fall into four broad groups with some degree of overlap. Table 2 documents the current survival following liver transplantation for a sample of specific indications.

Table 1. Some specific indications for liver transplantation.

1	Chronic liver disease	Primary biliary cirrhosis
		Biliary atresia
		Chronic active hepatitis
		Sclerosing cholangitis
2	Primary hepatic malignancy	Hepatocellular carcinoma
		Cholangiocarcinoma
3	Acute/subacute liver failure	Hepatitis A,B, non A non B
		Idiosyncratic drug reactions
		Amanita, halothane
4	Metabolic disorders	Wilson's disease
		α_1 Antitrypsin deficiency
		Primary hyperoxaluria

Table 2. Results for specific indications.

	2-Year actuarial survival (%)
Chronic liver disease	
Biliary atresia	68
Primary biliary cirrhosis	65
Primary hepatic malignancy	
Hepatocellular carcinoma	31
Acute liver failure up to 3 years	
(Cambridge/KCH)	65
(Pittsburgh)	50

RETRANSPLANTATION

Retransplantation of the liver may be indicated following acute or chronic allograft rejection or a vascular thrombosis in the early postoperative period or a poorly or non-functional first graft. The rate of retransplantation varies widely from centre to centre from approximately 25% in the Pittsburgh series to 8% in the Cambridge/Kings College Hospital series. Following retransplantation 1-year survival is between 40 and 50%.

CONCLUSION

In the last 5 years not only has liver transplantation become widely accepted as a therapeutic option for a widening spectrum of end stage liver diseases, it has become the treatment of choice in some specific situations for example fulminating or acute onset Wilson's disease, tyrosinosis, or severe pyridoxine-resistant primary hyperoxaluria. Models are currently being developed in primary biliary cirrhosis and in acute liver failure to identify poor prognostic factors and so help with the appropriate timing of transplantation. Early post-transplantation survival for malignancy remains excellent but at 2 years survival is poor due to the high rate of tumour recurrence (at least 70%). Clearing of B virus markers following transplantation is uncommon (10–15%). Recurrent chronic hepatitis B after transplantation is unpredictable but may occur in 15–20% of cases.

Ic Heart and Heart–lung Transplantation at Papworth Hospital

J. WALLWORK

Since Christian Barnard's arresting clinical experiment, now over 20 years ago, cardiac transplantation has become an accepted form of treatment for many patients with end stage cardiac failure (Wallwork, 1989). Much of this expansion has taken place since 1980, following the pioneering work of Shumway in Stanford. The demand for cardiac transplantation worldwide has increased rapidly as it has been shown to be an effective form of therapy. Improved survival has been largely, although not exclusively, due to the impact of the introduction of cyclosporin into immunosuppressive regimes. There are now about 150 centres in the United States and more than 50 in Europe. The worldwide activity for heart transplantation as recorded in the International Society for Heart Transplantation Register is shown in Figure 1a. Combined heart and lung transplantation is, by contrast, still in its developmental period, but over the last 5 years there has been a rapid increase in the number of heart–lung transplants performed (Figure 1b).

The place of single lung transplantation is still to be evaluated. The major current indication is for patients with fibrotic non-infected lung disease. However, developments in operative technique and a greater understanding of the physiology of single lung transplantation will make it an increasingly valuable addition to intrathoracic organ transplantation.

This report outlines the current experience of heart and heart–lung transplantation as illustrated by the activities at Papworth Hospital. Since the transplant programme began in 1979 there has been a steady increase in the numbers performed annually, although the planned activity of 110 transplants for the year 1988 was not fulfilled due to scarcity of suitable donor organs. As transplantation becomes more successful, both for heart and heart–lung recipients, the demands on the service outgrow our ability to provide for them and approximately 20% of patients can be expected to die on the waiting list. It is for this reason that recipients for heart and heart–lung transplantation are carefully selected in an attempt to make the best use of the available resources.

As the longer term survival has improved in adult patients, heart and heart–lung transplantation for children and infants has become a more attractive proposition. As a result, in the last 2 years we have begun to expand transplantation into the paediatric field in association with The Hospital for Sick Children at Great Ormond Street.

ORGAN TRANSPLANTATION: CURRENT CLINICAL AND
IMMUNOLOGICAL CONCEPTS   ISBN 0-7020-1393-5

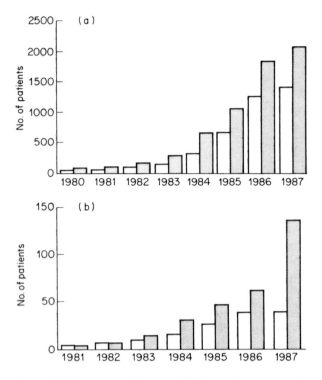

Figure 1. Number of (a) heart transplants and (b) heart–lung transplants performed in the United States (☐) only compared with the rest of the world (▦) from 1980–1987. From the International Society for Heart Transplantation.

HEART TRANSPLANTATION

Patients

Between November 1977 and October 1988, 1038 patients have been referred for transplantation. Of these, 617 have been assessed in hospital as being potentially suitable and 455 were accepted for transplantation. A subgroup of patients (40) were offered conventional cardiac surgery involving various conservative procedures.

As with all centres, our criteria for acceptance have been liberalized as results have improved. In particular, age limits have been relaxed so that patients are now accepted with an upper age limit of approximately 65 years. Many of the patients in their sixth decade have terminal cardiac failure as a result of severe coronary artery disease and this is now the single largest indication for heart transplantation. Patients with primary cardiomyopathy are the next largest group.

Of the 455 patients accepted for transplantation, 298 have received transplants. Eight have undergone a total of nine retransplants, one patient having been retransplanted twice after 3 and 6 years, for coronary occlusive disease on both occasions. The sex, age and diagnosis of the 298 patients transplanted are shown in Table 1.

Table 1. Cardiac transplantation, Papworth Hospital.
Patients transplanted by 31 October 1988.

Male	270
Female	28
Total	298
Age	
Mean	42
Range	6–63
Diagnosis	
Cardiomyopathy	138
Ischaemic heart disease	149
Other	11
Survival (15 days–8.8 years)	212

The Donor

The principal factor limiting cardiac transplant activity remains the supply of donor organs, and although access to suitable donor organs is increasing, the demand for cardiac transplantation is even greater. For this reason we have not felt it appropriate to accept patients from abroad for transplantation. Criteria for donor selection have also been relaxed as a result of demand and donors up to the age of 45 will now be considered for heart transplantation. Table 2 shows organs donated up to October 1988; over 50% of the donors in the UK are multi-organ donors. There is much current research directed towards better donor care. The recognition that major hormonal imbalances may occur along with massive fluid shifts following brain death is leading towards better donor management and the prospects of salvaging more hearts for transplantation. Nevertheless, despite improvements in preservation techniques over the years the upper limit for ischaemic time of the heart is still, for practical purposes, only 4 hours; early survival of patients receiving hearts with greater than 4 hours ischaemic time is less good.

Table 2. Cardiac transplantation, Papworth Hospital.
Donor organs harvested by 31 October 1988.

Donor organs	31st October 1988
Heart	307
Heart and lung	51
Kidney	695
Cornea	206
Liver	149
Pancreas	27
Lung	3

Some hearts are now becoming available for transplantation from patients receiving heart–lung transplantation, the so-called domino procedure. This increases the general organ pool and negates any criticism that heart–lung transplantation is denying patient access to the more established technique of heart transplantation.

Postoperative Management and Immunosuppression

The cardiac transplant operation itself has changed little in the last decade, and what used to be a service provided exclusively by consultants is now well within the capability of a trained senior registrar or chief resident. Postoperative management has been simplified and the need for barrier nursing in intensive care curtailed. At the beginning of the programme, 10 years ago, patients were expected to be barrier-nursed in the intensive care unit for some 4 weeks; this has now been reduced to 3 days. The majority of patients are able to leave hospital for intermediate care about 3 weeks following cardiac transplantation.

Table 3.   Cardiac transplantation, Papworth Hospital.

Patients	Immunosuppression
1–29	Azathioprine + steroids
30–89	Cyclosporin + low-dose steroids
90–150	Cyclosporin + steroids
	or
	Cyclosporin + azathioprine
151+	Triple therapy (see Figure 3)

There have been four distinct immunosuppressive protocols for cardiac transplantation since the programme began and these are shown in Table 3. The results have improved with each successive protocol and the current expected 1-year survival is 85% (Figure 2). Most cardiac transplant centres are adopting a protocol of triple therapy in an attempt to ameliorate the nephrotoxic effects of cyclosporin (Figure 3). All these protocols have included a prophylactic course of equine antithymocyte globulin, originally for 28 days but now for only 3.

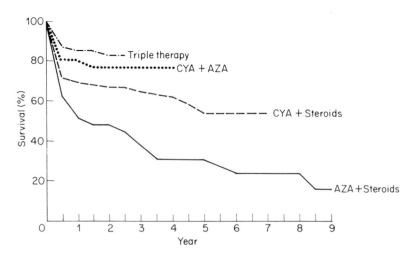

Figure 2.   Heart transplantation: patient survival according to the method of immuno-suppression.

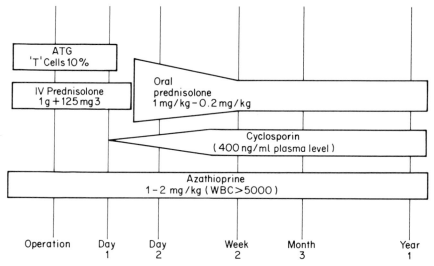

Figure 3.   Immunosuppression for cardiac transplantation.

Diagnosis of Rejection

The detection of rejection following cardiac transplantation relies on the histological appearances of endomyocardial biopsies. This technique introduced by Caves in 1973 has not been superseded by any reliable non-invasive methods. The use of echocardiography, sophisticated electrocardiogram measurements and cytoimmunological monitoring have all been used as adjuncts, but biopsies performed at decreasing frequency following transplantation remain the gold standard for the detection of rejection.

Results

The overall survival for heart transplantation in our series is shown in Figure 4. Since the

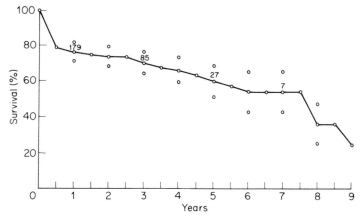

Figure 4.   Heart transplantation: patient survival in the Papworth series. Actuarial survival analysis has been performed on 298 patients available for follow-up: the indicated range is equivalent to twice the standard error.

introduction of cyclosporin, survival has improved (Figure 5). As previously illustrated (Figure 2), subgroups of patients treated with different cyclosporin-based regimens have shown an incremental improvement in survival with each regimen.

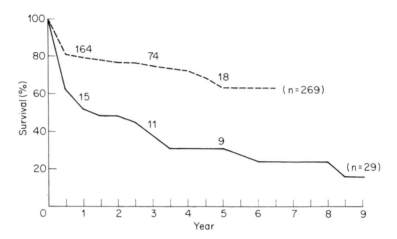

Figure 5.   Heart transplantation: patient survival depending on the type of immuno-suppression.

Table 4.   Cardiac transplantation at Papworth Hospital: causes of death (to 31 October 1988).

Causes of death	0–90 days	90 days–1 year	>1 year
		Time post-transplant	
Rejection	23	8	—
Infection	15	5	2
Coronary occlusive disease	—	1	13
Donor heart failure	5	—	—
Multifactorial	3	—	—
Pulmonary carcinoma	—	—	2
Lymphoma	1	—	—
Cerebrovascular event	4	1	—
Raised PVR	1		
Intestinal infarction	1		
Operative haemorrhage	1		
TOTAL	54	15	17

The causes of death are shown in Table 4. As might be anticipated, rejection and infection have been the principal causes of death during the first 3 months; indeed, it is during this period that most of the deaths occur. Both remain important causes of mortality during the remainder of the first year, but thereafter, accelerated coronary occlusive disease in the allografted heart becomes the most important determinant of survival. It is the incidence of this disease that will determine the long-term outlook for cardiac transplantation. Analysis of angiograms performed on an annual basis showed that the prevalence of significant angiographic coronary disease was 18% at 2 years and 25% at 5 years. Progressive coronary occlusion is an indication for retransplantation in appropriate patients. The aetiology of this condition is complex, but undoubtedly immunologically based; the incidence, time of onset, severity and rate of progress are variable and unpredictable. In some series, incidence has been related to the number of earlier rejection episodes and in a recent analysis at Stanford it has been related to the presence of cytomegalovirus (CMV) disease.

HEART–LUNG TRANSPLANTATION

Transplantation of the heart and lungs is progressing rapidly through its developmental phase, following the first successful operation in 1981. Since then there have been developments in distance procurement using both a simple pulmonary artery flush technique or cardiopulmonary bypass. In the last 2 years the development of an early, precise histological diagnosis of rejection using transbronchial biopsies has enabled patients to be better managed and has contributed to good survival (Wallwork, 1989).

Patients

There are three main groups of diseases for which heart–lung transplantation is appropriate: parenchymal lung disease, with or without secondary cardiac disease; primary cardiac disease associated with pulmonary hypertension (Eisenmenger's syndrome); and pulmonary vascular disease.

The criteria for patient acceptability have changed over the years. For instance, patients with cystic fibrosis are now accepted as potential candidates for heart–lung transplantation and may well form the single largest group of patients suitable for this surgery. The demand for heart–lung transplantation is large and increasing and thus recipients are selected carefully; moribund patients, or patients with pulmonary aspergillosis or multi-system disease, are not considered to be suitable candidates. In addition, because of the scarcity of suitable donor organs, emergency heart–lung transplantation is normally not available.

Since November 1982, 481 patients have been referred for heart–lung transplantation. Of these, 186 were admitted for a period of assessment and 118 were accepted as potential recipients. The diagnosis of the 51 patients who have been given transplants are shown in Table 5; in one of them a liver was transplanted simultaneously. Some 20% of patients have died awaiting a suitable organ. The upper age limit for acceptability for heart–lung transplantation has been arbitrarily set at 50 but even with this age limit the waiting list continues to lengthen.

Donors

Donors for heart–lung transplantation are even less available than donors for heart transplantation. Probably some 15–20% of donors suitable for heart transplantation would be suitable for heart–lung transplantation. The donor criteria for heart and lung donation are shown in Table 6. Rapid deterioration of the lungs can result from

Table 5.   Heart-lung transplantation, Papworth Hospital.
Diagnoses in patients transplanted April 1984 to 31 October 1988.

Age	
Mean	30
Range	11–53
Sex	
Male	24
Female	27
Diagnosis	
Eisenmenger's syndrome	14
Cystic fibrosis	11
Primary pulmonary hypertension	7
Thromboembolic pulmonary hypertension	2
Emphysema	3
Sarcoidosis	3
Fibrosing alveolitis	2
Histiocytosis X	2
Bronchiectasis	2
Systemic lupus erythmatosus + pulmonary hypertension	1
Cardiomyopathy + pulmonary hypertension	1
Pulmonary artery sarcoma	1
α_1 Antitrypsin deficiency	1
Primary biliary cirrhosis + pulmonary hypertension	1
Survival	37
Patients transplanted	51

Table 6.   Donor criteria in heart–lung transplantation.

Age <40 years (ideally)
ABO compatibility
Normal gas exchange
Good compliance and low ventilation pressures
Clear chest X-ray and no infections
Short period of ventilation
Appropriate size match for the recipient
Cytomegalovirus serology compatibility

inadequate monitoring of the donor and great care needs to be taken to avoid oedematous lungs. The quality of the donor lungs is extremely important in determining the ease of care in the immediate postoperative period, and, subsequently, the patient's chances of survival.

The sizes of the donor and recipient are matched according to the total lung capacity of the recipient measured at the time of assessment, and predicted values for the donor, based largely on the donor's height. The final comparison of chest X-rays is made at the donor hospital. A latex agglutination test for CMV is now used prospectively at the donor hospital to avoid primary CMV infection in the CMV-negative recipient by transplanting organs from a CMV-positive donor. As primary CMV disease has been a major cause of death in the early postoperative period we regard this as an important aspect of donor selection.

Until 1985 all donors for heart–lung transplantation were transported to the recipient hospital. Since then all donors in the UK have been obtained by long distance procurement. We have used a single flush technique, but others have used cardiopulmonary bypass and total body cooling for the donor. Using a single flush technique of extracellular fluid, combined with perioperative prostacyclin infusion, donor organ preservation has been satisfactory for up to 4 hours of ischaemia time. There have been no primary organ failures and early lung function has been poor in only two patients who received transplants from donors with oedematous lungs.

Postoperative Management and Immunosuppression

The operative techniques for heart–lung transplantation have been well described (Wallwork, 1989) and although this procedure is not yet as standard as heart transplantation and by its very nature more complex, the necessary stages of surgery are well worked out. The majority of patients are extubated within 24 hours following transplantation and a regimen similar to that described for heart transplantation is followed. The patients are barrier-nursed in the intensive care unit for 3 days and are often transferred to the ward before the end of the first week, where they will stay until their discharge at 3–4 weeks. Immunosuppression for heart–lung transplantation is based on cyclosporin and azathioprine, with steroids in reserve for rejection episodes. In addition, perioperative methyl prednisolone and a short, 3-day course of equine antithymocyte globulin is given (Figure 6).

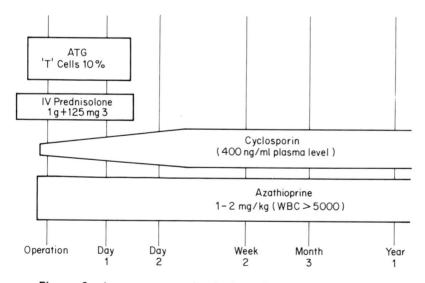

Figure 6.   Immunosuppression for heart–lung transplantation.

Diagnosis of Rejection

When clinical heart–lung transplantation began there was no reliable method of detecting lung rejection. This is no longer the case, thanks to developments at Papworth Hospital. Rejection is now diagnosed by a transbronchial biopsy: the indications for which include new clinical symptoms and signs, and alterations in chest X-ray or lung function. Transbronchial biopsies are also of use in distinguishing infection from rejection and in defining their coexistence. The routine use of endomyocardial biopsy has been shown to be of no value in the detection of rejection in heart–lung transplantation. It is likely that lung biopsy will be established as the gold standard against which less invasive methods of detecting rejection can be compared as they develop.

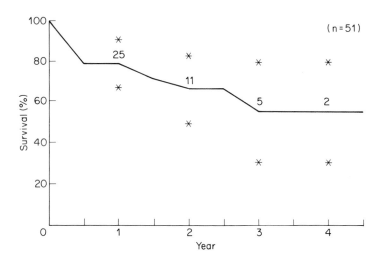

Figure 7.   Heart–lung transplantation: patient survival in the Papworth series; actuarial survival has been calculated on 51 patients who commenced therapy. The range indicated is two standard errors.

Table 7.   Heart–lung transplantation: causes of death to 31 October 1988.

Infection	
Cytomegalovirus	4
Other	2
Obliterative bronchiolitis	3
Infection/liver failure	1
Tracheal dehiscence	1
Cerebrovascular event	1
Infection/ruptured aorta	1
Small bowel infarction/Systemic lupus erythmatosus	1
TOTAL	14

Results

Fifty one patients have undergone heart–lung transplantation at Papworth Hospital and 37 are alive and well between 1 week and 54 months after surgery. The actuarial survival curve in Figure 7 shows a 78.7% 1-year survival rate. The causes of death are shown in

Table 7. The quality of life of these patients is good and comparable to patients having had heart transplants. The long-term complication of obliterative bronchiolitis, which is analogous to coronary occlusive disease in the donor heart in heart transplantation, is a continuing concern and will probably be the most important determinant of long-term survival. We believe that this condition is the result of persistent or undiagnosed rejection episodes and there are some indications that patients at risk can be diagnosed early in their postoperative period and have their immunosuppression enhanced accordingly. Nevertheless, the long-term results of heart-lung transplantation are as yet unknown.

REFERENCE

Wallwork J (ed.) (1989) *Heart and Heart–Lung Transplantation*. London: Grune & Stratton.

Id Summary of Clinical Data on Pancreas Transplants

DAVID E. R. SUTHERLAND
KAY C. MOUDRY-MUNNS

Pancreas transplantation as a treatment for diabetes mellitus has the following objectives: to establish a euglycaemic, insulin-independent state in the recipient and thereby prevent or halt the progression of complications of diabetes that afflict the eyes, nerves, kidneys and other organ systems. Abundant evidence supports the concept that the lesions developing in these systems after many years of diabetes are, indeed, secondary to disordered metabolism (Tchobroutsky, 1978).

Unlike heart and liver transplantation, pancreas transplants are not performed to save a life, but to improve the quality of life. The practice is akin to kidney transplantation, where the objective is to obviate the need for dialysis and to prevent the complications of chronic uraemia in patients with end-stage renal disease. Rejection of a kidney can be followed by a return to dialysis, just as rejection of a pancreas can be followed by a return to exogenous insulin therapy.

Pancreas transplants have been performed in diabetic patients since 1966 (Kelly et al, 1967). The earliest cases showed that a successful graft could establish a euglycaemic, insulin-independent state for many years, if not indefinitely (Lillehei et al, 1976; Gliedman et al, 1978). This state is achieved, however, at the cost of chronic immunosuppression. The need to provide anti-rejection therapy has limited the application of pancreas transplantation to recipients whose complications of diabetes are more serious than the potential side-effects of the immunosuppressive drugs, or to patients who are already immunosuppressed because of a previous or a simultaneous kidney transplant. Most pancreas transplant recipients receive a kidney transplant, but the number of non-uraemic, non-kidney transplant recipients has increased in recent years, particularly at the University of Minnesota (Sutherland et al, 1988a).

In this review of the current status of pancreas transplants, data are presented in three sections: (i) The Pancreas Transplant Registry – the results of pancreas transplants performed in all types of recipient worldwide; (ii) the Minnesota series which is the biggest series from a single centre currently available; (iii) a summary of the limited evidence from selected centres in which the effects of pancreas transplantation on diabetic sequelae have been studied.

ORGAN TRANSPLANTATION: CURRENT CLINICAL AND
IMMUNOLOGICAL CONCEPTS   ISBN 0-7020-1393-5

PANCREAS TRANSPLANT REGISTRY DATA

From December 1966 to July 1988, 1549 pancreas transplants were reported to the International Pancreas Transplant Registry (Figure 1). Patient and graft survival rates were calculated by actuarial techniques (Sutherland et al, 1988a). For the entire series, 1-year actuarial patient and graft survival rates were 80% and 40% (Sutherland et al, 1989). The results, however, have progressively improved with time (Figure 2). The one year actuarial patient and graft survival rates for 762 cases reported since 1985 were 88% and 55% respectively, significantly higher ($p < 0.01$) than in all previous periods examined.

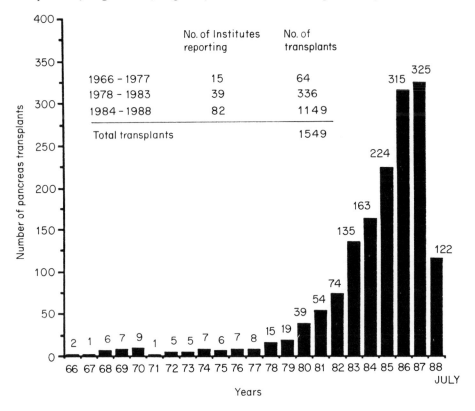

Figure 1. Number of pancreas transplants by year reported to the Registry from 17 December 1966 to 30 June 1988.

The effect of multiple variables on pancreas transplant results were determined in 1149 pancreas transplants performed from 1 January 1984 to 30 June 1988. The 1-year recipient and graft survival rates were 85% and 49% for all cases during this period.

A variety of surgical approaches have been used for management of the pancreatic duct and graft exocrine secretions, including duct-injection with a synthetic polymer, enteric drainage into the stomach or intestine, or urinary drainage into the ureter or bladder. When all 1984–88 cases were analysed, the functional survival rate curves for grafts transplanted by either of these approaches were not significantly different (Figure 3). However, when the least used techniques, drainage into the stomach or ureter, were

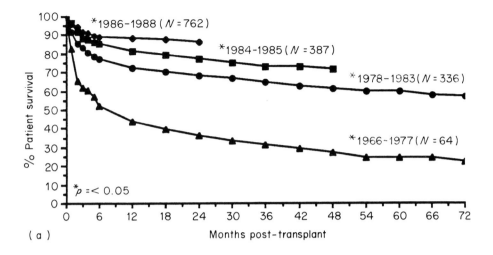

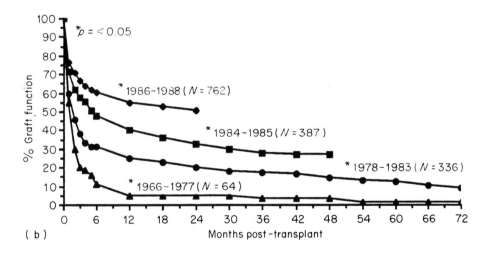

Figure 2. (a) Patient and (b) graft functional (insulin-independent) survival rates for pancreas transplant cases reported to the Registry according to era.

eliminated from the analysis, the most popular technique, bladder drainage was associated with a significantly higher ($p < 0.05$) functional survival rate (51% at 1 year) than was the third most popular, intestinal drainage (45% at 1 year); neither, however, differed significantly when compared to the second most popular technique, polymer injection (53% at 1 year). The functional survival rates were similar whether segmental or whole pancreas grafts were transplanted (50% v. 48% at 1 year), and there were no significant differences within the duct management categories for outcome according to type of graft (whole or segmental).

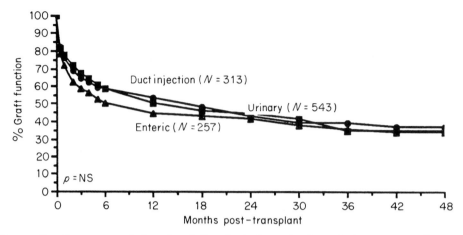

Figure 3. Pancreas graft functional (insulin-independent) survival rates according to the type of duct management for 1984–88 Registry cases.

Graft survival rates for 1984–88 cases, calculated according to preservation times, were 50%, 47%, 43% and 78% at 1 year for those stored for less than 6 hours ($n = 706$), 6–12 hours ($n = 243$), 12–24 hours ($n = 95$) and greater than 24 hours or more ($n = 9$). The results were not significantly different and preservation no longer seems to be a limiting factor in pancreatic transplantation (Abouna et al, 1987), especially with the advent of preservation solutions specifically designed for this organ (Florak et al, 1982; Wahlberg et al, 1987).

Immunosuppresive regimens that included both cyclosporin and azathioprine were associated with significantly ($p < 0.05$) higher graft survival rates than those that included only one or other of these drugs (Figure 4). The 1-year functional survival rates of technically successful grafts (those that did not fail for thrombosis, local infection bleeding or similar problems) were, respectively, 66, 56 and 47% in patients treated with azathioprine plus cyclosporin, cyclosporin without azathioprine, and azathioprine without cyclosporin.

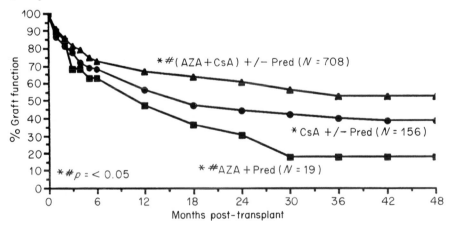

Figure 4. Pancreas graft functional (insulin-independent) survival rates according to immunosuppressive regimen for 1984–88 technically successful Registry cases. AZA, azathioprine; CsA, cyclosporin A; Pred, prednisone.

Minimizing the number of HLA antigen mismatches between the donor and recipient enhances cadaver pancreas graft survival rates (Squifflet et al, 1988). For technically successful 1984–88 cases, the functional survival rate was significantly ($p < 0.05$) higher for grafts mismatched for three or less HLA-A, -B and -DR antigens compared with grafts mismatched for four or more antigens (68% v. 59% at 1 year). The beneficial effect of minimizing mismatches was greatest at the DR loci (Figure 5). At 1 year the graft survival rates were 78% for cases with no DR mismatch versus 62% for 1 and 58% for 2 DR mismatches ($p < 0.02$).

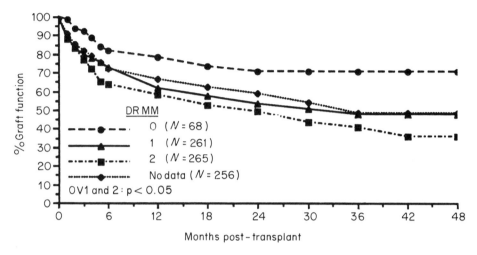

Figure 5. Pancreas graft functional (insulin-independent) survival rates according to number of HLA-DR mismatches (DR MM) with the recipient for 1984–88 technically successful cadaver donor Registry cases.

Pancreas graft survival rates for the 1984–88 Registry cases also differed according to whether a kidney was or was not transplanted and according to the timing of the kidney transplant. Thus, pancreas graft survival was 56, 42 and 32% at 1 year, respectively, for cases in which a kidney was transplanted simultaneously ($n = 763$), previously ($n = 197$), or not at all ($n = 189$). Functional survival rates were significantly higher ($p < 0.05$) for pancreatic grafts transplanted simultaneously with a kidney to patients with end-stage diabetic nephropathy (ESDN) (a) than for those transplanted to patients with ESDN who had received a kidney prior to the pancreas (b) or those transplanted to non-uraemic, non-kidney transplant patients as a pancreas graft alone (c). However, patient survival rates in these three categories were 82% (a), 91% (b), and 92% (c) at 1 year, the first differing significantly from the other two categories ($p < 0.05$). Within these three groups there appears to be a converse relationship between pancreas transplant success and patient mortality: the patient survival rates are the lowest in that group which has the highest graft survival rate, namely the recipients of simultaneous kidney transplants. In recipients of simultaneous pancreas and kidney transplants in the entire 1984–88 period ($n = 761$), the overall 1-year kidney graft survival rate was 72%. Loss of pancreas function with continuation of kidney function was more common than vice versa (Sutherland and Moudry, 1987). Within each of the major duct management categories, the pancreas graft functional survival rates were highest for recipients of a simultaneous kidney transplant (Table 1). The same relative differences were seen as in the overall 1984–88 analysis.

The results of pancreas transplantation continue to improve. In an analysis of all cases reported to the Registry for 1986–88 ($n = 762$), the 1-year patient and graft survival rates were 96 and 36%, respectively, for non-uraemic, non-kidney transplant recipients of a pancreas transplant alone ($n = 120$); 93 and 48% for recipients of a pancreas after a kidney ($n = 123$); and 85 and 61% for uraemic recipients of a simultaneous pancreas/kidney ($n = 519$). In the latter group the 1-year *kidney* graft survival rate was 78%, similar to that reported for cyclosporin-treated uraemic diabetic recipients of kidney transplants alone by the UCLA Kidney Transplant Registry (see Terashita and Cook, 1987).

Table 1. Cadaveric pancreas graft survival rates according to duct management techniques and recipient category for cases reported to the registry from 1 January, 1985 to 30 June, 1988.

	Bladder drainage		Intestinal drainage		Polymer injection	
	No. cases	1 yr function	No. cases	1 yr function	No. cases	1 yr function
All cases						
Pancreas + kidney	323	59%[a,b]	137	56%[c,d]	263	57%[f]
Pancreas after kidney	140	44%[a]	40	33%[c]	15	53%
Pancreas alone	72	33%[b]	80	32%[d]	35	29%[f]
Technically successful cases						
Pancreas + kidney	275	70%[g,h]	103	71%[i]	213	70%[i]
Pancreas after kidney	106	58%[g]	23	56%	8	88%
Pancreas alone	56	43%[h]	53	48%[i,k]	29	36%[i,k]

$p < 0.05$ for comparisons indicated by letter superscripts, i.e: a v. a: $p < 0.05$; b v. b: $p < 0.05$, etc.

RESULTS OF PANCREAS TRANSPLANTATION AT THE UNIVERSITY OF MINNESOTA

The differences in transplant outcome according to recipient status, surgical approach and donor source are illustrated by an analysis of results at one institution with a relatively large experience in all categories (Sutherland et al, 1988b). From July 1978 to July 1988, 230 pancreas transplants were performed at the University of Minnesota; 71 grafts are currently functioning, the longest for 10 years. Since October 1984, a uniform immuno-suppressive protocol has been used: antilymphocyte globulin, cylcosporin, azathioprine, and prednisone initially and the last three drugs for maintenance anti-rejection therapy. During this period 130 transplants were performed, 67 in non-uraemic, non-kidney recipients, 33 in recipients of a previous kidney, and 30 in recipients of a simultaneous kidney; 84 grafts were anastomosed to the bladder and 43 to the bowel; and 26 were from related and 104 from cadaver donors. The overall patient survival rate at 1 year was 91%, and there were no significant differences between the various categories and subcategories created by combinations of recipient characteristics and techniques used for transplantation.

Graft survival rates, however, differed between the various categories and subcategories. With bladder drainage, 1 year insulin-independent rates were 48% in recipients of a pancreas transplant alone ($n = 36$), 48% with a pancreas after a kidney ($n = 20$), and 71% following a simultaneous pancreas–kidney transplant ($n = 28$). With enteric drainage, 1-year insulin-independent rates were 38% for pancreas transplants alone ($n = 32$) and 36% for the pancreas after a kidney graft ($n = 11$) (enteric drainage was not done in the double transplant patients). Because of the high propensity for rejection episodes of grafts from cadaver donors, and an inability to diagnose rejection episodes early with enteric drainage, this approach is no longer used for cadaveric transplants. The best results were in recipients of bladder-drained cadaver donor and enteric or bladder-drained related donor grafts, and these approaches are currently being applied exclusively. Bladder drainage allows for early diagnosis and successful treatment of rejection based on urinary amylase monitoring (Sollinger et al, 1984; Prieto et al, 1987a). The incidence of rejection episodes is much lower for transplants from related donors and enteric drainage can be applied with a high success rate in this specific situation, but with cadaver donors the results at the University of Minnesota were clearly better with bladder drainage for recipients of pancreas transplants alone (Prieto et al, 1987b).

Table 2. Patient and graft functional survival rates at 1 year for pancreas transplants performed at the University of Minnesota from October 1984 to January 1988 by techniques in current use*.

Category	No. transplants	No. transplants	Patient survival	Graft survival	
				All[†]	TS[‡]
Pancreas + kidney	28	26	91%	71%	77%
Pancreas after kidney	27	14	87%	47%	85%
Pancreas alone	52	41	96%	48%	62%
TOTAL	107	81	93%	54%	71%

* Bladder drainage for all cadaver donor transplants ($n = 81$) and enteric drainage ($n = 23$) or bladder drainage ($n = 3$) for related donor segmental transplants.
[†] All cases, with successful cases and cases that failed for either rejection or technical reasons (thrombosis, infection, etc.) included in the analysis.
[‡] Technically successful cases (cases that failed for technical reasons not included in analysis–see text).

The results of an analysis of 107 pancreas transplants performed at the University of Minnesota since October 1984 by the approaches in current use are shown in Table 2. The functional survival rates are highest in uraemic recipients of simultaneous kidney transplants, but with quadruple immunosuppressive therapy long-term function can be achieved in nearly half of non-uraemic recipients of pancreas transplants alone.

THE COURSE OF PRE-EXISTING SECONDARY COMPLICATIONS OF DIABETES FOLLOWING SUCCESSFUL PANCREAS TRANSPLANTATION

Information on the course of secondary complications after pancreas transplantation is only just beginning to emerge. Most of that data are difficult to interpret because the majority of pancreas transplant recipients have also received a kidney at the same time, and uraemia as well as diabetes were simultaneously corrected; without a control group of kidney transplants alone the effect of the pancreas transplant *per se* on retinopathy and neuropathy in this group cannot be discerned.

In a study from Stockholm (Solders et al, 1987), electrophysiological measurements showed minimal improvement in neuropathy in diabetic recipients of kidney transplants, regardless of whether they received a simultaneous pancreas transplant. However, the Stockholm group also found that the development of microscopic lesions of diabetic nephropathy in kidneys transplanted to diabetic recipients was prevented by simultaneous transplantation of a pancreas (Bohman et al, 1985). Similar observations have been made at the University of Minnesota (Bilous et al, 1988). Patients who received a kidney followed by pancreas transplant had no or minimal lesions of diabetic nephropathy in follow-up biopsies of the transplanted kidney, in contrast to the uniform development of recurrence of disease in recipients of a kidney transplant alone (Mauer et al, 1983).

Studies at the University of Minnesota have, likewise, shown an objective improvement in nerve conduction velocities following pancreas transplantation in patients who were non-uraemic at the time of the transplant (Van der Vliet et al, 1988). With regard to retinopathy, patients with early failure of their pancreas transplant (<3 months) were compared with those with a functional (>1 year) graft (Ramsay et al, 1988). The progression of retinopathy during the first 2 years post-transplant did not differ in the two groups, but over a longer period (>3 years) the patients with functioning pancreas grafts appeared to be more stable. Finally, studies of microscopic lesions of diabetic nephropathy in native kidneys of non-uraemic, non-kidney recipients of pancreas transplants alone showed a reduction in glomerular mesangial volume at 2 years in patients with functioning grafts (Bilous et al, 1987).

These studies show that establishment of a euglycaemic state by pancreas transplantation has a favourable influence on the course of diabetic neuropathy and early nephropathy, and the beneficial effect is seen within the first 2 years of transplantation. Further, there appears to be a beneficial effect on the course of retinopathy, but the stabilizing influence of euglycaemia is not seen until more than 2 years post-transplant.

COMMENTS

Pancreas transplantation is currently the only method of treatment that can establish a constant euglycaemic state in a diabetic patient. The surgical risk has progressively decreased, and it is now so low that many centres now routinely perform pancreas transplants in diabetic individuals who are already committed to immunosuppression, namely kidney transplant recipients (Corry et al, 1986; Sollinger et al, 1987; Tyden et al, 1987; Cosimi et al, 1988; Sutherland et al, 1988b). Its application to non-uraemic, non-kidney transplant recipients is more limited (University of Michigan, 1988), and is generally restricted to diabetic patients who have problems of diabetes more serious than the potential side-effects of the immunosuppressive therapy (Sutherland, 1988). Rejection continues to be a problem, particularly in non-uraemic, non-kidney transplant recipients, but the bladder drainage technique, introduced at the University of Wisconsin a few years ago (Sollinger et al, 1984), allows an early diagnosis to be made based on urinary amylase excretion (Sollinger et al, 1984; Prieto et al, 1987a). This innovation, coupled with improved immunosuppressive regimens (combination therapy with low doses of cyclosporin, azathioprine, and prednisone for maintenance immunosuppression and the use of antilymphocyte globulin or OKT3 monoclonal antibody for treatment of rejection), have dramatically improved the results of pancreatic transplantation. Pancreas transplantation will be applicable to the general diabetic population, including those who have not yet shown themselves to be prone to complications, but only when totally effective, non-toxic anti-rejection strategies are available. For the time being, the restrictions described above should be applied, but this still leaves a substantial number of diabetic patients, both uraemic and non-uraemic, who are appropriate candidates for pancreas transplantation.

REFERENCES

Abouna GM, Sutherland DER, Florack G & Najarian JS (1987) Function of transplanted human pancreatic allografts after preservation in cold storage for 6–26 hours. *Transplantation* **43**: 630–635.

Bilous RW, Mauer SM, Sutherland DER & Steffes MW (1987) Glomerular structure and function following successful pancreas transplantation for insulin-dependent diabetes mellitus. *Diabetes* **36**: 43A.

Bilous RW, Mauer SM, Sutherland DER et al (1989) The effects of pancreas transplantation on the glomerular structure of renal allografts in patients with insulin-dependent (type I) diabetes mellitus. *New England Journal of Medicine* **321**: 80–85.

Bohman SO, Tyden G & Wilezek A (1985) Prevention of kidney graft diabetic nephropathy by pancreas transplantation in man. *Diabetes* **34**: 306.

Corry RJ, Nghiem DD, Schulak JA, Beutell WD & Gonwa TA (1986) Surgical treatment of diabetic nephropathy with simultaneous pancreatic duodenal and renal transplantation. *Surgery Gynecology and Obstetrics* **162**: 547–555.

Cosimi AB, Auchiniloss H, Delmonico F et al (1988) Combined kidney and pancreas transplantation in diabetics. *Archives of Surgery* **123**: 621–628.

Florack G, Sutherland DER, Heil J, Zweber B & Najarian JS (1982) Long term preservation of segmental pancreas autografts. *Surgery* **92**: 260–269.

Gliedman ML, Tellis VA, Soberman R et al (1978) Long-term effects of pancreatic transplant function in patients with advanced juvenile onset diabetes. *Diabetes Care* **1**: 1–9.

Kelly WD, Lillehei RC, Merkel FK, Idezuki Y & Goetz FC (1967) Allotransplantation of the pancreas and duodenum along with the kidney in diabetic nephropathy. *Surgery* **61**: 827.

Lillehei RC, Ruiz JO, Acquino C & Goetz FC (1976) Transplantation of the pancreas. *Acta Endocrinologica* **83** (supplement 205): 303.

Mauer SM, Steffes MW, Connett J et al (1983) Development of lesions in glomerular basement membrane and mesangium after transplantation of normal kidneys to diabetic patients. *Diabetes* **32**: 948–952.

Prieto M, Sutherland DER, Goetz FC, Rosenberg & Najarian JS (1987a) Pancreas transplant results according to technique of duct management: bladder versus enteric drainage. *Surgery* **102**: 680–691.

Prieto M, Sutherland DER, Fernandez-Cruz L, Heil J & Najarian JS (1987b) Experimental and clinical experience with urine amylase monitoring for early diagnosis of rejection in pancreas transplantation. *Transplantation* **43**: 71–79.

Ramsay RC, Goetz FC, Sutherland DER et al (1988) Progression of diabetic retinopathy after pancreas transplantation for insulin-dependent diabetes mellitus. *New England Journal of Medicine* **318**: 208–214.

Solders G, Gunnarsson R, Persson A et al (1987) Effects of combined pancreatic and renal transplantation on diabetic neuropathy: a two-year follow-up study. *Lancet* **ii**: 1232–1235.

Sollinger HW, Cook K, Kamps D et al (1984) Clinical and experimental experience with pancreaticocystostomy for exocrine pancreatic drainage in pancreas transplantation. *Transplantation Proceedings* **16**: 749–751.

Sollinger HW, Stratta RJ, Kalayoglu M et al (1987) Pancreas transplantation with pancreatico-cystostomy and quadruple immunosuppression. *Surgery* **102**: 674–679.

Squifflet JP, Moudry K & Sutherland DER (1988) Is HLA matching relevant in pancreas transplantation? *Transplant International* **1**: 26–29.

Sutherland DER (1988) Who should get a pancreas transplant? *Diabetes Care* **11**: 681–685.

Sutherland DER & Moudry KC (1987) Report of the International Pancreas Transplantation Registry. In Terasaki PI (ed.) *Clinical Transplants*, pp 63–101. Los Angeles: UCLA Tissue Typing Laboratory.

Sutherland DER, Kendall DM, Moudry KC et al (1988a) Pancreas transplantation in nonuremic, type I diabetic recipients. *Surgery* **104**: 453–464.

Sutherland DER, Goetz FC, Moudry KC & Najarian JS (1988b) Pancreatic transplantation – a single institution's experience. *Diabetes, Nutrition and Metabolism* **1**: 57–66.

Sutherland DER, Moudry KC & Fryd DS (1989). Pancreas Transplant Registry Report. *Transplantation Proceedings* **21**: 2759–2762.

Tchobroutsky G (1978) Relation of diabetes control to development of microvascular complications. *Diabetologia* **15**: 143–152.

Terashita GY & Cook JD (1987) Original disease of the recipient. In Terasaki PI (ed.) *Clinical Transplants*, pp 373–379. Los Angeles: UCLA Tissue Typing Laboratory.

Tyden G, Brattstrom C, Lundgren G et al (1987) Improved results in pancreatic transplantation by avoidance nonimmunological graft failures. *Transplantation* **43**: 674–676.

University of Michigan Pancreas Transplant Evaluation Committee (1988) Pancreatic transplantation as treatment of 1 DDM: Proposed candidate evaluation before end stage diabetic nephropathy. *Diabetes Care* **11**: 669–675.

van der Vliet JA, Navarro X, Kenedy WR et al (1988) The effect of pancreas transplantation on diabetic polyneuropathy. *Transplantation* **45**: 368–370.

Wahlberg JA, Lowe R, Landegaard L et al (1987) 72 Hour preservation of the canine pancreas. *Transplantation* **43**: 5–7.

le Allogeneic Bone Marrow Transplantation

F.E. ZWAAN   J.M.J.J. VOSSEN
W.E. FIBBE   E.C. GORDON-SMITH
T. de WITTE   J.M. GOLDMAN

In recent decades, marrow transplants from genetically non-identical (allogeneic) donors have been used to treat patients with a variety of haematological disorders and inborn errors of metabolism (Table 1) (Buckner and Clift, 1984; Gluckman et al, 1984; O'Reilly et al, 1984; Speck et al, 1984; Storb et al, 1984; Zwaan and Jansen, 1984). Most human bone marrow donors are HLA-identical siblings. More recently, selected patients received transplants from HLA-partially matched related donors (Beatty et al, 1985) or matched unrelated donors (Gingrich et al, 1985). The basic principles of bone marrow transplantation have been extensively reviewed (O'Reilly, 1983) and will not be discussed in this chapter. A number of regimens, most of them including the use of cyclophosphamide, have been designed to induce sufficient immunosuppression of the recipient in order to allow optimal engraftment (Van Bekkum, 1984). Chemotherapy and radiation produce a dose-dependent anti-tumour effect. The highest tolerated dose can be substantially escalated, however, if followed by transplantation of normal bone marrow to restore haematopoiesis. There is also evidence that transplantation of allogeneic bone marrrow may confer an immune-mediated graft-versus-leukaemia effect (Gale and Champlin, 1984).

Table 1. Current indications for bone marrow transplantation.

Acute non-lymphoblastic leukaemia
Acute lymphoblastic leukaemia
Chronic myeloid leukaemia
Hairy-cell leukaemia
Hodgkin's and non-Hodgkin's lymphoma
Multiple myeloma
Aplastic anaemia; Fanconi anaemia
Thalassaemia
Severe combined immune deficiencies
Inborn errors of metabolism
Myelodysplastic syndromes (e.g. preleukaemia)
Miscellaneous (e.g. myelofibrosis, chronic lymphoid leukaemia)

ORGAN TRANSPLANTATION: CURRENT CLINICAL AND
IMMUNOLOGICAL CONCEPTS   ISBN 0-7020-1393-5

Table 2. Potential complications of allogeneic bone marrow transplantation.

Toxicity of the pre-transplant conditioning regimen
Graft rejection or failure
Acute graft-versus-host disease
Chronic graft-versus-host disease
Interstitial pneumonitis
Post-transplant immune deficiency
Opportunistic infections

Bone marrow transplantation is an effective treatment modality for various diseases; it does, however, carry substantial risks for the recipient and is associated with a number of serious potential complications (Table 2) (Champlin and Gale, 1984; Sullivan et al, 1984). The cumulative transplant related mortality varies between 25 and 35%. Therefore the ultimate results of marrow transplantation, in terms of disease-free survival, must be carefully compared with more conventional approaches of treatment (Gale and Champlin, 1983).

We will summarize the current results of allogeneic bone marrow transplantation for its major indications. Most of the references relate to review articles.

RESULTS

Clinical Results of Allogeneic Bone Marrow Transplantation for Acute Leukaemia

Marrow grafting has emerged as an important therapy for *acute myeloid leukaemia (AML)*, and is the treatment of choice for selected patients with defined circumstances. The initial transplants for AML were performed in patients with advanced disease. Several centres reported 10–20% long-term ($\geq$ 5 years) disease-free survival in resistant AML patients receiving transplants from HLA-identical siblings (Thomas, 1969; Zwaan and Jansen, 1984). Improved results are achieved when bone marrow transplantation is performed in remission (Zwaan et al, 1984a,b; Doney et al, 1987). The rationale for this approach is to perform the transplantation when the leukaemia cell burden is low and before the development of resistant disease. From the available data, obtained from large single-centre studies and from large registry data (International Bone Marrow Transplant Registry [IBMTR], European Cooperative Group for Bone Marrow Transplantation [EBMT]), the representative results are summarized in Table 3 (Gale et al, 1982; Gratwohl et al, 1987, 1988).

Adults in the age of 20–50 years have substantially poorer results in bone marrow transplantation than patients under the age of 20 (Zwaan et al, 1985). Therefore in adults it remains unclear whether bone marrow transplantation, especially in first remission, is superior to post-remission intensive chemotherapy (Champlin and Gale, 1987).

Results have also been improved for patients with *acute lymphoblastic leukaemia (ALL)* using bone marrow transplantation in first or second remission (Gale et al, 1983; Herzig et al, 1987; Ringden et al, 1987). In patients with more advanced disease, actuarial relapse rates continue to exceed 60%, and the 2–4 years disease-free survival rate is approximately 25%.

Table 3. Results of allogeneic bone marrow transplantation from HLA-identical siblings for AML*.

Disease status	Disease-free survival[†] (%)	Relapse[‡] (%)
1st remission <20 years old	50 (40–70)	30 (15–45)
1st remission ≥20 years old	35 (30–50)	30 (15–45)
2nd or later remission	25 (15–50)	50 (40–70)

* Determined from literature review.
[†] Three-year disease-free survival probability.
[‡] Actuarial relapse probability.

Patients in first or second remission have a lower relapse rate, approximately 30%, and 30–50% are alive at 2–4 years post-transplant. The IBMTR analysed individuals with high-risk factor at diagnosis (B- or T-cell ALL, age >21 years, white blood cell count >50 × 10^9/l, central nervous system-leukaemia, or chromosomal abnormalities associated with an adverse prognosis [t(9;22); t(4;11)] who were transplanted in first versus second remission (Herzig et al, 1987). Actuarial survival was 60% for patients transplanted in first remission compared with 45% in these high-risk patients transplanted in second remission. Actuarial relapse rates were 20% and 60%, respectively.

Children with ALL associated with standard risk factors have a relatively good prognosis with chemotherapy and should not be considered for bone marrow transplantation in first remission. It is controversial whether adult ALL patients should receive bone marrow transplants in first remission or whether it should be reserved for patients with a relapse.

There is a clear need for prospective controlled trials of chemotherapy versus transplantation in ALL before definitive conclusions are possible.

Clinical Results of Allogeneic Bone Marrow Transplantation for Chronic Myeloid Leukaemia

The clinical results are relatively consistent between different centres using different transplant protocols (Goldman, 1987) and can be summarized best by reference to data collected by the European and International Registries. In 1986 the IBMTR compared results of BMT performed in different phases of *chronic myeloid leukaemia (CML)*. The actuarial probability of survival and disease-free survival were higher and of relapse lower for patients transplanted in chronic phase than for those transplanted in later phases of the disease (Table 4). It is notable, however, both in the IBMTR data and in the results reported independently from Seattle, that about 15% of patients transplanted in blastic transformation become long-term, disease-free survivors.

The IBMTR has recently analysed results of BMT performed for 405 patients transplanted in chronic phase in 82 centres in 27 countries (Goldman et al, 1988). The actuarial probabilities for survival and relapse for the whole group were 55 ± 5% (mean ± 95% confidence interval) and 19 ± 8% respectively (Table 4). The major determinants of relapse were the use of T cell depletion of donor marrow and the absence of chronic graft-versus-host disease (GVHD). These collected results are consistent with the data reported from individual centres with one notable exception. Thus the Seattle group has reported a significant relationship between the interval between diagnosis and transplant and the probability of survival post-transplant (Thomas et al, 1986).

Table 4. Results of HLA-identical sibling transplants in chronic myeloid leukaemia analysed by phases of disease at time of transplant.

| Phase | No. | Four-year actuarial probability* of | | |
		Relapse	Survival	LFS
Chronic	405	19 ± 8	55 ± 5	46 ± 6
Accelerated	292	47 ± 12	33 ± 6	25 ± 7
Blastic	69	53 ± 19	15 ± 10	15 ± 9

*Data are expressed as mean percentage values ±95% confidence interval. The data were collected and analysed by the International Bone Marrow Transplant Registry and presented in 1987.
LFS, leukaemia-free survival.

Given then the fact that the transplant should be performed before the onset of acceleration or transformation, the question remains of *when* within the chronic phase. If the risk of a patient entering transformation in any given year on the one hand and the risk of death as a complication of the transplant procedure on the other could both be estimated for a given patient, one could then construct a model that predicts the point after diagnosis when the former risk will begin to exceed the latter. In practice there must be many caveats to this approach into clinical decision-making and other more subjective factors must also be considered.

There is still considerable uncertainty as to the optimal conditioning regimen for the patient with CML in chronic phase. The majority of patients have been transplanted after treatment with high-dose cyclophosphamide and total body irradiation (TBI) but the use of single dose versus fractionated TBI may give comparable results. Whether the patient's spleen should be removed, irradiated or left unmolested before transplant is not yet resolved.

T-cell depletion of donor marrow reduces the incidence and severity of GVHD, as it does after transplantation for acute leukaemia, but is associated with a highly significant increased risk of relapse (Goldman et al, 1988). Preliminary results using unmanipulated donor marrow and the combination of cyclosporin and methotrexate for GVHD prophylaxis look encouraging (Storb et al, 1986).

Interest has focused recently on the possibility that the use of matched unrelated donors might yield clinical results comparable to those achieved with HLA-identical sibling donors. At the Hammersmith Hospital in London in 1985 a programme was initiated in which patients received increased immune suppression (involving infusion of anti-T-cell monoclonal antibodies pre-transplant and addition of total lymphoid irradiation), increased anti-leukaemic therapy and transfusion of marrow cells from an HLA-identical unrelated donor that were depleted of T cells. Thus far 16 patients have received such transplants and 12 survive at a median follow-up of 9 months. These results are sufficiently encouraging to warrant continuation of the study. While the methodology for identifying unrelated donors is still in its infancy and consequently slow, CML is the ideal disease for this approach because there is often no immediate urgency to transplant.

Clinical Results of Allogeneic Bone Marrow Transplantation for Myelodysplastic Syndromes

An increasing incidence of myelodysplastic syndromes (MDS) has been observed in younger patients, mainly following irradiation or chemotherapy (Pedersen-Bjergaard et al, 1981). The results of chemotherapy in leukaemias secondary to MDS have been disappointing with reported remission rates of about 10% (Kantarjian et al, 1986) and short median survival time.

Young patients with a histocompatible sibling are potential candidates for allogeneic bone marrow transplantation. Marmont and Tura (1986) reviewed the recent literature and they described seven cases, including two new patients. Six patients received a transplant as primary therapy for their disease. All achieved a complete remission and no relapse had occurred at the time of writing. Five out of the six patients had refractory anaemia or refractory anaemia with excess of blasts (RAEB). Appelbaum et al (1987) reported the results in 23 patients with refractory anaemia or RAEB, treated with TBI and cyclophosphamide, followed by allogeneic bone marrow transplantation. Twelve of the patients were alive and disease-free at the time of reporting. Two patients with RAEB had recurrent disease. In the City of Hope Hospital in Duarte, 20 patients were transplanted for advanced preleukaemic conditions (O'Donnell et al, 1987). Increased marrow blasts ($> 10\%$) seemed to have a negative impact on disease-free survival. Three of four relapses were in this group; only two of ten patients with this pretransplant characteristic survive, as compared with six of ten patients who had less than 10% marrow blasts when preparation for bone marrow transplantation was begun.

Recently the Leukaemia Working Party of the EBMT conducted a survey in patients transplanted for MDS or secondary AML (De Witte et al, 1988). Data were collected on 44 patients from 17 centres. Intensive chemotherapy with the option to induce remission prior to transplantation was given to 17 patients. A complete remission was achieved in seven patients; the remaining ten patients were transplanted during hypoplasia or when a partial remission was achieved. Table 5 summarizes the disease status at transplant and the results.

Table 5. Allogeneic bone marrow transplantation in myelodysplastic syndromes and secondary leukaemia.

Disease status at BMT	No.	Relapse	Transplant-related mortality	Alive in CCR
Complete remission	7	0	3	4
Partial remission	2	1	1	0
Hypoplasia	8	3	3	2
AML	8	3	4	1
RAEBt*	8	1	1	6
RAEB†	5	1	2	2
RA‡	6	1	1	4

* Refractory anaemia with excess of blasts in transformation.
† Refractory anaemia with excess of blasts.
‡ Refractory anaemia.

From these results and those from the literature it can be concluded that allogeneic bone marrow transplantation in young patients with MDS is feasible. This treatment approach is associated with a good prognosis when the transplant is performed during the 'preleukaemic' phase. Transplantations performed during overt AML, or AML not in complete remission after transformation to overt leukaemia, have a relatively poor prognosis comparable to relapsed de novo AML. However, bone marrow transplantation performed after induction of complete remission with intensive chemotherapy results in excellent disease-free survival comparable to bone marrow transplantation for de novo AML in complete remission. This does not necessarily imply that each patient with AML secondary to MDS should receive intensive chemotherapy prior to the conditioning of bone marrow transplantation. Especially secondary leukaemias with hypocellular or myelofibrotic bone marrow are not likely to respond favourably to intensive chemotherapy.

Clinical Results of Allogeneic Bone Marrow Transplantation for non-Hodgkin's Lymphoma

In the majority of patients failing to respond to primary treatment or those with relapsed lymphoma, long-term disease-free survival cannot be obtained with salvage regimens. In these patients the use of high-dose chemotherapy and/or TBI followed by infusion of previously cryopreserved autologous bone marrow seems a promising approach, provided that no tumour involvement of the bone marrow is present. In particular, patients in second or with a responding relapse do well after such a therapy and appear to have a 2-year survival rate of approximately 40% (Philip et al, 1987). In patients with bone marrow involvement, allogeneic bone marrow transplantation performed in first or subsequent remission represents an alternative approach. This applies particularly to patients with high-grade malignant lymphoma, who often have primary bone marrow involvement. In a recent survey of the EBMT a total number of 85 patients (including children) were reported to have received an allogeneic marrow graft from an HLA-identical sibling donor (Dr P. Ernst, personal communication, 1988). The characteristics of these patients are summarized in Table 6. All but two patients received TBI as part of the conditioning regimen, in 65% of cases in combination with cyclophosphamide. Of the 22 patients transplanted in partial response or at relapse of the disease 15 (68%) entered complete remission after transplantation; four of these (27%) subsequently relapsed and died. Since in these patients the toxic death rate is also high, the overall outcome is poor (Table 7). In patients with high-grade lymphoma, transplantation in first or second remission appears to be a promising approach, particularly for patients with bone marrow involvement.

For patients with intermediate grade lymphoma with bone marrow involvement, allogeneic transplantation can be considered as salvage treatment in second remission or in responsive relapse. In the absence of bone marrow involvement autologous bone marrow transplantation may also be considered. Very few patients with low-grade lymphoma have undergone allogeneic bone marrow transplantation during the indolent phase of the disease. However, there are not yet sufficient data to evaluate this approach critically.

Table 6.   Allogeneic bone marrow transplantation in lymphoma (EBMT); patient characteristics.

			No.	%
Median age (yr)	22	Stage at diagnosis		
Range	3–43			
		I	2	2
Sex (male/female)	58/27	II	4	5
		III	10	12
Bone marrow involvement		IV	69	81
before BMT				
No. of patients	45	Disease category		
%	53	Intermediate grade	6	7
		Lymphoblastic	50	59
Central nervous system		Burkitt	11	13
involvement before BMT		Other high grade	18	21
No. of patients	11	malignant lymphoma		
%	13			
Median time interval				
from diagnosis to BMT				
(months)	7			
Range	2–50			

Table 7.   Results of allogeneic bone marrow transplantation in lymphoma (EBMT).

Disease status at BMT	No.	%	Toxic death (%)	Relapse (%)	Alive and well (%)	5 years DFS* (%)
1st remission	38	45	13	21	66	70
2nd remission	19	22	16	26	58	55
>3rd remission	6	7	17	33	50	18 at 30 months
Partial response + relapse	22	26	41	50	9	

* DFS, disease-free survival.

Clinical Results of Allogeneic Bone Marrow Transplantation for Multiple Myeloma

Multiple myeloma represents a disseminated haematologic malignancy for which curative chemotherapy is not yet available. With standard treatment, such as melphalan, prednisone, responses can be obtained in 50–60% of untreated patients resulting in a median survival of approximately 30 months (Bergsagel et al, 1979).

Allogeneic bone marrow transplantation has been performed in a limited number of patients with multiple myeloma. Within the EBMT, 36 patients have been transplanted (Dr G. Gahrton, personal communication, 1988). Seven patients were in first-line chemotherapy and 29 were receiving salvage treatment at the time of bone marrow transplantation. In one patient the conditioning regimen for transplantation consisted of melphalan only, all other patients received cytotoxic drugs and TBI. The results are summarized in Table 8. Lytic bone lesions persisted after transplantation in the majority of patients, also in those who had no other signs of active myeloma. The optimal timing for transplantation cannot be concluded from these data, although it is likely that transplantation at an earlier stage than in the present material would improve the results. These preliminary data suggest that a small subset of patients with multiple myeloma may benefit from allogeneic bone marrow transplantation. Important issues to be resolved remain the selection of optimal preparative regimens to eliminate the malignant clone, and the optimal timing for transplantation.

Table 8. Allogeneic bone marrow transplantation in multiple myeloma (EBMT).

			No. of patients
No. of patients	36	Complete remission after BMT*	18
		Early death	13
Median age (yr)	39	Transplant-related death	11
Range	29–53	Persistent disease	5
		Relapse	3
Disease status at BMT (Stage)			
I	7		
II	7		
III	22		
			Months
Median time interval from	19	Median survival	32
diagnosis to BMT (months)		Median disease-free survival	15
Range	3–80		

* Disappearance of monoclonal immunoglobulin in serum, light chains in urine and abnormal plasma cells in bone marrow aspirates.

Clinical Results of Allogeneic Bone Marrow Transplantation for Aplastic Anaemia

Before the introduction of allogeneic bone marrow transplantation for aplastic anaemia by the Seattle group (Storb et al, 1974, 1976), the only treatment for the disease, apart from support with blood products and antibiotics was the use of androgens. Patients with aplastic anaemia can be divided into two groups, those with severe aplastic anaemia (SAA) who had a 10% chance of recovery (Camitta et al, 1975), and those with non-severe aplastic anaemia where recovery approached 50%. The introduction of antilymphocyte globulin (ALG) treatment for aplastic anaemia has improved the survival of patients with SAA (Speck et al, 1977; Champlin et al, 1983). Nevertheless, it is possible to identify a group of patients with very severe aplastic anaemia (VSAA), who have a very poor chance of surviving. These are patients with the criteria of SAA but in whom the neutrophil count is particularly severely depressed ($0.2 \times 10^9/l$) and who are infected at the time treatment is started (Bacigalupo et al, 1987). In some ways the success of ALG

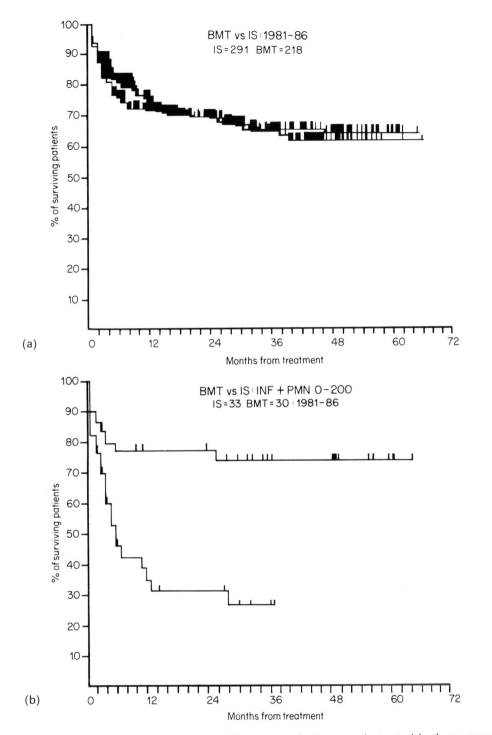

Figure 1. (a) Survival of patients with severe aplastic anaemia treated by bone marrow transplantation or immunosuppression reported to the EBMT registry. (b) Patients with severe aplastic anaemia infected at the time of treatment. Upper curve: bone marrow transplantation (BMT), lower curve: immunosuppression (IS).

treatment has made the selection of patients for bone marrow transplantation more difficult. On the one hand bone marrow transplantation carries a high risk of treatment related death (20–25%), on the other hand failure of immunosuppressive treatment may produce a patient sensitized to blood products and possibly infected at the time of transplantation, each of which diminishes the chance of success of bone marrow transplantation. Figure 1 illustrates the problem; the survival of patients with SAA in the European experience is the same in the immunosuppressed group and the transplanted group (Bacigalupo et al, 1987), but the characteristics of the patients who die in each group are different.

Apart from their neutropenia patients with aplastic anaemia are immunocompetent, indeed exposure to multiple blood transfusions stimulates the immune response. Therefore it is not surprising that these patients have a higher incidence of graft rejection compared with leukaemic patients. Also transplantation with marrow other than HLA-matched marrow greatly increases the chances of rejection in these patients (Gordon-Smith et al, 1987).

The introduction of cyclosporin for post graft immunosuppression greatly reduced the graft rejection rate in these patients (Hows et al, 1982). Even so graft rejection remains high at about 10%. Late graft failure may be seen after cyclosporin is withdrawn and the oral drug should be continued for at least a year after the transplant.

Other measures have been used to further reduce graft failure including thoracoabdominal irradiation (TAI) (Gluckman et al, 1979) and total lymphoid irradiation (TLI) (Ramsey et al, 1980). Each of these additional manoeuvres reduces graft rejection, but survival has not improved possibly because the introduction of irradiation increases GVHD, particularly chronic GVHD. Apart from HLA-matching and immunosuppression the number of cells infused appears to be particularly important in establishing a successful graft in SAA (Storb et al, 1977). A cell dose in excess of 3.0×10^8 cells/kg body weight of the recipient should be achieved.

T-cell depletion of aplastic anaemia transplants as prevention of acute GVHD leads to a high incidence of graft failure when only cyclophosphamide is used for immunosuppression. Increasing the immunosuppression with TLI with or without antilymphocyte monoclonal antibodies may improve the graft take, though the number of patients treated in this way is too small as yet to identify the effects on long-term survival.

Most published series of patients transplanted for SAA have been transplanted using cyclophosphamide with methotrexate or cyclosporin. In most series, including the collected EBMT data and the IBMTR, a long-term survival of 65–75% is achieved. Untransfused patients have a long-term survival of 80% (Storb et al, 1984).

Patients with VSAA should be transplanted as a first option. Patients under 20 with criteria of SAA should also be offered bone marrow transplantation in the first instances. For other patients a trial of ALG should be considered before proceeding to transplantation.

Clinical Results of Allogeneic Bone Marrow Transplantation for Inherited Immunodeficiencies, Infantile Osteopetrosis and Lysosomal Storage Disorders

Until the end of 1987 more than 200 infants and children, suffering from inherited immunodeficiencies, and 19 infants with the autosomal recessive form of osteopetrosis

Table 9. Results of bone marrow transplantation for immunodeficiencies and osteopetrosis[*].

Disease	Total patients grafted	HLA-identical		HLA-mismatched	
		Patients grafted	Sustained engraftment[†]	Patients grafted	Sustained engraftment[†]
Severe combined immunodeficiencies	124				
Reticular dysgenesis	4	1	1	3	1
ADA deficiency	23	6	5	17	6
Absence of T lymphocytes	61	24	18	37	24
Alymphocytosis	27	14	8	13	5
Non-functional T and B lymphocytes	9	7	6	2	1
Combined immunodeficiencies	35				
HLA class II deficiency	15	6	1	9	3
PNP deficiency	1	1	0		
Others	19	8	7	11	5
Wiskott–Aldrich syndrome	24	9	6	15	5
Phagocytic cell disease	27				
Chediak–Higashi	8	6	5	2	0
Lymphohistiocytosis	6	4	1	2	0
Agranulocytosis	5	3	2	2	1
Chronic granulomatous disease	2	2	0		
Leukocyte adhesion deficiency	6	3	2	3	3
Osteopetrosis	19	10	7	9	4

* Update of the European survey (Fischer and Landais, 1988).
† Sustained engraftment at ≥ 6 months after bone marrow transplantation.
ADA, adenosine deaminase; PNP, purine nucleoside phosphorylase.

were treated with bone marrow transplantation in Europe, and registered in the Paris Data Bank of the European Group for Immunodeficiency (EGID) and the Working Party on Immunology and Inborn Errors of the EBMT. A European survey of the results was recently updated up to the end of 1987 (Fischer and Landais, 1988). From June 1980 onwards, when a patient with Hurler disease was given a bone marrow graft (Hobbs et al, 1981), approximately 100 children with lysosomal storage disorders have been grafted until the end of 1987. The data reported in the literature were evaluated and will be summarized.

Table 9 summarizes the results of HLA-identical and HLA-mismatched bone marrow transplantation in 210 infants and children with inherited immunodeficiencies and in 19 infants with osteopetrosis, as updated until the end of 1987 (Fischer and Landais, 1988). The success rate is high, with an overall actuarial disease-free survival of 54%, ranging from about 60 to 65% for HLA-identical bone marrow transplantation in severe combined immunodeficiencies (SCID) and combined immunodeficiency, to about 35 to 40% for HLA-mismatched bone marrow transplantation in non-SCID patients. Besides disease-related or transplant-related complications, graft failure was one of the major causes of lack of success. Second grafts were performed in 56 patients with SCID and combined immunodeficiency, and in 28 patients with other immunodeficiencies and osteopetrosis, using a more intensive preparative treatment, and resulted in successful engraftment in about one third of the cases. All-in-all a remarkable success rate was obtained by bone marrow transplantation for inherited immunodeficiencies and osteopetrosis.

Unfortunately, many reports on bone marrow transplantation for lysosomal storage disorders are very incomplete and/or preliminary, e.g. in the form of short communications or meeting abstracts, and can thus not be evaluated properly. We carefully scrutinized the literature for reports on bone marrow transplantation for lysosomal storage diseases until the end of 1987, and traced about 75 cases. The most relevant data are summarized in Table 10. Bone marrow transplantation for lysosomal storage diseases is only justifiable where the most prominent and debilitating abnormalities, e.g. early dementia, invalidating skeletal anomalies and joint contractures, life-threatening anomalies of heart and lungs, can either be corrected or at least their progression can be prevented at an early stage. The discrepancy between the numbers of cases in which an improvement was claimed and the three children in whom this could be objectively documented, is in part due to misinterpretation of data and unfamiliarity with the natural course of the disease, and in part due to inadequate documentation. This is the more objectionable in view of the well-known heterogeneity in clinical expression of these disorders, even within the same type of disease and sometimes within one kinship. The three patients in whom an improvement was verifiable were, first, a boy with Hurler's disease (Hobbs et al, 1981; Hugh-Jones et al, 1984) whose psychomotor development improved slightly, although it was not definitely established whether this case was either a Hurler or a Hurler/Scheie compound disease; second, a girl with Maroteaux–Lamy disease (Krivit et al, 1982, 1984; McGovern et al, 1986) whose cardiopulmonary function improved dramatically following bone marrow transplantation, but who also had a tracheostomy prior to bone marrow transplantation; and third, a girl with Niemann–Pick disease type B, i.e. without neurological impairment, who had hepatosplenomegaly but was otherwise healthy, and whose liver and spleen decreased in size after bone marrow transplantation (Vellodi et al, 1987).

Table 10. Results of bone marrow transplantation for lysosomal storage disorders.

Disease	Total patients grafted	Effect of BMT	
		Claimed by authors	Clearly documented
Hurler	29	10	1
Hunter	7	1	0
Sanfilippo	7 (6)*	3	0
Morquio	5	4	0
Maroteaux-Lamy	2	2	1
Mannosidosis	1	0	0
Metachromatic leukodystrophy	5	2	0
Gaucher	11	4	0
GM1-gangliosidosis	2	0	0
Niemann–Pick	3	1	1
Wolman	1	0	0
Pompe	2	0	0
Total	75 (74)*	27	3

* The same patient is possibly incorporated into two reports.

In conclusion, claims of improvement following bone marrow transplantation for lysosomal storage disorders are hardly substantiated by facts. The case histories of two children, followed for several years after bone marrow transplantation and adequately documented, illustrate the danger of drawing premature conclusions as to a possible beneficial effect of bone marrow transplantation for lysosomal storage disorders in the long run. A girl with the 'late infantile type' of metachromatic leukodystrophy seemed to have a more stable and much more prosperous course after bone marrow transplantation than her older untreated sister (Lipton et al, 1986; Krivit et al, 1987). However, on accurate observation of the hard facts (Krivit et al, 1987) it can be seen that her course is progressively deteriorating. Also a girl with type III Gaucher disease, clinically a very heterogeneous type, was reported to be less tired and to have an increased growth rate after bone marrow transplantation, which was preceded by a splenectomy (Lundgren et al, 1984; Svennerholm et al, 1984; Groth et al, 1985). However, the most recent report (Ringden et al, 1988) shows that she is getting slightly worse and the history of her disease is in fact compatible with what one might expect to be the natural course. Proper documentation and long-term follow-up are urgently needed in order to assess the potential role of bone marrow transplantation for lysosomal storage disorders.

SUMMARY

Allogeneic bone marrow transplantation offers a reasonable proportion of curation in patients with acute and chronic leukaemia if the transplant is performed in an early stage of the disease. This holds also true for selected patients with Hodgkin's or non-Hodgkin's lymphoma and myelodysplastic syndromes. Marrow grafting for multiple myeloma is still in an experimental phase; the long-term results are still unknown. For aplastic anaemia patients, especially children, allogeneic bone marrow transplantation is the therapy of choice. For older patients with aplastic anaemia comparable results can be achieved with antilymphocyte globulin treatment.

For children with immunodeficiencies the results are extremely good. However, the indication for allogeneic bone marrow transplantation in lysosomal storage disorders is very doubtful. Although some prospective randomized trials have been performed, more studies are necessary to prove the ultimate value of allogeneic bone marrow transplantation.

Acknowledgement

The secretarial assistance of Ms J. Kooreman is gratefully acknowledged.

REFERENCES

Appelbaum FR, Storb R, Ramberg RE et al (1987) Treatment of preleukemic syndromes with marrow transplantation. *Blood* **69**: 92–96.

Bacigalupo A, Gordon-Smith EC, Van Lint MT et al (1987) Bone marrow transplantation (BMT) vs immunosuppression (IS) in the management of severe aplastic anaemia. *Bone Marrow Transplantation* **2** (supplement 1): 99.

Beatty PG, Clift RA, Mickelson EM et al (1985) Marrow transplantation from related donors other than HLA-identical siblings. *New England Journal of Medicine* **313**: 765–771.

Bergsagel D, Phil D, Bailey AJ et al (1979) The chemotherapy of plasma-cell myeloma and the incidence of acute leukemia. *New England Journal of Medicine* **301**: 743–748.

Buckner CD & Clift RA (1984) Marrow transplantation for acute lymphoblastic leukemia. *Seminars in Hematology* **21**: 43–47.

Camitta BM, Rappeport JM, Parkman R & Nathan DG (1975) Selection of patients for bone marrow transplantation in severe aplastic anemia. *Blood* **45**: 355–363.

Champlin RE & Gale RP (1984) The early complications of bone marrow transplantation. *Seminars in Hematology* **21**: 101–108.

Champlin RE & Gale RP ('1987) Bone marrow transplantation for acute leukemia: recent advances and comparison with alternative therapies. *Seminars in Hematology* **24**: 55–67.

Champlin RE, Ho W & Gale RP (1983) Antilymphocyte globulin treatment in patients with aplastic anaemia. *New England Journal of Medicine* **30**: 113–116.

De Witte T, Zwaan F, Gratwohl A et al (1988) Allogeneic bone marrow transplantation in secondary leukemias and myelodysplastic syndromes. *Bone Marrow Transplantation* **3** (supplement 1): 142–143.

Doney K, Buckner CD, Kopecky KJ et al (1987) Marrow transplantation for patients with acute lymphoblastic leukemia in first marrow remission. *Bone Marrow Transplantation* **2**: 355–363.

Fischer AF & Landais P (1988) Bone marrow transplantation for immunodeficiencies and osteopetrosis. A report of the EBMT Immunodeficiency Working Party. *Bone Marrow Transplantation* **3** (supplement 1): 46–47.

Gale RP & Champlin RE (1983) Bone marrow transplantation in leukemia: critical analysis and controlled clinical trials. In Gale RP (ed.) *Recent Advances in Bone Marrow Transplantation*, pp 71–94. New York: Alan R Liss.

Gale RP & Champlin RE (1984) How does bone marrow transplantation cure leukemia? *Lancet* **ii**: 28–30.

Gale RP, Kay HEM, Rimm AA et al (1982) Bone marrow transplantation for acute leukemia in first remission: Report of the International Bone Marrow Transplant Registry. *Lancet* **ii**: 1006–1008.

Gale RP, Kersey JH, Bortin MM et al (1983) Bone marrow transplantation for acute lymphoblastic leukemia. *Lancet* **ii**: 663–667.

Gingrich R, Howe C, Giekin N et al (1985) Successful bone marrow transplantation with partially matched unrelated donors. *Transplantation Proceedings* **17**: 450–452.

Gluckman E, Devergie A, Dutreix A et al (1979) Total body irradiation in bone marrow transplantation. Hopital Saint-Louis results. *Pathologie et Biologie* (Paris) **27**: 349–352.

Gluckman E, Berger R & Dutreix J (1984) Bone marrow transplantation for Fanconi anemia. *Seminars in Hematology* **21**: 20–26.

Goldman JM (1987) Bone marrow transplantation for chronic myeloid leukaemia. *Hematological Oncology* **5**: 265–279.

Goldman JM, Gale RP, Horowitz MM et al (1988) Bone marrow transplantation for chronic myelogenous leukemia in chronic phase: increased risk of relapse associated with T-cell depletion. *Annals of Internal Medicine* **108**: 806–814.

Gordon-Smith EC, Hows J, Bacigalupo A et al (1987) Bone marrow transplantation for severe aplastic anaemia (SAA) from donors other than matched siblings: a report of the EBMT working party. *Bone Marrow Transplantation* **2** (supplement 1): 100.

Gratwohl A, Hermans J, Lyklema A & Zwaan FE (1987) Bone marrow transplantation for leukemia in Europe. Report from the Leukaemia Working Party 1987. *Bone Marrow Transplantation* **2** (supplement 1): 15–18.

Gratwohl A, Hermans J, Barrett AJ et al (1988) Allogeneic bone marrow transplantation for leukaemia in Europe. Report from the Working Party on Leukaemia, European Group for Bone Marrow Transplantation. *Lancet* **i**: 1379-1382.

Groth CG, Lundgren G, Nillson O et al (1985) Biochemical recovery in juvenile Gaucher's disease after bone marrow transplantation. *Transplantation Proceedings* **17**: 453–454.

Herzig RH, Bortin MM, Barrett AJ et al (1987) Bone marrow transplantation in high risk acute lymphoblastic leukaemia in first and second remission. *Lancet* **i**: 786–789.

Hobbs JR, Hugh-Jones K, Byrom N et al (1981) Reversal of clinical features of Hurler's disease and biochemical improvement after treatment by bone marrow transplantation. *Lancet* **ii**: 709–712.

Hows JM, Palmer S & Gordon-Smith EC (1982) The use of cyclosporin in allogeneic bone marrow transplantation for severe aplastic anaemia. *Transplantation* **33**: 382–386.

Hugh-Jones K, Hobbs J, Chambers D et al (1984) Bone marrow transplantation in mucopolysaccharidosis. *Proceedings of the Conference on the Molecular Basis of Lysosomal Storage Disorders, Bethesda, 1983*, p. 411. New York: Academic Press.

Kantarjian HM, Keating MJ, Walters RS, et al (1986) Therapy-related leukemia and myelodysplastic syndrome: clinical, cytogenetic, and prognostic features. *Clinical Oncology* **4**: 1748–1757.

Krivit W, Kersey J, Tsai M et al (1982) Bone marrow transplantation as treatment for Maroteaux–Lamy syndrome (type VI) mucopolysaccharidosis. *Blood* **60** (supplement): 170a.

Krivit W, Pierpont ME, Ayaz K et al (1984) Bone marrow transplantation in the Maroteaux–Lamy syndrome (mucopolysaccharidosis VI). *New England Journal of Medicine* **311**: 1606–1611.

Krivit W, Lipton ME, Lockman LA et al (1987) Prevention of deterioration in metachromatic leukodystrophy by bone marrow transplantation. *American Journal of Medical Sciences* **294**: 8–85.

Lipton ME, Lockman LA, Ramsay NKC et al (1986) *Bone Marrow Transplantation for Treatment of Lysosomal Storage Diseases*. New York: Alan R Liss, 57 pp.

Lundgren G, Eriksson A, Gahrton G et al (1984) Bone marrow transplantation in juvenile Gaucher's disease. *Experimental Hematology* **12** (supplement 15): 99–100.

Marmont AM & Tura S (1986) Bone marrow transplantation for secondary leukemia. Report of two cases. *Bone Marrow Transplantation* **1** (supplement 1): 191–192.

McGovern MM, Ludman MD, Short MP et al (1986) *Bone Marrow Transplantation for Treatment of Lysosomal Storage Diseases*. New York: Alan R Liss, 41 pp.

O'Donnell MR, Nademanee AP, Snyder DS et al (1987) Bone marrow transplantation for myelodysplastic and myeloproliferative syndromes. *Journal of Clinical Oncology* **5**: 1822–1826.

O'Reilly RJ (1983) Allogeneic bone marrow transplantation: Current status and future directions. *Blood* **69**: 941–964.

O'Reilly RJ, Brochstein J, Dinsmore R & Kirkpatrick D (1984) Marrow Transplantation for congenital disorders. *Seminars in Hematology* **21**: 188–221.

Pedersen-Bjergaard J, Philip B, Mortensen BT et al (1981) Acute nonlymphocytic leukemia, preleukemia, and acute myeloproliferative syndrome secondary to treatment of other malignant diseases. Clinical and cytogenetic characteristics and results of in vitro culture of bone marrow and HLA-typing. *Blood* **57**: 712–723.

Philip T, Armitage JO, Spizer G et al (1987) High-dose therapy and autologous bone marrow transplantation after failure of conventional chemotherapy in adults with intermediate-grade or high-grade non-Hodgkin's lymphoma. *New England Journal of Medicine* **316**: 1493–1498.

Ramsey NK, Kim TH, McGlave P, et al (1980) Total lymphoid irradiation and cyclophosphamide conditioning prior to bone marrow transplantation for patients with severe aplastic anaemia. *Blood* **62**: 622–628.

Ringden O, Zwaan FE, Hermans J & Gratwohl A, for the Leukaemia Working Party of the European Group for Bone Marrow Transplantation (1987) European experience of bone marrow transplantation for leukemia. *Transplantation Proceedings* **19**: 2600–2604.

Ringden O, Groth CG, Erikson A et al (1988) Long-term follow-up of the first successful bone marrow transplantation in Gaucher disease. *Transplantation,* (in press).

Speck B, Gluckman E, Haak HL & Van Rood JJ (1977) Treatment of aplastic anaemia by antilymphocyte globulin with or without bone marrow infusion. *Lancet* **ii**: 1145–1148.

Speck B, Gratwohl A, Osterwalder B & Nissen C (1984) Bone marrow transplantation for chronic myeloid leukemia. *Seminars in Hematology* **21**: 48–52.

Storb R, Thomas ED, Buckner CD et al (1974) Allogeneic marrow grafting for treatment of aplastic anaemia. *Blood* **43**: 157–180.

Storb R, Thomas ED, Weiden PL et al (1976) Aplastic anemia treated by allogeneic bone marrow transplantation: a report on 49 new cases from Seattle. *Blood* **48**: 817–841.

Storb R, Prentice RL & Thomas ED (1977) Marrow transplantation for aplastic anaemia. An analysis of factors associated with graft rejection. *New England Journal of Medicine* **296**: 61–66.

Storb R, Thomas ED, Buckner CD et al (1984) Marrow transplantation for aplastic anemia. *Seminars in Hematology* **21**: 27–35.

Storb R, Deeg HJ, Whitehead J et al (1986) Methotrexate and cyclosporin compared with cyclosporin alone for prophylaxis of graft-vs-host disease after marrow transplantation for leukemia. *New England Journal of Medicine* **314**: 729–735.

Sullivan KM, Deeg HJ, Sanders JE et al (1984) Late complications after marrow transplantation. *Seminars in Hematology* **21**: 53–63.

Svennerholm L, Mansson N, Nilsson O & Tibblin E (1984) Bone marrow transplantation in the norrbottnian form of Gaucher disease. *Proceedings of the Conference on the Molecular Basis of Lysosomal Storage Disorders, Bethesda, 1983*, p. 441. New York: Academic Press.

Thomas, ED (1969) The role of bone marrow transplantation for eradication of malignant disease. *Cancer* **10**: 1963–1969.

Thomas ED, Clift RA, Fefer A et al (1986) Marrow transplantation for the treatment of chronic myelogenous leukemia. *Annals of Internal Medicine* **104**: 155–163.

Van Bekkum DW (1984) Conditioning regimens for marrow grafting. *Seminars in Hematology* **21**: 81–90.

Vellodi A, Hobbs JR, O'Donnell NM, Coulter BS & Hugh-Jones K (1987) Treatment of Niemann–Pick disease type B by allogeneic bone marrow transplantation. *British Medical Journal* **295**: 1375–1376.

Zwaan FE & Jansen J (1984) Bone marrow transplantation in acute nonlymphoblastic leukemia. *Seminars in Hematology* **21**: 36–42.

Zwaan FE, Hermans J, Barrett AJ & Speck B (1984a) Bone marrow transplantation for acute nonlymphoblastic leukaemia: a survey of the European Group for Bone Marrow Transplantation (E.G.B.M.T.). *British Journal of Haematology* **56**: 645–653.

Zwaan FE, Hermans J, Barrett AJ & Speck B (1984b) Bone marrow transplantation for acute lymphoblastic leukaemia: a survey of the European Group for Bone Marrow Transplantation (E.G.B.M.T.). *British Journal of Haematology* **58**: 33–42.

Zwaan FE, Hermans J & Lyklema A (1985) Bone marrow transplantation for leukemia in Europe. Factors influencing the possibility of long term survival. *Experimental Hematology* **13** (supplement 17): 3–5.

If   Corneal Grafting

D. L. EASTY   C. A. ROGERS*
W. J. ARMITAGE   S. M. GORE*
S. J. MOSS   B. A. BRADLEY*

The World Health Organisation returns show that corneal disease accounts for more blindness than any other form of eye disease. It is in countries where such blindness is most common that the practice of corneal grafting is limited because of the lack of technical resources or of available donor tissue. In developed countries grafting is frequently performed for a variety of indications. In spite of many advances in recent years, most corneal surgeons agree that grafts still fail and research into the treatment and avoidance of operative and postoperative complications is required.

The cornea is an avascular membrane serving as a protective coat and a refractive lens, the function depending on its transparency, and the integrity of the surface epithelium and the overlying tear film. Structurally, the epithelium is composed of five cell layers supported by a basement membrane. Where epithelium is damaged, cells first slide into position to fill the deficit, and then start to replicate. The stroma underlies the epithelium and accounts for about 95% of the thickness. Transparency depends upon the orthogonal arrangement of collagen fibrils, that are equal in diameter and equidistant from each other, forming a lattice. The arrangement is lost in many corneal diseases and so vision deteriorates.

Endothelium lines the inner surface, its nutrition depending upon normal circulation of aqueous humour. The importance of this layer is that it is a metabolic pump that maintains the stroma in deturgescence. Where there has been damage there is no renewal of the layer by cell replication, the remaining cells enlarging to maintain deturgescence. This layer is made visible with specular photography, and it is known that normal cell counts amount to $2000-3000/mm^2$, younger people having higher counts than the elderly. A count of less than 500 cell/mm^2 is associated with failure of the endothelial pump, swelling and opacification of the cornea, and loss of vision.

It had first been thought that because the cornea was avascular it was immunologically privileged and that allograft rejection would be an unlikely cause of failure. It was later realised that a substantial number of grafts are prone to rejection, and clear-cut syndromes are now recognized. Each corneal layer is capable of inducing host sensitization and rejection when manipulated in the rabbit model (Khodadoust and Silverstein,

* On behalf of the Corneal Transplant Follow-up Study

ORGAN TRANSPLANTATION: CURRENT CLINICAL AND
IMMUNOLOGICAL CONCEPTS   ISBN 0-7020-1393-5

1969). Epithelial and endothelial 'rejection' lines can be seen originating at a leash of ingrowing blood vessels, the latter leading to corneal oedema and graft failure if treatment is not introduced immediately. Stromal rejection induces focal opacities that can also affect the visual outcome (Krachmer and Alldredge, 1978).

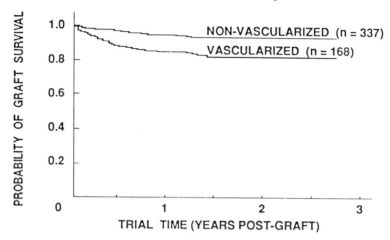

Figure 1.   Effect of host corneal vascularization on graft survival. From Williams et al (1988), with permission.

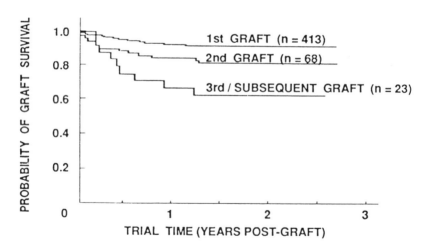

Figure 2.   Effect of the number of grafts on survival in the ipsilateral eye. From Williams et al (1988), with permission.

Class I MHC antigens are expressed on epithelial, stromal and endothelial cells, and class II on epithelial and stromal cells (Mayer et al, 1983; Treseler et al, 1984; Whitsett and Stulting, 1984). It has been demonstrated that class I can act as effective targets for both humoral and cellular immune responses in genetically well-defined animal models. Class II antigens are thought to be important (Braude and Chandler, 1983), particularly when carried by passenger cells within the stroma (Volker-Dieben et al, 1982a; Williams et al, 1985). Cell culture of human stromal and endothelial cells in the presence of human γ-interferon-induced expression of HLA-DR antigens (Young et al, 1985). Corneal grafts fail for a number of reasons, some being related to factors within the recipient, including the presence of vascularization (Figure 1), a history of previous graft failure (Figure 2), the presence of glaucoma, decreased corneal sensation, a history of intraocular inflammation (Figure 3), or associated disease of the external eye such as the dry eye syndrome, eyelid disease or abnormal conjunctiva (Volker-Dieben et al, 1982a; Volker-Dieben, 1984; Williams et al, 1988).

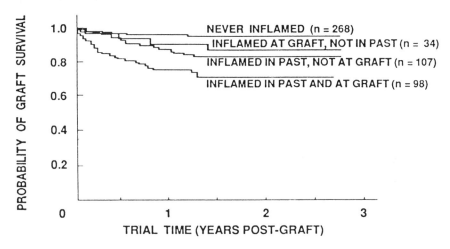

Figure 3. The effect of intraocular inflammation on graft survival. From Williams et al (1988), with permission.

Corneal allograft rejection, a common cause of graft failure, can be witnessed at an early stage with the slit-lamp microscope, and so presents an opportunity to study factors that influence the immune response of the host against the donor tissue. Several studies have reported the influence of HLA matching on the prognosis of penetrating keratoplasty (Batchelor et al, 1976; Stark, 1980; Volker-Dieben et al, 1982b; Foulks et al, 1983; Volker-Dieben, 1984; Sanfillipo et al, 1986) (Figure 4). These studies have been inconclusive mainly because they were retrospective, and because the follow-up was short. The studies have generally indicated a beneficial effect from matching. Thus in one study, out of 38 patients receiving corneas with good HLA matches (two or more antigens), 21% had graft rejection, compared with 49% in patients with poor matches (no or one antigen) (Sanfillipo et al, 1986). The influence of presensitization by HLA-A and -B antigens has been investigated with unclear results (Stark et al, 1973; Ehlers et al, 1981). Incompatibility of ABO-blood group antigens expressed on human cornea, seemingly contribute to the corneal allograft reaction, although this has yet to be confirmed (Treseler et al, 1986).

Generally allograft rejection can be reversed with topical corticosteroid. Prophylactic treatment carries a risk of inducing secondary cataract or glaucoma. The use of matched tissue, if of proven value, will hopefully reduce the need for steroid therapy. Other methods of treatment have met with little success. Cyclosporin has not yet been formulated as a topical preparation, although laboratory studies indicate that it could be of value (Bell et al, 1982; Shepherd et al, 1982).

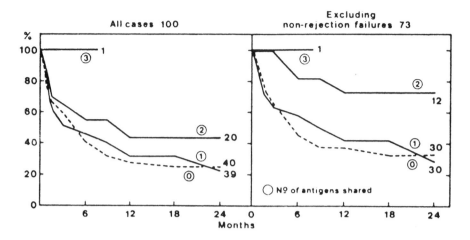

Figure 4. Survival of grafts in cases with severe vascularization. Graft survivals are plotted according to the number of HLA antigens shared by donor and recipient. From Batchelor et al (1976), with permission.

Donor factors are of considerable significance. The health of the corneal endothelium is critical to the success of the transplant. With new techniques the quality of donor tissue can be precisely documented, and the result in the recipient can be assessed. Thus new methods of corneal storage can be assessed prior to and following transplantation.

In September 1983 a national corneal transplant service (CTS) was launched by the United Kingdom Transplant Service (UKTS) with financial support from the Iris Fund for the Prevention of Blindness (Bradley, 1986). The purpose was to improve the availability of corneal tissue in the UK by widening the field of potential donors, co-ordinating the use of available corneas, and, where applicable, by reducing the incidence of rejection by the provision of tissue matched corneas. The CTS also aimed to standardize the transportation of eyes in moist chambers and supplied McCarey Kaufman medium for short-term storage of corneo-scleral discs. A further objective was to increase the awareness of the need for donors. UKTS runs a redistribution scheme for corneas which aims to avoid wastage of tissue by providing 24-hour on-call matching and transport facilities. It maintains a national waiting list for patients who require a transplant, and it also provides statistical analyses for administrative and scientific purposes. The waiting list for corneal tissue rose from 246 in June 1985 to 600 by January 1988. More than 150 centres have now registered patients with UKTS. The number of corneal transplants reported to UKTS has risen from 770 in 1986 to 1059 by 30th September 1988 (Table 1).

In collaboration with the Department of Ophthalmology at the University of Bristol, the Corneal Transplant Service Eye Bank (CTSEB) was established in 1986. The success of this enterprise depends upon storage of corneas for periods of up to 30 days by organ culture at 34C (Doughman et al, 1976; Pels and Schuchard, 1983; Easty et al, 1986). This means that material is always available for emergency grafts anywhere in the UK and increases the opportunity for surgeons to schedule routine grafts well in advance. Table 1 demonstrates the increasing use of the CTSEB employing corneas stored by organ culture, and lists the reasons why tissue was not used for transplantation.

Table 1. Tissue stored in the Corneal Transplant Service Eye Bank.

	Year		
	1986	1987	1988*
Corneas stored			
Carried over from previous year	1	20	50
Received	147	571	1095 (1460)
TOTAL STORED	148	591	1145
Current stock[†]			68
Contributing hospitals	40	85	107
Corneas transplanted			
Penetrating keratoplasty	57	407	713
Lamellar keratoplasty	1	9	23
TOTAL TRANSPLANTED	58	416	736 (981)
Recipient transplant centres	11	66	95
Corneal grafts reported to UKTS	770	974	1059 (1412)
Percentage supplied through CTS Eye Bank	8	43	69
Corneas discarded			
Supplied to centre but not used	1	10	13
Not suitable for grafting[‡]	17	59	202
No HIV or hepatitis B tests	1	8	15
Positive HIV or hepatitis B tests	2	0	0
Contaminated	16	39	70
Outdated	0	7	39
Research	33[§]	2	2
TOTAL DISCARDED	70	125	341 (454)
Discard rate[‖]	55%	22%	32%

* Data for 1 January to 30 September 1988. The figures in brackets are projected totals for the whole of 1988.
[†] Current stock = Total stored − (Total transplanted + Total discarded).
[‡] Donor's cause of death was a contraindication or corneal endothelium was inadequate.
[§] These corneas were used for establishing the methods of corneal storage and evaluation used in the CTS Eye Bank. They could not be placed by UKTS for immediate use and would otherwise have been wasted.
[‖] Discard rate = 100 × Total discarded/(Total transplanted + Total discarded).

The future objectives are to create a database to identify the important influences, be they donor, technical, or immunological, on success rates. Such multicentre studies are mounted in the USA and Australia (Williams et al, 1988). To this end UKTS has established a multicentre Corneal Transplant Follow-up Study (CTFS) in collaboration with the MRC Biostatistics Unit in Cambridge. It is anticipated that over a period of about 3 years, sufficient data will be collected to provide information about the value of prospective matching of donor and recipient. Table 2 lists the diagnoses in 436 patients who have undergone keratoplasty. Keratoconus, where the corneal curvature is conical and not spherical, is the most common indication. Poor endothelial function, as in pseudophakic and aphakic bullous – a complication of cataract extraction, or in the

Table 2. Diagnosis and recipient sex in 436 CTFS patients who have undergone kerato-plasty. Note the relatively high percentage of females with Fuch's dystrophy and males with keratoconus.

Diagnosis in order of relative frequency		Total recipients	% Female
Keratoconus	(24%)	105	39
Bullous keratopathy	(24%)		
Pseudophakic		61	48
Aphakic		44	55
Fuch's dystrophy	(13%)	57	74
Herpes simplex	(11%)	50	46
Inflammation	(13%)		
chronic		42	60
acute		12	67
Stromal dystrophy	(5%)	23	43
Secondary endothelial failure	(3%)	12	
Trauma	(3%)	11	
Congenital malformation	(2%)	9	49
Congenital dystrophy	(1%)	5	
Contact lens related	(1%)	4	
Other	(<1%)	1	—
TOTAL		436	52

Table 3. Frequency of previous grafts in 485 patients.

Number of previous grafts	Frequency	%
0	396	82
1	61	13
2	20	4
3	4	<1
4	3	<1
5+	1	<1
TOTAL	485	

Table 4. Known reasons for failure of 82 previous first grafts.

Cause	Frequency	%
Rejection	25	30
Endothelial decompensation	19	23
Disease recurrence	17	21
Technical	10	12
Infection	4	5
Other	7	9

elderly patient where it seemingly occurs spontaneously, accounted for 37% of grafts. Table 3 shows there were a number of regrafts, the most frequent cause of failure being rejection (Table 4). Other causes were endothelial decompensation probably due to the use of imperfect donor material, recurrence of the original disease (such as in the dystrophies – lattice dystrophy is the most common), and technical causes of failure, for example loss of the anterior chamber via inadequate apposition of the interface between donor and recipient.

Table 5. Number of corneal grafts performed with HLA typing of donor or recipient or both, or neither (July 1987–May 1988).

		Number of grafts	%
Recipient untyped	donor untyped	365	43
Recipient typed	donor untyped	27	3
Recipient untyped	donor typed	222	26
Recipient typed	donor typed	238	28
TOTAL		852	

A key objective is to determine the influence of HLA-A and -B matching on graft prognosis: Table 5 documents the number of grafts performed with typing of donor only, recipient only, both donor and recipient, and neither. It is anticipated that a substantial database will be collected that will help in defining further the value of tissue typing and matching in corneal grafting. Data already shows that there is little difference between the visual outcome using tissue stored for short periods of up to four days and tissue stored for up to 30 days in organ culture (Tables 6 and 7).

Table 6. Preoperative visual acuity in 506 CTFS patients who have undergone keratoplasty, categorized according to method of storage (i.e. 4C storage for up to 4 days, or organ cultured for up to 30 days).

	Method of storage			
Visual acuity	Organ culture	4C	Total	
No perception of light	0	0	0	
Light perception	17	10	27	(5%)
Hand movements	66	43	109	(22%)
Counting fingers	126	59	185	(37%)
6/60	51	24	75	(15%)
6/36	25	12	37	(7%)
6/24	16	15	31	(6%)
6/12	26	9	35	(7%)
6/6	4	3	7	(1%)
TOTAL	331	175	506	

No difference in the distribution of visual acuities was expected pre-transplant between those recipients receiving cultured tissue and those not, nor is there any.

Table 7. Postoperative visual acuities at 3 months following keratoplasty in 211 CTFS patients categorized according to whether cultured or non-cultured corneas were used.

Visual acuity	Method of storage		Total
	Organ culture	4C	
No perception of light	0	1	1 (<1%)
Light perception	1	0	1 (<5%)
Hand movements	4	1	5 (2%)
Counting fingers	23	8	31 (15%)
6/60	22	13	35 (17%)
6/36	14	12	26 (12%)
6/24	19	9	28 (13%)
6/12	36	23	59 (28%)
6/6	17	8	25 (12%)
TOTAL	136	75	211

Less than 20% of recipients have a visual acuity of CF or less at 3 months post-graft compared to 64% pre-transplant. 53% of recipients have a visual acuity of 6/24 or better.

REFERENCES

Batchelor JR, Casey TA, Werb A et al (1976) HLA matching and corneal grafting. *Lancet* **i**: 551–554.

Bell TAG, Easty DL & McCullogh KG (1982) A placebo controlled blind trial of cyclosporin A in prevention of corneal graft rejection in rabbits. *British Journal of Ophthalmology* **66**: 303–308.

Bradley BA (1986) Corneal supply in the United Kingdom. *Transactions of the Ophthalmological Societies of the United Kingdom* **105**: 397–400.

Braude LS & Chandler JW (1983) Corneal allograft rejection. The role of the major histocompatibility complex. *Survey of Ophthalmology* **27**: 290–305.

Doughman DJ, Hams JE & Schmitt MK (1976) Penetrating keratoplasty using 37°C organ cultured corneas. *Transactions of the American Academy of Ophthalmology and Otolaryngology* **81**: 778–793.

Easty DL, Carter CA & Lewkowicz-Moss SJ (1986) Corneal cell culture and organ storage. *Transactions of the Ophthalmological Societies of the United Kingdom* **105**: 385–396.

Ehlers N, Olsen T & Hohnson HE (1981) Corneal graft rejection probably mediated by antibodies. *Acta Ophthalmologica* **59**: 119–125.

Foulks GN, Sanfillipo FP, Locascio JA III, McQueen JM & Dawson DV (1983) Histocompatibility testing for keratoplasty in high risk patients. *Ophthalmology* **90**: 239–243.

Khodadoust AA & Silverstein AM (1969) The survival and rejection of epithelium in experimental corneal transplants. *Investigative Ophthalmology and Visual Science* **8**: 169–179.

Krachmer JH & Alldredge OC (1978) Subepithelial infiltrates. *Archives of Ophthalmology* **96**: 2234–2237.

Mayer DJ, Daar AS, Casey TA & Fabre JW (1983) Localisation of HLA-A, B, C and HLA-DR antigens in the human cornea. *Transplantation Proceedings* **15**: 126–129.

Pels E & Schuchard Y (1983) Organ culture preservation of human corneas. *Documenta Ophthalmologica* **56**: 147–153.

Sanfillipo F, MacQueen BA, Vaughan WK & Foulks GN (1986) Reduced graft rejection with good HLA-A and B matching in high risk corneal transplantation. *New England Journal of Medicine* **315**: 29–35.

Shepherd WF, Coster DJ, Chinfook T, Rice NS & Jones BR (1982) Effect of cyclosporin A on the survival of corneal grafts in rabbits. *British Journal of Ophthalmology* **64**: 148–153.

Stark WJ (1980) Transplantation immunology of penetrating keratoplasty. *Transactions of the American Ophthalmological Society* **78**: 1079–1117.

Stark WJ, Opelz G, Newsome D et al (1973) Sensitisation of human lymphocyte antigens by corneal transplantation. *Investigative Ophthalmology and Visual Science* **12**: 639–645.

Treseler PA, Foulks GN & Sanfillippo F (1984) The expression of HLA antigens by cells in the human cornea. *American Journal of Ophthalmology* **98**: 763–772.

Treseler PA, Foulks GN & Sanfillipo F (1986) Expression of ABO blood groups, haemopoietic, and other cell-specific antigens by cells in the human cornea. *Cornea* **4**: 157–168.

Volker-Dieben HJ (1984) The effect of immunological and non-immunological factors on corneal graft survival – a single centre study. *Documenta Ophthalmologica* **16**: 57(1–2): 1–151.

Volker-Dieben HJ, Kok-Van Alphen CC, Lansberger Q & Persin GG (1982a) Different influences on corneal graft survival in 539 transplants. *Acta Ophthalmologica* **60**: 190–202.

Volker-Dieben HJ, Kok-Van Alphen CC, Lansberger Q & Persin GG (1982b) The effect of prospective HLA-A and -B matching on corneal graft survival. *Acta Ophthalmologica* **60**: 203–212.

Whitsett CF & Stulting RD (1984) The distribution of HLA antigens on human corneal tissue. *Investigative Ophthalmology and Visual Science* **25**: 519–524.

Williams KA, Ash JK & Coster DJ (1985) Histocompatibility antigen and passenger cell content of normal and diseased human cornea. *Transplantation* **39**: 265–269.

Williams KA, Sawer MA, White MA, Mahmood M & Coster DJ (1988) *The Australian Graft Registry Report.* Dept Ophthalmology, Flinders Medical Centre, Adelaide.

Young E, Stark WJ & Prendergast RA (1985) Immunology of corneal allograft rejection: HLA-DR antigens on human corneal cells. *Investigative Ophthalmology and Visual Science* **26**: 571–574.

II The Incidence of Renal Failure Worldwide and National Statistics for Treatment by Transplantation

ROBERT A. SELLS
ANTONY J. WING

A detailed account of the incidence of end-stage renal disease (ESRD) in different countries is outside the scope of this chapter; however an approximate indication of the recurrent load of new patients suitable for treatment in the West can be derived from careful analyses carried out in the UK and the USA. A study of Glamorgan hospital records in 1966–1968 (Branch et al, 1971) revealed an incidence of 39 patients per million population (pmp) who suffered chronic renal failure before the age of 60, and who were suitable for dialysis and transplantation. A similar analysis in Scotland (Pendreigh et al, 1972) revealed an incidence of 52 cases pmp. Caucasian populations exhibit a similar annual incidence of ESRD cases in developed countries, but genetic and environmental factors have a dramatic influence on the prevalence of terminal renal disease: Rostand et al (1982) claimed an overall incidence of 91 cases of ESRD per million population using data from patients referred for treatment in Alabama USA; stratification of their sample revealed an incidence of 44.4 in white patients, and 188.4 in blacks.

Apart from these studies, reliable data on the incidence of disease requiring dialysis and for transplantation is lacking, and one can only speculate that renal failure is even more common in many countries where genetic susceptibility combines with dietary deficiency, widespread parasitic and microbial disease, and lack of adequate primary care facilities. Thus, unpublished observations in Kenya led to the conclusion that between 80 and 100 patients per million population died of renal failure in 1978 to 1979, none of whom were offered treatment. It is likely that at least 50 000 patients die annually of end-stage renal disease on the Indian subcontinent (Chugh, 1979). In a large post mortem series from Nigeria, 45% of deaths were associated with evidence of progressive glomerulonephritis (Edington and Mainwaring, 1966).

The registry of the European Dialysis and Transplant Association (EDTA) has attempted over the years to collect data on the demography of ESRD in 34 European countries, but these data do not give the true incidence because they include only the treated population.

ORGAN TRANSPLANTATION: CURRENT CLINICAL AND
IMMUNOLOGICAL CONCEPTS   ISBN 0-7020-1393-5

The causes of end-stage renal disease recorded by the EDTA registry are illustrated in Figure 1 (a and b). Data are provided for patients aged 15–65 years and for those over 65 years who commenced treatment for ESRD in 1986, in all countries combined. The aetiology of chronic renal failure was uncertain in 13% of the 15–65 year olds, and in 20% over 65 years. The older age group had larger proportions of patients with pyelonephritis and vascular or hypertensive renal disease, but smaller proportions with glomerulonephritis and cystic kidney disease. Congenital diseases were not reported in the older patients, and diabetes (12%) and multisystem diseases (8%) accounted for the same proportion in both age groups.

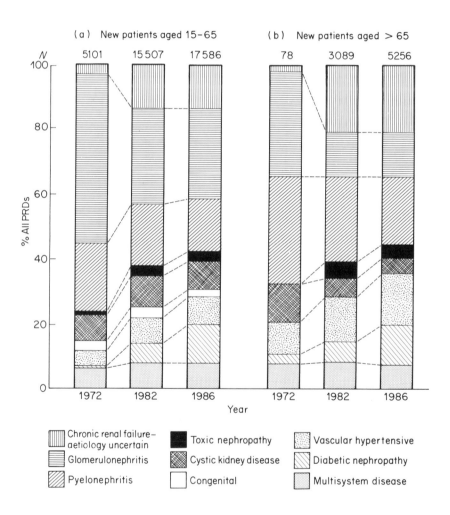

Figure 1. Proportions of causes of end stage renal failure in the treated European population. (a) New patients aged 15–65. (b) New patients aged >65.

The diseases represented amongst the older patients will become increasingly important as this group is growing most rapidly: between 1983 and 1986 the number of treated patients aged 65 and over increased by 70% whereas those aged 15–65 increased by only 13%. Figure 1 shows patients grouped according to nine causes of end-stage renal failure: for additional breakdown of these groups the reader is referred to other publications of the EDTA Registry (e.g. Broyer et al, 1986).

End-stage renal disease is a universal and common life-threatening condition, afflicting most commonly middle-aged and elderly patients. Chronic renal disease often progresses insidiously, and early detection and appropriate treatment may be difficult or impossible in those countries where facilities for primary care and screening are not well-developed. Where it is possible, early diagnosis may be beneficial in at least delaying ESRD; treatment of reversible and potentially non-progressive renal lesions includes the control of hypertension, eradication of infection, treatment of obstruction, the removal of stones, and improved control of diabetes mellitus. Recent evidence that dietary restriction of protein and phosphorus may result in a slowing of renal decompensation (Brenner, 1983) indicates the possibility of delaying the need for dialysis, although not of preventing it. Although early diagnosis and treatment may considerably improve the quality of life, the majority of patients with established renal failure will proceed to the stage of renal decompensation requiring dialysis.

The twin technologies of renal dialysis and transplantation have developed in parallel during the last two decades; since disposable dialysers and peritoneal dialysis (particularly continuous ambulatory peritoneal dialysis (CAPD)) on the one hand, and safer immuno-suppression and cadaveric kidney grafts, on the other, have become more widely deployed, the two have become increasingly interdependent. The reasons for this are partly clinical and partly economic: successful transplant recipients have a considerably better quality of life, consume less state allowances, have a higher employment rate and, therefore, probably pay more taxes than chronic dialysis patients; maintenance costs per year of life with a transplant are less than those for dialysis: these factors have favoured the development of transplantation. Furthermore, patients themselves increasingly seek the opportunity of transplantation in view of the lower complication rate and reduced mortality with current immunosuppressive regimens.

FACTORS INFLUENCING PREVALENCE AND AVAILABILITY OF KIDNEY TRANSPLANTATION

Statistics in this section are derived from several sources: the European Dialysis and Transplant Association Registry (1987) provided most of the information on dialysis and transplant rates, and population and Gross National Product figures come from the 1988 updated World Bank Atlas.

Table 1 presents the numbers of renal transplants performed in 38 countries (listed with their populations). In Table 2 are listed the nations that form the basis of the EDTA reports, having more than 100 patients per million population (pmp) alive on all forms of treatment for ESRD, with the different modalities of treatment given.

In 18 years there has been rapid growth in the acceptance rate for dialysis and transplantation, as is shown in Figure 2. Longer survival and more provision for dialysis

Table 1.   Population statistics for countries studied by EDTA. From the 1988 update of the World Bank Atlas.

Country	Population in millions	Gross national product per capita 1986 (US$)
Algeria	22.6	2 570
Australia	16.0	11 910
Austria	7.6	10 000
Belgium	9.9	9 230
Bulgaria	9.0	Not known
Canada	25.7	14 100
Cyprus	0.7	4 360
Czechoslovakia	15.5	Not known
Denmark	5.1	12 640
Egypt	49.7	760
Federal Republic of Germany	60.9	12 080
Finland	4.9	12 180
France	55.4	10 740
German Democratic Republic	16.6	Not known
Greece	10.0	3 680
Hungary	10.6	2 010
Iceland	0.2	13 370
Ireland	3.6	5 080
Israel	4.3	6 210
Italy	57.2	8 570
Japan	121.4	12 850
Libya	3.9	Not known
Luxembourg	0.4	15 920
Morocco	22.5	590
Netherlands	14.5	10 050
New Zealand	3.3	7 110
Norway	4.2	15 480
Poland	37.5	2 070
Portugal	10.3	2 230
South Africa	33.2	1 800
Spain	38.9	4 840
Sweden	8.4	13 170
Switzerland	6.5	17 840
Tunisia	7.3	1 140
Turkey	51.4	1 110
United Kingdom	56.6	8 920
United States of America	241.3	17 500
Yugoslavia	23.3	2 300

have allowed more dialysis for older patients in the early 1980s compared with the early 1970s, a trend also seen in the increasing age of patients receiving transplants. A more recent study (Wing et al, 1988) reveals a striking increase in the number of patients over 55 years who received kidney transplants, notably in Britain and the Scandinavian countries. This trend may reflect the improvement in the availability and quality of cadaver organs, as well as safer and more successful immunosuppressive regimens since the advent of cyclosporin in 1980.

Table 2. Summary of the number of patients per million population who were being treated for end-stage renal disease in 1986. The figures represent the 'stock' of patients in each category of treatment. Numbers are given for each country studied by the European Dialysis and Transplantation Registry.

Country	Haemodialysis	Peritoneal dialysis	Total dialysis 'stock'	Functioning graft	Total live patient 'stock'
Japan	587	17	604	Not known	604
USA	321	59	380	170	550
Luxembourg	274	3	277	107	384
Israel	223	79	302	73	374
Belgium	238	18	256	115	371
Canada	115	61	176	165	341
Federal Republic of Germany	273	9	272	50	332
Switzerland	179	41	220	78	298
Netherlands	141	29	170	127	297
Australia	104	40	144	150	294
Italy	235	23	258	33	290
Cyprus	211	0	211	78	289
Spain	212	18	239	53	283
Sweden	103	24	127	156	283
France	225	19	244	32	277
Austria	200	6	206	67	272
Finland	56	41	97	169	266
Denmark	108	46	154	108	261
Norway	45	10	55	203	259
New Zealand	70	51	121	128	250
United Kingdom	71	51	122	118	240
Portugal	197	2	199	24	223
Yugoslavia	167	6	173	20	194
Ireland	70	12	82	108	191
Greece	127	18	145	28	172
Iceland	29	50	79	79	158
German Democratic Republic	113	1	114	36	150
Bulgaria	124	<1	124	4	128
Czechoslovakia	75	<1	75	31	107

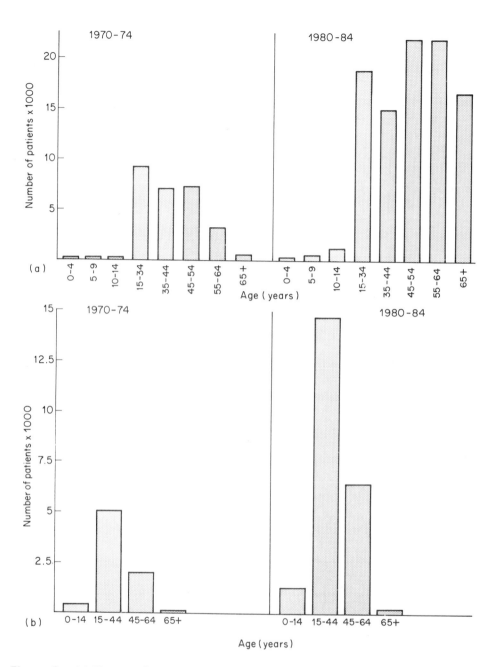

Figure 2. (a) The rate of acceptance of patients for treatment of end-stage renal disease by all therapies, according to age, during two decades. Data from all countries studied are included. (b) The number of patients receiving renal transplants, by age, during two decades. Data from all countries studied are included.

The availability of dialysis and transplantation is very significantly affected by the financial resources available. In Figure 3 we relate the number of patients pmp who received treatment by dialysis and were alive with functioning transplants in 1986 (i.e. the 'stock' of live, treated patients) to the per capita Gross National Product (GNP) for the year. No account is taken of the variable proportion of each country's GNP that is spent on healthcare, but there appears to be an association between national wealth and the availability and success of treatment.

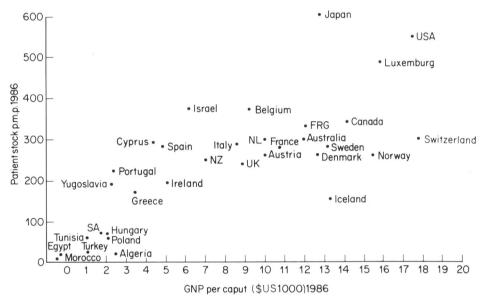

Figure 3.   The relationship between the total number of patients alive on all forms of renal replacement therapy on 31 December 1986 and the gross national product (GNP) per capita in 33 individual countries. FRG, Federal Republic of Germany; NL, Netherlands; UK, United Kingdom; NZ, New Zealand; SA, South Africa; USA, United States of America.

The total number of patients treated pmp represents the 'stock' of cases alive in each country, some treated recently and others being long-term survivors on dialysis or with transplants. The size of the stock gives little indication of what proportion of patients requiring treatment actually receive it, nor does it tell us how each country is coping with the recurrent load of new cases that may arise each year.

In many countries healthcare strategies have recently been aimed at maximizing the use of dialysis and transplantation facilities in order to increase the number of patients treated and to improve the quality of their lives. Ideally, dialysis should be offered to all new cases who need it, but a high proportion of suitable patients on dialysis should be offered renal transplants. This principle of 'integrated therapies' has the benefit of generating vacancies for new cases each year; it allows the transfer of patients from the high cost modality of dialysis to the more cost-effective (though far from cheap) modality of a successful transplant. Most important, the majority of ESRD patients can be offered the opportunity of a normal life after suffering a life-threatening disease. The cost of setting up the 'integrated therapies' system is however very considerable: Figure 4 confirms that in 16 countries studied, the number of transplants performed is closely related to GNP. However, other factors, too, also determine the transplant rate in each country, the principal one being the availability of cadaveric and living related donor organs. For instance, although Japan has the largest stock of treated patients in the world, the transplant rate is allegedly very low due to religious and social restrictions that discourage the removal of organs from cadavers. In many countries where the stock of patients is small due to economic factors, the transplant rate is commensurately low: if a country cannot afford the infrastructure of adequate community and primary health care, and is short of skilled nurses, it is hardly surprising that the relatively expensive 'superstructure' of intensive care units (from which most organ donors originate) and transplant units cannot be provided.

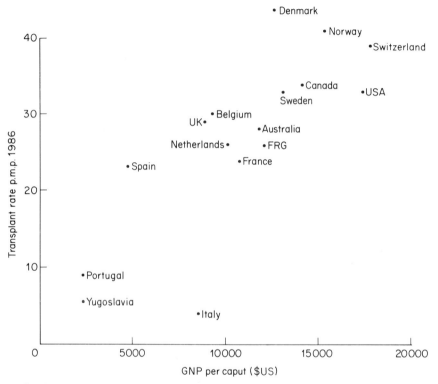

Figure 4. The transplant rate per million population, compared with the gross national product per capita in $US (1986). Fourteen representative countries studied. FRG, Federal Republic of Germany; UK, United Kingdom; USA, United States of America.

There is little information available to indicate the number of patients who would benefit from transplantation per annum. A questionnaire survey of British transplant units indicated that about 45 patients pmp per annum would be suitable for the operation (Sells et al, 1985). In 1986 only four countries approached this figure: Denmark (44.5), Sweden (41.7), Norway (41.3) and Switzerland (40.3). Norway achieved 41 transplants pmp by using live donors in 47%, and Sweden in 18%, of cases whereas Denmark used only 8% and Switzerland less than 2% live donors. Despite the fact that almost all the countries studied failed to achieve the 'ideal' number of transplants per year, there is evidence that the proportion of patients treated by transplantation is increasing, at least in Europe. Figure 5 shows that, whereas the number of 'stock' patients on dialysis stayed about the same in 1984 to 1985, a significant increase occurred in the number of patients alive with functioning renal transplants. This may well reflect a reluctance by European health departments and insurance bodies to continue unlimited funding of dialysis and a tendency to channel more resources into transplantation.

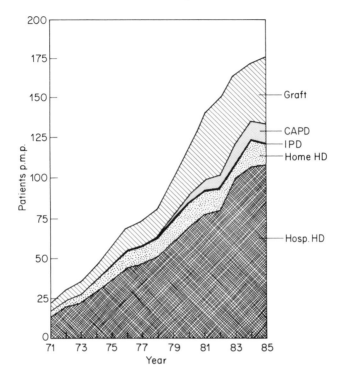

Figure 5.   The number of patients per million population in Europe alive on any method of renal replacement therapy on 31 December for each of the years, 1971–1985. CAPD, continuous ambulatory peritoneal dialysis; IPD, intermittent peritoneal dialysis; HD, haemo-dialysis.

The treatment of ESRD in the USA is now astonishingly prevalent: no less than one third of all the world's patients alive on treatment reside in the USA. The transplantation rate is at least 33 pmp per year, which is high by European standards but small compared to the rate of acceptance of new patients in the USA, which exceeds 100 pmp per year (Brunner et al, 1989). Medicare benefits for ESRD patients introduced in 1972 have greatly increased the take-on rate for dialysis and subsequent transplantation. Free access to dialysis in the USA has caused a pronounced shift in the age distribution in that only 7% of patients treated in 1967 were aged over 55, whereas in 1986 52% of newly enrolled patients were aged 60 years or more. Eleven per cent of American dialysis patients were awaiting a renal transplant in 1985, compared (for instance) with 44.9% in the UK (Tufveson et al, 1989). The reduced preference for transplantation in the USA can be explained in part by the fact that funding for dialysis is available to virtually all

American citizens who require it and the economic pressure that favours transplantation in some European countries is not yet a major factor in determining American attitudes to therapy. The slightly more 'safe' option of dialysis is therefore preferred in the older age groups which, with blacks, comprise the minority of transplant recipients.

Figure 6 compares annual acceptance rate for all forms of therapy of ESRD in 1986 with the annual transplant rate for each country studied. Most countries accepting more than 30 patients pmp for treatment have developed transplant facilities to supplement their dialysis services, and in 18 of the 26 at least 22 patients pmp received transplants in 1986. Of the remaining eight countries, where transplant rates were 10 pmp per year or less, suitable transplant recipients were mostly sent to other countries for their operation.

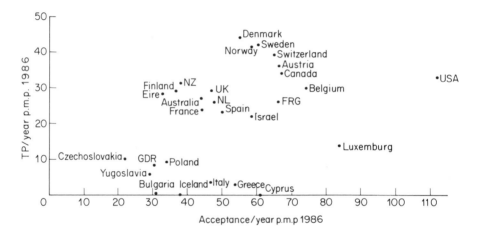

Figure 6. The annual acceptance rate of patients for all forms of therapy (per million population) *versus* the annual transplant rate per million population for 1986. FRG, Federal Republic of Germany; GDR, German Democratic Republic; NL, Netherlands; NZ, New Zealand; UK, United Kingdom; USA, United States of America.

We conclude this review by addressing in more detail the correlation between the stock of patients (that is, the number on dialysis) and transplantation, and the relationship (which may be permissive or inhibitory) between per capita GNP and the proportion of patients transplanted per annum.

The size of the dialysis population is likely to influence the number of transplants performed: not only does a larger dialysis pool attract more and better matched cadaveric grafts from national and international organ sharing agencies, but the economic arguments are likely to favour significantly the development of transplantation in national treatment strategies. This 'pressure' effect of the size of the dialysis stock on transplant rates can be crudely measured by defining a 'transplant probability index' represented by:

$$\frac{\text{Number of transplants per year}}{\text{Stock of dialysis patients per year}} \times 100$$

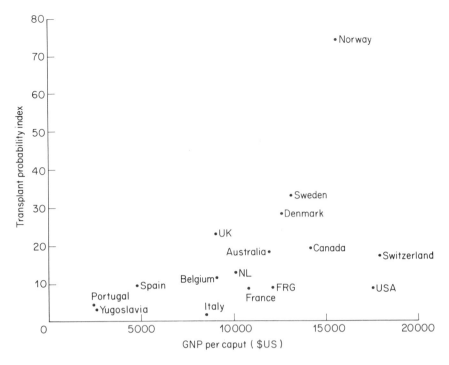

Figure 7. The 'transplant probability index' compared with the gross national product per caput in $US. Data is presented for 16 selected countries. FRG, Federal Republic of Germany; NL, Netherlands; UK, United Kingdom; USA, United States of America.

The Transplant Probability Index for 1986 is compared with per capita GNP in Figure 7, and several interesting points emerge. In Switzerland and the USA, the two wealthiest countries studied here, there were very large numbers of patients on dialysis with only a modest fraction of the stock of dialysis patients being transplanted each year, although the actual transplant rates in 1986 in these two countries were 39 and 33 patients pmp respectively (see also Figure 6). Norway, however, had a small dialysis pool (55 pmp) and a well-organized donor programme (based on a high proportion of live donors), with an ensuing high transplant rate (41 patients pmp) and thus a very high transplant probability index. So in these three wealthy countries a high GNP allowed the development of either a transplant-based or a predominantly dialysis-based health-care plan for ESRD patients. One might expect that the financial pressure of a sizeable dialysis stock would increase the transplant probability index in poorer countries, but this is not so: Portugal, Yugoslavia and Spain exhibit relatively low transplant rates despite large numbers of dialysis patients (199, 173, and 230 pmp respectively). In Italy, many patients emigrate to other countries for transplantation, so that the low probability index given in Figure 7 may be misleading. In the UK, the dialysis budget allocated by the Government Health Service has been restrained for some years, and the swing towards a relatively high transplant rate was predictable and perhaps inevitable. This is reflected in the large stock of transplanted British patients alive in 1986 compared with other countries of similar size (see Table 3).

Table 3. Numbers of patients alive with functioning transplants in 1986 in selected countries. From the Combined Report on Regular Dialysis and Transplantation in Europe.

Country	Patients alive	Population (millions)	Patients alive (pmp)
France	3993	55.1	72.6
Italy	2121	56.9	37.3
Federal Republic of Germany	3035	61.1	49.7
Spain	3056	38.7	30.0
United Kingdom	6638	56.5	117.5

Although the existence of a stock of patients on long-term dialysis influences to some degree national transplantation policies, Figure 7 provides no information about the proportion of *recently accepted* patients who are transplanted. We have therefore defined another index, which relates the transplants done per year to the number of patients accepted for treatment during that year; because this formula relates to the dynamic flow of patients rather than the static patient stock, we term this the 'transplant flow index':

$$\frac{\text{Number of patients transplanted per year}}{\text{Number of new patients starting treatment per year}^*} \times 100$$

This index, which reflects the yearly transplant activity as a proportion of annual 'take-on' rate, may allow us to predict the 'pressure effect' of accumulated dialysis stock, and the effect of GNP on contemporary transplant policies. In Figure 8 the transplant flow index for 1986 is plotted against patient dialysis stock for those countries in which transplant facilities allow more than ten patients pmp to be transplanted per annum. We have not attempted a linear correlation of the values for these two parameters because any statistically coherent relationship would be meaningless for those countries with a large stock of dialysis patients; nevertheless, there seems to be a trend suggesting that in countries with low dialysis stocks referral rates for transplant patients are high, and vice versa. Figure 9 examines the effect of per capita GNP on the transplant flow index, and we conclude that although GNP may affect the availability of gross resources, national wealth does not affect referral rates for transplantation in terms of the percentage of new cases accepted annually for treatment.

CONCLUSIONS

Because transplantation depends on the existence of adequate primary care services to permit diagnosis and referral, as well as on dialysis technology and transplant services,

---

* The great majority of patients accepted for treatment commence dialysis prior to transplantation; the very few who are transplanted without prior dialysis have not been separately identified in this analysis and are therefore included in the denominator.

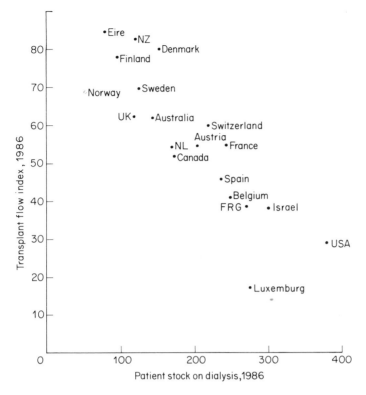

Figure 8. The 'Transplant flow index' for 1986 compared with the patient stock on dialysis for that year. Only those countries are included in which more than ten patients are transplanted per annum per million population. FRG, Federal Republic of Germany; NL, Netherlands; NZ, New Zealand; UK, United Kingdom; USA, United States of America.

this mode of therapy at present is almost entirely limited to those developed countries wealthy enough to pay for it. Of 330 000 patients alive on treatment for ESRD worldwide in 1986, 91% resided in the USA, Europe and Japan. There is little evidence to suggest that countries in the Third World and Eastern Europe have made much significant progress in the treatment of their patients. Twenty one per cent of all treated patients survive with a functioning transplant. Recent evidence suggests that, as not even the wealthiest countries can afford an open-ended 'free for all' dialysis strategy, the proportion of cases transplanted is rising accordingly. It has been calculated (Bone JM, personal communication) that for a region containing one million people in the UK, and with a transplant rate of 60 per million per annum and a failure rate at one year of 20% (excluding mortality), a dialysis pool of 100 spaces would be necessary for every new case of ESRD to be treated. The revenue cost of such a programme could well exceed US$ 3 million per year per million population. Three-quarters of the world's population lives in countries with a per capita GNP of less than US$ 2700 per annum. For the hundreds of thousands of people in these countries suffering from ESRD there can be little hope of treatment in the foreseeable future.

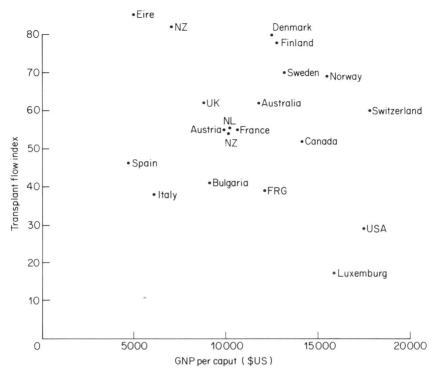

Figure 9. The relationship between transplant flow index and the wealth of individual countries as judged by the gross national per capita product in $US. Those countries are included that report more than ten patients transplanted per annum per million population. FRG, Federal Republic of Germany; NL, Netherlands; NZ, New Zealand; UK, United Kingdom; USA, United States of America.

REFERENCES

Branch RA, Clarke GW, Cochrane A et al (1971) Incidence of uraemia and requirements for maintenance haemodialysis. *British Medical Journal* **1**: 249.

Brenner B (1983) Dietary protein intake and the progressive nature of kidney disease. *New England Journal of Medicine* **307**: 652.

Broyer M, Brunner FP, Brynger H et al (1986) Demography of Dialysis and Transplantation in Europe 1984. *Nephrology, Dialysis and Transplantation* **1**: 1–8.

Brunner FP, Wing AJ, Dykes SR et al (1989) International Review of Renal Replacement Therapy: Strategies and Results. In J Maher (ed.) *Replacement of Renal Function by Dialysis*, pp 697–719. Dordrecht: Kluwer Academic Publishers.

Chugh KS (1979) Management of Renal Failure in India. Proceedings of the second meeting of the International Society for Artificial Organs (ISAO) New York, 1979. *Journal of Chronic Diseases* **26**: 237.

Edington GM & Mainwaring AR (1966) Nephropathies in West Africa. In FK Mostofi & DE Smith (eds) *The Kidney*, p. 488. Baltimore: Williams and Wilkins.

Pendreigh DM, Heasman MA, Howitt LF et al (1972) Survey of chronic renal failure in Scotland. *Lancet* **i**: 304.

Rostand SG, Kirk K, Rutsky E et al (1982) Racial differences in the incidence of treatment for end-stage renal disease. *New England Journal of Medicine* **306**: 1276.

Sells RA, MacPherson S & Salaman JR (for the British Transplantation Society) (1985) *Lancet* **i**: 195–196.

Tufveson G, Geerlings W, Broyer M et al (1989) EDTA Registry Centre Survey 1986. *Nephrology, Dialysis, Transplantation* **4**: 161–171.

Wing AJ, Broyer M, Brunner FP et al (1988) Demography of Dialysis and Transplantation in Europe in 1985 and 1986: Trends over the previous decade. *Nephrology, Dialysis and Transplantation* **3**: 714–727.

III Notes on the History of Tissue and Organ Transplantation

L. BRENT
ROBERT A. SELLS

CONTENTS

Introduction
Adoptive transfer of transplantation immunity
Allograft rejection as an immunological phenomenon
Antilymphocyte serum
Artificial kidney
Criteria of brain death
Cytotoxic effector cells
Discovery of the HLA system and tissue typing
Experimental bone marrow transplantation and radiation chimeras
First successful human renal transplant in modern times
First long-surviving human kidney transplants
First experience with whole body irradiation for immunosuppression in man
First human recipients treated with cyclosporin A (cyclosporine; Sandimmune)
First attempts at clinical bone marrow transplantation
First clinical pancreas transplants
First liver transplants in man
First heart transplants in man
Graft-versus-host disease
Immunological enhancement
Immunological tolerance
Immunologically privileged sites
Kidney preservation for more than 24 hours
Minor histocompatibility and MHC restricted responses
Mixed lymphocyte reaction and discovery of Ia and D region antigens
Mouse monoclonal anti-human CD3 globulin
Thymus and bursa of Fabricius: T and B lymphocytes
6-Mercaptopurine and azathioprine (Imuran)

INTRODUCTION

The transplantation of tissues and organs has fascinated surgeons for centuries, but human allotransplantation was not seriously attempted until the nineteenth century (for reviews see Hamilton, 1988; Silverstein, 1989). The results of these efforts were variable: kidney grafts, though they sometimes appeared to remain viable for remarkably long periods, usually failed, but it was often claimed that skin homografts, as they were then known, were accepted. Documentation was generally poor and, with skin grafts, it was easy enough to be deceived by the insidious replacement of the graft epidermis by native epithelium. We nevertheless owe these early and intrepid surgeons, E. Ullman, A. Carrel and C. H. Guthrie among them, a great debt in initiating some of the surgical techniques used in the transplantation of organs such as the kidney.

Modern transplantation has its roots in the work done in the 1920s and 1930s on tumour transplantation, and a number of workers at that time realized that there was a genetic, and possibly an immunological, cause for the failure of allogeneic tumours in experimental animals. Nevertheless, a clear understanding of the immunological nature of graft rejection had to await the pioneering studies of P. A. Gorer, G. D. Snell and P. B. Medawar, and modern transplantation immunology is largely based on their fundamental observations, even though the phenomena that they studied have proved to be infinitely more complex than was realized at the time. These pioneering studies in transplantation immunology led directly to the era of cellular immunology and thus made a profound contribution not only to transplantation immunology but to the development of the field of immunology in general.

Rather than attempt to write a history we have selected here a number of phenomena, discoveries and techniques that have made a substantial impact on the development of tissue and organ transplantation, and provided short notes on them. Such a list must inevitably be selective and, to some degree, subject to the prejudices of the authors, and we acknowledge that there may be significant omissions in the topics selected and in our attributions. We wish to thank Dr Elizabeth Simpson and Professors J. R. Batchelor, H. Festenstein and A. N. Mitchison for their helpful comments.

General historical references

Hamilton D (1988) Kidney transplantation: a history. In Morris, P.J. (ed.) *Kidney Transplantation*, pp 1–13. New York: Grune & Stratton.
Silverstein AM (1989) Transplantation and Immunogenetics. In *A History of Immunology*. New York: Academic Press.

ADOPTIVE TRANSFER OF TRANSPLANTATION IMMUNITY

Mitchison NA (1954) Passive transfer of immunity. *Proceedings of the Royal Society of London, Series B* **142**: 72–87.
Billingham RE, Brent L & Medawar PB (1954) Quantitative studies on tissue transplantation immunity. II. The origin, strength and duration of actively and adoptively acquired immunity. *Proceedings of the Royal Society of London, Series B* **143**: 58–80.

Earlier studies had shown that resistance to a tumour can be passively transferred by means of antibody (W. H. Woglom, 1933–1937) and that delayed-type hypersensitivity can be transiently transferred by means of cells (K. Landsteiner and M. W. Chase, 1945). Both groups of workers used non-inbred animals, thus making the demonstration of passive transfer, especially with cells, very difficult.

Mitchison was the first to use inbred strains of mice in this context and to show that resistance to an allogeneic lymphosarcoma can be passively transferred with minced lymph nodes, but not with serum, to non-susceptible mice, and he established the principle that this kind of experiment demands that the lymphoid cell donor and the recipient belongs to the same inbred strain.

Billingham et al extended this concept to skin allografts and went on to show that draining lymph node cells, even in suspended form, are capable of transferring immunity but that spleen cells are less active in this respect following skin graft sensitization. Blood leukocytes, contralateral lymph nodes and serum were found to be inactive. They coined the term 'adoptive transfer' to distinguish it from antibody-mediated transfer of immunity, and they showed that adoptive transfer can be successfully carried out as long as 30 days after active sensitization. These findings led them to liken transplantation immunity to delayed-type hypersensitivity, a concept that has survived.

ALLOGRAFT REJECTION AS AN IMMUNOLOGICAL PHENOMENON

Little CC & Tyzzer EE (1916) Further experimental evidence on the inheritance of susceptibility to a transplantable tumour, carcinoma (J.W.A.) of a Japanese Waltzing mouse. *J. Exp. Res.* **33**: 393–427.

Gorer PA (1937) The genetic and antigenic basis of tumour transplantation. *Journal of Pathology and Bacteriology* **44**: 691–697.

Gorer PA, Lyman S & Snell GD (1948) Studies on the genetic and antigenic basis of tumour transplantation: linkage between a histocompatibility gene and 'fused' in mice. *Proceedings of the Royal Society of London, Series B* **135**: 499–505.

Snell GD (1948) Methods for the study of histocompatibility genes. *Journal of Genetics* **49**: 87–103.

Medawar PB & Gibson T (1943) The fate of skin homografts in mice. *Journal of Anatomy, London* **77**: 299–310.
Medawar PB (1944) The behaviour and fate of skin autografts and homografts in rabbits. *Journal of Anatomy, London* **79**: 157–176.

Little and Tyzzer were the first to demonstrate that susceptibility and resistance of mice to certain tumour transplants could be explained by Mendelian genetics, and they postulated that '. . . susceptibility to a transplantable tumor is based on a factor complex or on the coexistence of a number of inherited factors in the individual.' They thought the number of factors to be 'rather large'.

Gorer's important early contribution was to correlate susceptibility and resistance to the growth of a transplantable sarcoma (which arose spontaneously in A strain mice, and was therefore transplantable within that strain, but rejected by C57 mice) with the absence or presence of an antigen that he termed 'antigen II'. (Antigens I and III had been identified in other studies; all three were found on murine red blood cells but antigen II was also shown to be expressed by other kinds of cells.) The A mice possessed antigen II whereas C57 mice did not; the latter not only rejected the tumour but also generated antibodies that agglutinated A strain red cells. This was the first 'iso-antibody' (which we would now call an alloantibody) to be identified in mice. Gorer unfortunately died in 1961, aged only 54.

Snell's enormous contribution to transplantation immunology and genetics was to develop a number of congenic strains, i.e. inbred strains differing at only a single genetic locus from the strain of origin. Using such strains Snell discovered a locus that seemed to determine allogeneic tumour graft rejection, and he called this the H-locus (for histocompatibility). Gorer, Snell and their colleagues then went on to show that antigen II was coded for by the H locus, and H-2 – the major histocompatibility locus of the mice, as it turned out to be – thus became known and much studied.

Meanwhile Medawar and Gibson, spurred on by the exigencies of war-torn Britain and the need to find a better treatment for badly burnt patients, carried out their classical study on a single burnt patient by transplanting auto- and homografts (the latter now called allografts) and closely studying their fate using serial biopsies. This limited but incisive experiment clearly illustrated the difference between the two kinds of grafts, pointed to the existence of a latent period before the onset of rejection, failed to find, curiously enough, much evidence of cellular involvement, and left no doubt at all that second-set grafts undergo rejection more rapidly than first-set grafts. They concluded that the homografts were rejected as a result of 'active immunisation'.

Medawar followed up these observations with more detailed but equally elegant studies in the rabbit, the first published in 1944 and the second a year later in the same journal. These experiments, which not only confirmed the human data but also established the specificity of graft rejection and drew attention to the cellular infiltrates that characterize rejection, left no doubt whatever that allograft rejection was an immunological event. The modern era of transplantation immunology had begun.

ANTILYMPHOCYTE SERUM

Metchnikoff M (1899) Étude sur la resorption des cellules. *Annals of the Institute Pasteur* **13**: 737, 760.
Chew WB & Lawrence JS (1937) Anti-lymphocyte serum. *Journal of Immunology* **33**: 271–278.
Woodruff MFA & Anderson NF (1963) Effect of lymphocyte depletion by thoracic duct fistula and administration of anti-lymphocyte serum on the survival of skin homografts in rats. *Nature* **200**: 702.
Levey RH & Medawar PB (1966) Some experiments on the action of anti-lymphoid antisera. *Annals of the New York Academy of Sciences* **129**: 164–177.

Metchnikoff was the first to prepare antilymphocyte serum (ALS) by the injection of guinea pigs with rat and rabbit lymph node preparations. The sera thus obtained were shown to be agglutinating and cytotoxic. Further in vitro studies by Chew and Lawrence showed that ALS caused complement-dependent cytotoxicity and leukoagglutination; they also first suggested that the rapid disappearance of the lymphopenic effect of ALS was due to the immune response of the recipients to the heterologous protein. The experiments from Woodruff's laboratory were the first to demonstrate successful prolongation of skin allografts from albino donors placed on hooded rats treated with ALS. Untreated recipients rejected their grafts within 8 days whereas recipients treated by a combination of thoracic duct fistula and rabbit anti-rat ALS showed graft survival for up to 75 days. Subsequent authors, especially Medawar's group, demonstrated similar or even better protective effects of ALS alone in various rodent models, including the depression of secondary antibody response and the prolongation of 'second-set' skin grafts. They also showed that the optimal immunosuppressive effect on murine skin allograft rejection occurred when ALS was given during the first few days after grafting.

THE ARTIFICIAL KIDNEY

Kolff WJ (1946) *The Artificial Kidney* N.V. Kampen (Holland): J.H. Kok.

After 16 fruitless attempts to treat patients with his novel artificial kidney machine, Kolff achieved success with this 17th patient. She had cholecystitis, jaundice and anuria due to hepatorenal syndrome and was admitted to hospital on 3 September 1945. There she developed oedema, hypertension and coma, and 8 days later she underwent eleven and a half hours of dialysis, 60 g of urea being removed from her blood. The timing of this intervention was propitious: two days later she passed 800 ml of urine and the blood urea peaked and then fell to normal levels within a week. Seven months later the patient was fit and the blood urea and blood pressure were normal. The gall bladder had not been removed.

CRITERIA OF BRAIN DEATH

Report of the Ad Hoc Committee of the Harvard Medical School to examine the definition of brain death (1968) *Journal of the American Medical Association* **205**: 339–340.

Cadaveric organ transplantation focused attention on the need for an infallible method of determining death of the donor. Transplant surgeons in the early 1960s were in a quandary because clear advice from neurologists was lacking on this crucial issue: was the patient with brain death truly dead whilst the heart was still beating? The *ad hoc* committee (comprising six neurological scientists, a lawyer, a psychiatrist, a sociologist, a theologian and two transplant physicians) drew up the criteria of irreversible coma. They were, in summary: unreceptivity and unresponsiveness; no movements or breathing; no reflexes; and a flat electroencephalogram. Further enquiry on the fate of people suffering irreversible coma, and a very extensive retrospective study of the case material of brain-injured patients requiring intensive care, made possible a firmer declaration by the profession in the UK on the definition of death in heart-beating donors. Thus, in 1976 the conference of Royal Colleges of the United Kingdom published a list of minimal criteria of brain death that excluded a flat EEG. In 1979 the conference went further in affirming that the state of brain death can be equated with actual death. Despite a damaging attack in 1981 by a British television programme on these criteria, these rules for establishing brain death have been reaffirmed, they endure as the ethical and professional benchmark in the UK and they have been adopted by intensive care physicians and transplant surgeons in many other countries.

CYTOTOXIC EFFECTOR CELLS

Vainio T, Koskimies O, Perlmann P, Perlmann H & Klein G (1964) In vitro cytotoxic effect of lymphoid cells from mice immunized with allogeneic tissue. *Nature* **204**: 453–455.

Wilson DB (1965) Quantitative studies on the behaviour of sensitized lymphocytes in vitro. I. Relationship of the degree of destruction of homologous target cells to the number of lymphocytes and to the time of contact in culture and consideration of the effect of isoimmune serum. *Journal of Experimental Medicine* **122**: 143–166.

Rosenau W & Moon HD (1966) Studies on the mechanisms of the cytotoxic effect of sensitized lymphocytes. *Journal of Immunology* **96**: 80–84.

Brunner KT, Mauel J, Cerrottini J-C & Chapuis B (1968) Quantitative assay of the lytic action of immune lymphoid cells on ⁵¹Cr-labelled allogeneic target cells in vitro; inhibition by isoantibody and drug. *Immunology* **14**: 181–196.

Wunderlich JR & Canty TG (1970) Cell mediated immunity induced in vitro. *Nature* **228**: 62–63.

Häyry P & Defendi U (1970) Mixed lymphocyte cultures produce effector cells: model in vitro for allograft rejection. *Science* **168**: 133–135.

Wagner H & Feldman M (1972) Cell-mediated immune response in vitro. I. A new in vitro system for the generation of cell-mediated cytotoxic activity. *Cellular Immunology* **3**: 405–420.

Alter BJ, Schendel D, Bach ML, Bach, FH, Klein J & Stimpfling JH (1973) Cell-mediated lympholysis. Importance of serologically defined H-2 regions. *Journal of Experimental Medicine* **137**: 1303–1309.

Cantor H & Boyse EA (1975) Functional subclasses of T lymphocytes bearing different Ly antigens. I. The generation of functionally distinct T-cell subclasses is a differentiation process independent of antigen. *Journal of Experimental Medicine* **141**: 1376–1389.

Cytotoxic T lymphocytes, with specificity for the stimulator cells, are generated during the course of mixed lymphocyte culture (MLC or MLR). However, even before the discovery of the MLR, Vainio et al had become interested in the effect of lymphoid cells from specifically sensitized animals on target cells bearing the appropriate MHC antigens. Using inbred strains of mice, they showed that target cells obtained from the trypsinization of fetal or adult tissues were lysed by in vivo sensitized lymphoid cells. They concluded that the cytotoxic action of the cells was not brought about by antibodies though they felt unable to exclude their participation.

Wilson carried out extensive studies on the in vitro destruction of target cells by direct contact with sensitized lymphoid cells. He concluded that '... the destruction of homologous target cells ... occurs as a two step process. First, the attacking lymphocytes attach to their targets via a non-toxic cell-bound substance having an immunologic specificity, and then, destruction of the target cells followed the result of some process dependent on the metabolic activity of the attacking lymphoid cells'. Rosenau and Moon, like Vainio et al and Wilson before them, ruled out the participation of antibodies in the in vitro destruction of target cells and related this event to a 'functional modification of lymphocytes'.

The basis of the cell-mediated lympholysis (CML) assay was laid by the work of Brunner et al, in that they developed an in vitro method for measuring the level of cytotoxicity generated by in vivo sensitization of mice with alloantigens. Cytotoxicity was estimated by the release into the medium of ⁵¹Cr, with which the target cells were labelled. Working likewise with mice, Wunderlich and Canty and, quite independently Häyry and Defendi, showed that specific cytotoxic lymphocytes could be generated in vitro during the course of an MLR. The latter concluded that 'in view of the specificity for both the afferent and the efferent responses, it is possible to consider the MLI (mixed lymphocyte interaction) a complete in vitro model for allograft rejection'. Wagner and Feldman provided a quantitative assay that was both reproducible and sensitive, using a 5-day MLR and a 6-hour cytotoxic assay. In the following year Alter et al demonstrated decisively that the target molecules for cytotoxic lymphocytes were the H-2 serologically defined (SD) antigens (now called class I): cells from strains of mice with identical SD antigens did not generate a cytotoxic response. Finally, it was left to Cantor and Boyse to demonstrate that there are different subclasses of T lymphocytes with different functions. Thus, Ly-23 + cells on their own could not provide 'help' but generated cytotoxic activity for target cells, whereas Ly-1$^+$ cells give good helper responses but were unable on their own to generate cytotoxic activity. The difference between T helper and T cytotoxic lymphocytes thus became established: we would now term these subpopulations CD4 and CD8 positive, respectively.

Although the CML assay is frequently accepted as an in vitro analogue of allograft rejection, it must be remembered that it measures primarily the reactivity of CD8$^+$ cytotoxic cells directed against, or restricted by, MHC class I antigens and not CD4$^+$ helper cells, which likewise participate in graft rejection.

DISCOVERY OF THE HLA SYSTEM AND TISSUE TYPING

Dausset J (1958) Iso-leuco anticorps. *Acta Haematologica* **20**: 156–166.

Dausset J, Ivanyi P & Ivanyi D (1965) Tissue alloantigens in humans: identification of a complex system (Hu-1). *Histocompatibility Testing* **11**: 51–62.

Van Rood JJ & van Leeuwen A (1963) Leucocyte grouping, a method and its application. *Journal of Clinical Investigation* **42**: 1382–1390.

Hamburger J, Vaysse J, Crosnier, J, Auvert J, Lalannae ClM & Hopper J (1962) Renal transplantation in man after radiation of the recipient. Experience with 6 patients since 1959. *American Journal of Medicine* **32**: 854–871.

Dausset J, Rapaport FT, Ivanyi P & Colombani J (1965) Tissue alloantigens and transplantation. *Histocompatibility Testing* **11**: 63–72.

Vredevoe DL, Terasaki PI, Mickey MR, Glassock R, Merrill JP & Murray JE (1965) Serotyping of human leucocyte antigens. III. Long term kidney homograft survivors. *Histocompatibility Testing* **11**: 25–36.

Patel R, Mickey MR & Terasaki PI (1968) Serotyping for homotransplantation. XVI. Analysis of kidney transplants from unrelated donors. *New England Journal of Medicine* **279**: 501–506.

Batchelor JR & Voysey VC (1969) Influence of HL-A incompatibility on cadaveric renal transplantation. *Lancet* **ii**: 790–793.

Morris PJ, Kincaid-Smith P, Ting A, Stocker JW & Marshall VC (1968) Prospective leucocyte typing in cadaver renal transplantation. *Lancet* **ii**: 803–805.

Dausset was the first to describe serum alloantibodies reacting with human leucocytes, defining an antigen that he called Mac, and he postulated that such an antigen may have a role to play in histocompatibility responses. Mac later turned out to be HLA-A2, interestingly enough the first HLA antigen to be subjected to X-ray crystallography (1987). Dausset, who was later to share a Nobel Prize for his discovery, went on with his colleagues to define further antigens making up a system they termed Hu-1.

Van Rood and van Leeuwen and their colleagues made major contributions to our knowledge of what is now known to be an extremely complex major histocompatibility system, initially by defining the first allelic leukocyte antigens, which they called 4a and 4b. They introduced the idea of using serum from pregnant women for the identification of leukocyte antigens, and they enabled the field to advance rapidly by the use of computer analysis. In their 1963 paper they concluded, following family studies, that the two antigens identified (now BW4 and BW6) were inherited in simple Mendelian fashion as autosomal co-dominant alleles.

The remarkably speedy unravelling of the HLA system was assisted by the work previously done on the H-2 complex, its murine counterpart (see notes on allograft rejection), but the most decisive factors were the use of computers and the regularly held Histocompatibility Workshops. Many workers apart from Dausset and van Rood and their colleagues and those listed in the references made significant contributions: for example, Rose Payne, R. Ceppellini, D. B. Amos, R. L. Walford, F. Kissmeyer-Nielsen,

J. G. and W. F. Bodmer, H. Balner, E. Thorsby, A. Ting, and H. Festenstein. The first Histocompatibility Workshop was held in 1964 and it became a regular event, enabling tissue typers and immunogeneticists to compare their reagents directly against the same panels of cells, to discuss the implications of their findings and to resolve problems of nomenclature.

The first glimmer that matching for major histocompatibility antigens may be beneficial came from a retrospective study of a small group of patients by Hamburger's group as early as 1962. Three out of six of their cadaveric kidney recipients, irradiated with 430–460 rads, were long-term survivors who had a better antigen match for the few antigens known at the time than those who had rejected their kidneys soon after transplantation. This was followed by a more comprehensive study by Vredevoe et al on long-term kidney allograft survivors who had received kidneys from living related donors: the numbers of mismatches were generally, though not always, less than would be expected from random chance. Dausset et al demonstrated in the same volume that human volunteers strongly sensitized against ten leukocyte antigens (Hu-1) generally rejected well-matched skin allografts more slowly than poorly matched skin grafts, and these workers concluded that Hu-1 antigens were 'transplantation antigens'.

A detailed retrospective analysis of HLA matching and *cadaveric* kidney transplants came from Terasaki's group in 1968. They identified five major antigens and found that well-matched patients had a better creatinine clearance and fewer rejection crises and were generally clinically superior compared with poorly matched patients – findings that were confirmed by Batchelor and Joysey. The first *prospective* attempt at HLA matching for cadaveric kidney recipients seems to have been made by Morris et al, who matched for eight antigens and showed that poorly matched patients fared badly compared with well matched individuals. (For information on HLA-D/DR, see notes below on the mixed lymphocyte reaction.)

EXPERIMENTAL BONE MARROW TRANSPLANTATION AND RADIATION CHIMERAS

Jacobson LO, Simmons EL, Marks EK & Eldridge J (1951) Recovery from radiation injury. *Science* **113**: 510–511.

Lorenz E, Uphoff D, Reid TR & Shelton E (1951) Modification of irradiation injury in mice and guinea pigs by bone marrow injections. *Journal of the National Cancer Institute* **12**: 197–201.

Cole LJ, Fishler MC & Bond VP (1953) Subcellular fractionation of mouse spleen radiation protection activity. *Proceedings of the National Academy of Sciences, USA* **39**: 759–772.

Barnes DWH & Loutit JF (1954) What is the recovery factor in spleen? *Nucleonics* **12**: 68–71.

Barnes DWH & Loutit JF (1955) The radiation recovery factor: preservation by the Polge–Smith–Parkes technique. *Journal of the National Cancer Institute* **15**: 901–905.

Lindsley DL, Odell TT & Tausche FG (1955) Implantation of functional erythropoietic elements following total-body irradiation. *Proceedings of the Society for Experimental Biology and Medicine* **90**: 512–515.

Main JM & Prehn RT (1955) Successful skin homografts after the administration of high dosage X irradiation and homologous bone marrow. *Journal of the National Cancer Institute* **15**: 1023–1028.

Ford CE, Hamerton JL, Barnes DWH & Loutit JF (1956) Cytological identification of radiation-chimaeras. *Nature* **177**: 452–454.

Makinodan T (1956) Circulating rat cells in lethally irradiated mice protected with rat bone marrow. *Proceedings of the Society for Experimental Biology and Medicine* **92**: 174–179.

Nowell PC, Cole LJ, Habermeyer JG & Roan PL (1956) Growth and continued function of rat marrow cells in X-irradiated mice. *Cancer Research* **16**: 258–261.

Vos O, Davids JG, Weyzen WWH & van Bekkum DW (1956) Evidence for the cellular hypothesis in radiation protection by bone marrow cells. *Acta Physiologica et Pharmacologica Néerlandica* 4: 482–486.

van Bekkum DW, Vos O & Weyzen WH (1956) Homo- et hétérogreffes hématopoiétiques chez la souris. *Revue d'Hématologie* 11: 477–485.

Mitchison NA (1956) The colonisation of irradiated tissue by transplanted spleen cells. *British Journal of Experimental Pathology* 37: 239–247.

The 1950s saw a great upsurge of interest in radiation biology and attempts to mitigate radiation-induced injury to the haemopoietic system. Attempts were made to counter radiation injury by the injection of allogeneic (then known as homologous) or xenogeneic (heterologous) bone marrow or spleen cells immediately after the administration of a lethal or near-lethal dose of whole body irradiation. (For the early work on graft-versus-host reactivity as an explanation for secondary disease see notes on 'Graft-versus-host disease'; for references on the first attempts to apply bone marrow transplantation to man, see notes below on 'The first attempts at clinical bone marrow transplantation').

Jacobson and his colleagues were among the first to propose that the haemopoietic tissue of an irradiated mouse recovers by the production of a soluble factor. Their early experiments were based on partial shielding of various tissues during irradiation with lethal doses of X-rays. They found that shielding of the spleen protected the majority of mice and that, even without shielding, the intraperitoneal implantation of whole spleens from young mice of the same strain led to recovery in about 40% of animals. They thought it 'unlikely' that cells would migrate out of the shielded tissues and proposed the production of a soluble factor. This erroneous notion held sway until the mid-1950s; Cole et al thought they had shown that isolated nuclei protected quite well and they suggested, wrongly as it turned out, that nucleoprotein might be involved. Lorenz et al tentatively suggested as early as 1951 that intravenously administered bone marrow cells in both mice and guinea-pigs cause the generation of 'new areas of hematopoiesis, contrary to the assumption of Jacobson of a humoral factor'; it seems surprising that more weight was not given to this notion of cellular repopulation at the time.

Arguably the first serious consideration of the cell repopulation concept came from Barnes and Loutit in 1954. They reviewed the evidence favouring the humoral hypothesis and found much of it equivocal and some of it more in keeping with a cellular hypothesis. Their own data, based on the injection of cells after various treatments, suggested that the viability of the transplanted cells was the all-important factor, favouring the idea that donor cells repopulate the damaged host bone marrow. In 1955 they showed that bone marrow cells could be frozen in a glycerol-containing medium and kept at $-70°C$ for many weeks without losing their protective properties after rapid thawing.

Proof of the repopulation hypothesis now came thick and fast. Lindsley et al injected rat bone marrow into mice given an LD_{50} dose of irradiation and, using red cell antigens as markers, were able to show the persistence of rat red blood cells for many months. This was soon followed by several other equally convincing demonstrations. Ford et al, using the mouse donor strain carrying the T6 translocation, showed that virtually all dividing cells in the bone marrow, lymph nodes and thymus carried the T6 marker; Makinodan demonstrated that 100% of red blood cells in irradiated mice inoculated with rat bone marrow were of rat origin by day 65, an observation that was likewise made by Nowell et al using an alkaline phosphatase assay identifying rat blood and bone marrow leukocytes, and confirmed by van Bekkum's group. Finally, Mitchison identified donor cells in the tissues of lethally irradiated mice protected by allogeneic spleen cells from 8-day-old donors, and showed that there was enhanced antibody production by the host's spleen cells if the donor cells had been taken from mice sensitized by Salmonella typhi (H) antigen. It was Mitchison who coined the term 'radiation-chimaera'. Meanwhile, Main and Prehn had demonstrated the specific survival of donor strain skin allografts in surviving radiation chimeras. The work on radiation chimeras was undoubtedly influenced by the tolerance work of Billingham et al, first published in 1953, which showed that tolerant mice were cellular chimeras.

THE FIRST SUCCESSFUL HUMAN RENAL TRANSPLANT IN MODERN TIMES

Hufnagel C (1947), in Moore FD (1972) *Transplant: The Give and Take of Tissue Transplantation,* pp 40–41. New York: Simon and Schuster.

The first renal transplant that succeeded in its therapeutic objective was described by Hufnagel and his colleagues who, in 1946, transplanted a cadaveric kidney to the *arm* of a woman suffering from septicaemia and anuria. The operation was noteworthy, too, for having been performed in the ward (the patient having been too ill to be moved to the operating theatre) and by the assistance of two other distinguished clinical scientists – D. Hume and E. Landsteiner. The kidney was rejected after 3 days, but the patient's own kidneys had by then begun to function satisfactorily. Shortly after this event dialysis became more widely available, and short-term transplants such as this were not pursued with much vigour thereafter.

THE FIRST LONG-SURVIVING HUMAN KIDNEY TRANSPLANT

Merrill JP, Murray JE, Harrison JH & Guild WR (1956) Successful homotransplantation of the human kidney between identical twins. *Journal of the American Medical Association* **160**: 277–282.

Murray developed the modern clinical renal transplant operation, which has been adopted by transplant surgeons since it was first put into practice in a historic operation by Murray, Harrison and others at the Peter Bent Brigham Hospital, Boston, on 23 December 1954. The donor kidney was removed from the patient's identical twin and transplanted to the iliac fossa; the renal artery was joined to the internal iliac artery, the vein to the external iliac vein, and the ureter to the bladder. The kidney functioned immediately, and the patient recovered promptly from his uraemia. He lived for a further 8 years but succumbed eventually to recurrent disease (glomerulonephritis) in the graft. This surgical achievement signalled the beginning of organ transplantation. Further isogeneic kidneys were transplanted successfully within the next few years and renal allografts soon followed.

THE FIRST EXPERIENCE WITH WHOLE BODY IRRADIATION FOR IMMUNOSUPPRESSION IN MAN

Merril JP, Murray JE, Harrison JH, Friedman EA, Dealy JB Jnr & Dammin GJ (1960) Successful homotransplantation of the kidney between non-identical twins. *New England Journal of Medicine* **262**: 1251–1260.

Hamburger J, Vayesse J, Crosnier J, Tubiana M, Lalanne C-M, Antoine B, Auvert J, Soulier J-P, Dornot J, Salmon Ch, Maisonnet M & Amiel J-L (1959) Transplantation d'un rein entre jumeaux non monozygotes après irradiation du receveur; bon fonctionnement au quatrième mois. *Presse Medicale* **67**: 1771–1775.

After their success with identical twin donors, the Brigham team had many cases of renal failure referred to them where non-identical relatives had offered to donate kidneys. At that time pharmacological immunosuppression was not available, and a potentially lethal dose of X-irradiation was given followed by a bone marrow transplant from the donor in an attempt to 'rescue' the recipient from the destruction of their own marrow. Five patients died when the marrow grafts failed to 'take', although histologically their kidney grafts showed little or no signs of rejection. The sixth patient, who suffered from chronic renal failure due to glomerulonephritis with superimposed infection, was given a preliminary skin graft from the putative donor. This was not rejected, probably because of uraemia, and a renal transplant was inserted 8 days after a sublethal dose of 450 roentgen of total body irradiation, without a precautionary marrow graft. The transplant functioned well, but life-threatening septicaemia set in from the patient's own infected kidney 11 days after surgery. The risks of leaving his own kidneys in situ at a time of X-ray induced leukopenia and immunological inertia were even greater than the hazardous operation of bilateral nephrectomy. Harrison proceeded to remove both kidneys, and the patient recovered quickly. Nine months thereafter a renal biopsy revealed a rejection crisis, which was reversed with cortisone and further small doses of X-rays. This patient and his transplant survived for more than 10 years.

Three areas of new ground were broken in this historic case: (i) Early rejection was first prevented by prophylactic irradiation (a technique that was not found uniformly to be successful in subsequent trials). (ii) A rejection episode was reversed by deliberate if limited doses of X-rays and cortisone. (iii) A courageous and timely surgical intervention for sepsis in an immunologically incompetent patient helped to overcome the infection and saved the patient's life.

At or around the same time as this American case, Hamburger's group in Paris transplanted a fraternal non-identical twin's kidney to a patient suffering from chronic glomerulonephritis. A preoperative dose of 450 roentgen units of whole body radiation was administered to the recipient, who developed a typical rejection crisis (pyrexia and oliguria) some days after transplantation. More irradiation was given and the rejection was reversed. This first successful European recipient of a clinical renal allograft was well and active 10 years after his transplant.

FIRST HUMAN RECIPIENTS TREATED WITH CYCLOSPORIN A (CYCLOSPORINE; SANDIMMUNE)

Borel JF, Feurer C, Gubler HU & Stähelin H (1976) Biological effects of Cyclosporin A: a new antilymphocytic agent. *Agents and Actions* **6**: 468–475.

Calne RY, White DJG, Thiru S, Evans DB, McMaster P, Dunn DC, Craddock GN, Pentlow BD & Rolles K
(1978) Cyclosporin A in patients receiving renal allografts from cadaver donors. *Lancet* ii: 1323–1327.
Powles RL, Barnett AJ, Clink H, Kay HEM, Sloane J & McElwain TD (1978) Cyclosporin A for the treatment
of graft-versus-host disease in man. *Lancet* ii: 1327–1331.

Cyclosporin A is a fungal metabolite that was found to have potent immunosuppressive
properties without significantly depressing bone marrow function. Borel had shown in
1976 that cyclosporin A suppresses skin graft rejection and graft-versus-host disease in
mice as well as impairing delayed hypersensitivity, experimental allergic encephalomyelitis and adjuvant arthritis, and delaying the appearance of direct and indirect plaque-
forming cells in mice. After experiments in orthotopic heart transplantation in the pig had
shown that cyclosporin A therapy for 3 days caused significant graft prolongation
without bone marrow suppression, Calne and his colleagues in Cambridge, England,
demonstrated improved kidney graft survival in patients. Early problems with this drug
included lymphoma (a hazard which has receded with improved blood level monitoring
of the drug, and subsequent reduction in dosage) and nephrotoxicity, which has proved
to be reversible.

In the same volume Powles et al describe the first attempt to suppress human graft-
versus-host disease, following allogeneic bone marrow transplantation, with cyclosporin
A. Although the skin lesions resolved within days, four out of five patients died, with
liver damage.

FIRST ATTEMPTS AT CLINICAL BONE MARROW TRANSPLANTATION

Thomas ED, Lochte HL, Lu WC & Ferrebee JW (1957) Intravenous infusion of bone-marrow in patients
receiving radiation and chemotherapy. *New England Journal of Medicine* **257**: 491–496.
Humble JG & Newton KA (1958) Technique of human bone-marrow transplants. *Lancet* i: 142.
Thomas ED, Lochte HL & Ferrebee JW (1959) Irradiation of the entire body and marrow transplantation:
some observations and comments. *Blood* **14**: 1–23.
Mathé G, Bernard J, Schwarzenburger L, Larrieu MJ, Lalanne CM, Dutreix A, Denoix PF, Surmont J,
Schwarzmann V & Céora B. (1959) Essai de traitement de sujets atteints de leucémie aigue en rémission
par irradiation totale suivie de transfusion de moelle osseuse homologue. *Revue Française d'Études Cliniques
et Biologique* **4**: 675–704.
Jammet H, Mathé G, Pendić B, Duplan JF, Maupin B, Latarjet R, Kalić D, Schwarzenberger L, Djukić Z &
Vigne J (1959) Étude de six cas d'irradiation totale aigue accidentelle. *Revue Française d'Études Cliniques et
Biologique* **4**: 210–225.

The first clinical attempts were described by Thomas and his colleagues in 1957,
involving six patients with various malignancies who were given, prior to the intravenous inoculation of allogeneic bone marrow cells, doses of whole body irradiation
varying between 90 and 600 rads. Two of these patients showed signs of temporary
'take'. The authors felt that a higher level of immunosuppression would have been
desirable. In their following paper, discussing five further cases of acute leukaemia, they
concluded that only two of twelve patients in their total experience had shown
'significant clinical benefit'. Meanwhile Humble and Newton had transfused allogeneic
bone marrow cells into five patients suffering form malignant diseases; they avoided
whole body irradiation because of the parlous state of the patients' own bone marrow but
irradiated the pelvis and the lumbar vertebrae. Only two patients showed any improvement.

A number of other papers were published in 1959 describing the transplantation of allogeneic or autologous bone marrow to leukaemic patients, among them that by Mathé's group. The case of the Yugoslav nuclear laboratory workers, who received high doses of neutron and gamma rays following an accident, is worth special mention (Jammet et al). Although the exact dose of radiation to which the patients had been exposed is controversial it would appear that several were within the lethal or near-lethal range. Having been kept in strict isolation for about 4 weeks, four of them were given allogeneic bone marrow cells (8.5×10^9 or 14×10^9 on two separate occasions). The appearance of donor-type erythrocytes was transient and within 2 months they had disappeared, suggesting that the foreign cells had been eliminated. It is a matter of conjecture whether the patients' survival, with good clinical and haematological recovery, owed anything to a transient protective effect from the transplants.

Influenced by experimental studies (see notes above on 'Experimental bone marrow transplantation and radiation chimeras'), current bone marrow transplantation programmes developed from these early attempts (see Chapter 6 and Appendix Ie).

FIRST CLINICAL PANCREAS TRANSPLANTS

Lillehei RC, Idezuki Y, Uchida H, Kelly WD, Najarian JS, Merkel FK & Goetz FC (1969) Pancreatic allotransplantation in the dog and man. *British Journal of Surgery* **56**: 699 (abstract).

Developing a safe technique of transplanting this difficult organ has not been easy. The Minneapolis group started by Lillehei pioneered and developed the model in man, involving the transplantation of the pancreas together with a piece of duodenum to the iliac fossa, with endocrine secretions drained heterotopically into the systemic circulation. The Minneapolis group has continued its programme energetically to this day (Najarian, Goetz and Sutherland), and pancreatic transplants are now carried out in many other centres.

FIRST LIVER TRANSPLANTS IN MAN

Starzl TE, Marchioro TL, Huntley RT, Rifkind D, Rowlands DT Jnr, Dickinson TC & Waddell WR (1964) Experimental and clinical homotransplantation of the liver. *New York Academy of Sciences* **120**: 739–765.

During 1964 the first six orthotopic liver transplants were performed in Denver by Starzl and his team. Immunosuppression consisted of azathioprine and steroids and the first donor liver was removed from a policeman who had a bullet injury to the brain. The recipient suffered from a massive secondary liver tumour thought at the time to be a primary hepatoma. The native liver was removed and the new orthotopically placed graft worked well for 10 days before the patient died of hepatic infarction and infection. The next five grafts fared little better, the longest surviving for 23 days. A moratorium on clinical transplants followed whilst further experimental work was done on the orthotopic model and on immunosuppression and liver preservation. In 1967 Starzl in Denver and R. Y. Calne in Cambridge, England, recommenced their clinical programmes. Credit goes to Calne for the world's first long-term survivor (Mrs W. S.), who received a child's liver at Newmarket Hospital on 11 February 1969, following excision of her own liver, which had a large primary hepatoma. She survived, well, until 1976.

FIRST HEART TRANSPLANT IN MAN

Barnard CN (1968) Human cardiac transplantation: an evaluation of the first two operations performed at the Groote Schuur Hospital, Cape Town. *Ann. Cardiol.* **22**: 284–596.

Although most of the work done with experimental heart grafts had been performed in Richmond (R. Lower and D. Hume) and Stanford (N. E. Shumway), the surgeon who was the first to transplant a human heart was Barnard. His first patient died early, but the second survived for 18 months; both the patient (Dr Blaiberg) and his surgeon became internationally fêted overnight and press coverage followed in which the sensational aspects of the operation were exploited to the full. The public interest, not to say hysteria, was enhanced by the zeal, and occasionally by the irresponsible enthusiasm, of some heart surgeons who attempted to emulate Barnard's feat. The results from this first wave of early operations were tragic: of 150 recipients given hearts in 1968–1970, 80% died soon after the operation. However, results have improved substantially over the last 20 years, largely thanks to the careful and systematic clinical and experimental work carried out by Shumway and his colleagues (see Appendix Ic for current results of cardiac transplantation).

GRAFT-VERSUS-HOST-DISEASE

Dempster WJ (1951) Problems involved in the homotransplantation of tissues, with particular reference to skin. *British Medical Journal* **2**: 1041–1049.

Dempster WJ (1953) Kidney transplantation. *British Journal of Surgery* **40**: 447–465.

Simonsen M (1953) Biological incompatibility in kidney transplantation in dogs. *Acta Pathologica et Microbiologica Scandinavica* **32**: 36–84.

Cock AO & Simonsen M (1958) Immunological attack on new born chickens by injected adult cells. *Immunology* **1**: 103–110.

Simonsen M (1957) The impact of the developing embryo and animals of adult homologous cells. *Acta Pathologica et Microbiologica Scandinavica* **40**: 480–500.

Billingham RE, Brent L & Medawar PB (1955) Acquired tolerance of skin homografts. *Annals of the New York Academy of Sciences* **59**: 409–415.

Billingham RE & Brent L (1957) A simple method for inducing tolerance of skin homografts in mice. *Transplantation Bulletin* **4**: 67–71.

Billingham RE & Brent L (1959) Quantitative studies on tissue transplantation immunity. V. Induction of tolerance in newborn mice and studies on the phenomenon of runt disease. *Philosophical Transactions of the Royal Society of London, B* **242**: 439–477.

Trentin JJ (1956) Mortality and skin transplantability in X-irradiated mice receiving isologous, homologous and heterologous bone marrow. *Proceedings of the Society for Experimental Biology and Medicine* **92**: 688–693.

Uphoff D (1957) Genetic factors influencing irradiation protection by bone marrow. I. The F_1 hybrid effect. *Journal of the National Cancer Institute* **19**: 123–130.

Barnes DWH, Ilbery PLT & Loutit JF (1958) Avoidance of 'secondary disease' in radiation chimaeras. *Nature* **181**: 488.

Graft-versus-host disease was discovered in two quite different experimental situations: in immunologically immature animals injected with allogeneic cells and in radiation chimeras. Both Dempster and Simonsen had suggested, before there was any experimental evidence, that grafts such as kidneys might be expected to produce a reaction against the antigens of the host. They concluded this from histological examination of allogeneic kidneys undergoing rejection. Dempster in his 1951 review noted that 'The infiltration may be a proliferation of already existing reticulo-endothelial cells in the kidney' and that the 'homostransplanted kidney reacts against the host'. This idea was further developed in his subsequent paper, again on histological grounds. Simonsen concluded likewise from histological examination of canine renal allografts, in which he too had observed pyroninophilic cells, that such cells in the interstitial tissue 'are taken to be of local origin and to represent the response of the renal mesenchyma to the recipient's individual-specific antibodies and antigens'. He went on to say that 'These findings underline the importance of regarding kidney and spleen transplantation as a parabiosis, in which the incompatible partners occur as both host and donor, which, according to antigenic differences, damage each other and react against the damaging substances'.

Although this notion may well have been based on a misinterpretation of the histology (we now know that host lymphocytes are to be found in perivascular sites in transplanted tissues and organs), convincing evidence came in 1957 that transplanted lymphoid cells may indeed react against the recipient's antigens in much the same way in which graft recipients reject their transplants. But even before this Billingham et al had shown (1955) that the transplantation of normal lymphoid cells syngeneic with a mouse carrying a tolerated allograft resulted in the destruction of the foreign graft, proof of the concept that transplants can react against the tissues of the host (although tissue, in this case, was the tolerated donor skin, adoptively rejected by the non-tolerant injected lymphocytes). Two years later Billingham and Brent reported that allogeneic cells administered intravenously to newborn mice brought about a delayed mortality that varied in extent in different strain combinations (100% in the C57Bl → A combination) and that the lymphoid organs of surviving tolerant mice frequently showed extensive involution. Many mice failed to thrive postnatally and were 'runted'. The authors excluded a possible infective cause and suggested that their data were consonant with the hypothesis that the mortality and pathological changes were caused by 'immunological reactions produced by the inoculated and adult spleen cells against the tissue antigens present in their young hosts', and that the organs overtly affected 'are those in which the cells have been shown to settle out electively and to establish themselves, i.e. the organs in which damage would be expected if such a graft-versus-host reaction occurred'. They pointed out the danger inherent in any attempts to make newborn babies tolerant by the injection of suspensions containing immunologically active cells or to restore reactivity to hypogammaglobulinaemic patients with allogeneic lymphoid cells. Further incontrovertible evidence that 'runt disease' was caused by a graft-versus-host reaction was provided in their full 1959 publication.

Simonsen had meanwhile injected adult chicken spleen and buffy coat cells intravenously into chick embryos 3 days prior to hatching, and found that the recipients developed severe splenomegaly and a positive Coomb's test. A histological study of the changes in the spleen, liver, thymus and bone marrow was 'fully compatible with the assumption that cell members of the transplant have by host antigens been stimulated to multiplication and antibody formation. In doing so they largely destroyed and replaced the native cell population'. Together with Cock he later demonstrated that splenomegaly and hepatomegaly did not occur when F_1 hybrid donor cells were inoculated into F_1 hybrid chicks derived from pure lines, thus supporting his hypothesis of a graft-versus-host reaction as the cause of the pathological changes.

Almost simultaneously, evidence emerged from those working with radiation chimeras that 'secondary disease', the object of much puzzlement and controversy, is essentially a graft-versus-host reaction by the transplanted allogeneic cells against host histocompatibility antigens. Trentin was the first to point out that the degree and duration of protection after lethal doses of X-irradiation is directly related to the closeness of the relationship between the bone marrow donor and the recipient. He speculated that 'If the introduced foreign strain mouse or rat marrow survives and proliferates and produces cells capable of antibody formation, this . . . should be immunologically active against all the tissues of the irradiated host'. Uphoff, too, noted that secondary disease occurred when H-2 incompatibility was greatest and that the protection afforded by F_I hybrid donor bone marrow (i.e. a hybrid between the graft donor and recipient inbred mouse strains) provided much better protection than fully allogeneic tissue. She suggested that an immune response of the graft against the host was the cause of the irradiation syndrome, a point firmly established by the work of Barnes et al when they showed that fetal or newborn myeloid cells do not induce secondary disease.

IMMUNOLOGICAL ENHANCEMENT

Casey AE (1941) Experiments with a material from the Brown–Pearce tumor. *Cancer Research* **1**: 134–135.

Casey AE & Gunn J (1952) XYZ effect in strain of origin: E0771 carcinoma in C57Bl/6 mice. *Proceedings of the Society for Experimental Biology and Medicine* **80**: 610–613.

Snell GD, Cloudman AM, Failor E & Douglass P (1946) Inhibition and stimulation of tumor homoiotransplants by prior injections of lyophilized tumor tissue. *Journal of the National Cancer Institute* **6**: 303–316.

Snell GD (1952) Enhancement and inhibition of the growth of tumor homoiotransplants by pretreatment of the hosts with various preparations of normal and tumor tissue. *Journal of the National Cancer Institute* **13**: 719–729.

Kaliss N & Molumut (1952) Effect of prior injections of tissue antiserums on survival of cancer homoiografts in mice. *Cancer Research* **12**: 110–112.

Lee S (1967) An improved technique of renal transplantation in the rat. *Surgery* **61**: 771–773.

Stuart FP, Saitoh T & Fitch FW (1968) Rejection of renal allografts: specific immunologic suppression. *Science* **160**: 1463–1467.

French ME & Batchelor JR (1969) Immunological enhancement of rat kidney grafts. *Lancet* **ii**: 1103–1106.

Casey's first study on the so-called xyz factors was published as early as 1932. For references see Casey and Gunn, who defined these factors as 'specific agents in long-frozen or lyophilized tissue or fresh supernatant from certain malignant tumors' that rendered the hosts more susceptible to the same subsequently transplanted tumour. These experiments were done in an inbred strain, the C57Bl/6, and prior inoculation of these mice with frozen non-viable tumour (containing the mysterious xyz factors) caused the tumours to grow and the hosts to die more rapidly than in the untreated controls. They were thus *not* dealing with allografts, and it was Snell and Kaliss who applied the same kind of protocol to recipients of tumour allografts and who threw light on the factors involved. These turned out to be the major histocompatibility (H-2) antigens and lyophilization was shown to be highly beneficial in channelling the immune response of the hosts into a protective rather than a destructive mould. The vital contribution of Kaliss and Molomut was to demonstrate that enhanced growth of tumour allografts could likewise be obtained when hyperimmune antisera specific for the histocompatibility antigens of the tumour donor strain were given to the tumour recipients close to the time of transplantation. These and many other subsequent studies led to the hypothesis that enhancement is brought about by the coating of antigenic sites within the tumour grafts with specific antibody – a notion that we now know to have been simplistic.

It was believed for many years that the much studied phenomenon of enhancement was peculiar to certain kinds of solid tumours, for skin allografts transplanted to inbred mice treated in much the same way (either actively with lyophilized tissues or passively with specific antibodies) were shown by Billingham et al to survive, at best, for only a few extra days. This idea had to be abandoned when two groups of workers made use of the surgical innovations introduced by Lee in 1967, which made it possible to transplant kidney allografts to rats. Thus, Stuart et al persuaded inbred Lewis rats to accept (Lewis × Brown Norway) F_1 kidneys by inoculating the recipients with a combination of donor strain spleen cells and hyperimmune serum with antibodies directed against the histocompatibility antigens of the donor strain. The treatment was given 1 day before transplantation. French and Batchelor soon after observed the permanent survival of (AS × Aug)F_1 kidneys in AS rats that had received anti-donor strain hyperimmune serum only on the day of renal transplantation and for several days thereafter. The rats had virtually normal serum creatinine levels. Parental (homozygous) strain (i.e. Aug) kidneys showed only limited prolongation of survival, a finding that has been repeatedly made by many subsequent workers and that is attributed to a gene-dose effect.

Although these early observations were followed by an avalanche of other studies, mainly in the rat, the mechanism of enhancement is still not wholly understood, antibody, immune complexes and suppressor cells all having been proposed as effectors. The way seemed wide open for a major advance in transplantation surgery but so far it has not proved possible to translate the numerous animal models into clinical practice. It is possible that the advent of 'humanized' monoclonal antibodies will change this.

IMMUNOLOGICAL TOLERANCE

Owen RD (1945) Immunogenetic consequences of vascular anastomoses between bovine twins. *Science* **102**: 400–401.

Burnet FM & Fenner F (1949) *The Production of Antibodies.* Macmillan & Co., Melbourne, London.

Billingham RE, Lampkin GH, Medawar PB & Williams HL (1952) Tolerance to homografts, twin diagnosis, and the freemartin condition in cattle. *Heredity* **6**: 201–212.

Billingham RE, Brent L & Medawar PB (1953) Actively acquired tolerance of foreign cells. *Nature* **172**: 603–606.

Hasek M (1953) Vegetavní hybridisace živocichů spojením krevních obehů v embryonálním vývojhi (Vegetative hybridisation of animals by parabiosis during embryonic development). *Československá Biologie* **2**: 265–280.

Billingham RE, Brent L & Medawar PB (1956) Quantitative studies on tissue transplantation immunity. III. Actively acquired tolerance. *Philosophical Transactions of the Royal Society, Series B* **239**: 357–414.

Shapiro F, Martinez C, Smith JM & Good RA (1961) Tolerance of skin homografts induced in adult mice by multiple injections of homologous cells. *Proceedings of the Society for Experimental Biology and Medicine* **106**: 472–475.

Brent L & Gowland G (1962) Induction of tolerance in skin homografts in immunologically competent mice. *Nature* **196**: 1298–1301.

Mitchison NA (1965) Induction of immunological paralysis in two zones of dosage. *Proceedings of the Royal Society, London, Series B* **161**: 275–292.

It has long been known to, and taken for granted by, experimental embryologists that tissues such as avian limb rudiments transplanted from one embryo to the chorio-allantoic membrane of another survive and differentiate in their foreign environment. In 1945

Owen made the extraordinary observation that dizygotic cattle twins, which share a placental circulation in utero, possess not only their own red blood cells but also, in varying proportions, red cells patently derived from their partner. As such cattle twins were known to develop a placental vascular anastomosis fairly early in development Owen postulated that an exchange of blood-borne red cell precursors must have taken place. Burnet and Fenner were aware of this important discovery when they published their germinal monograph in 1949, in which they described Owen's discovery as 'a particularly interesting example of the tolerance of fetal tissues for foreign material' and developed their self-marker hypothesis. Though obscure in detail this postulated that the difference between the way the body sees 'self' and 'non-self' has its origin in embryonic development.

A few years later Billingham, Medawar and other colleagues took matters a step further by showing that cattle dizygotic twins, against all expectations on genetic grounds, will accept skin grafts transplanted from one to the other. This led Medawar's team to attempt to establish what they later called 'actively acquired tolerance' by the inoculation of viable allogeneic cells into mouse embryos and neonates, followed by the transplantation of skin, later in life, from an animal of the same donor strain. They showed the resulting unresponsiveness to be donor-specific, to be dependent on the immunological immaturity of the cell recipient, and (using an adoptive transfer protocol) to be brought about by the clonal elimination or inactivation of antigen-specific lymphocytes rather than by active suppression of responsiveness. Meanwhile Hasek, working initially in isolation, carried out experiments involving the parabiosis of avian embryos, in which the parabionts later in life displayed a defect in their ability to produce antibodies against the cells of their partner. Hasek believed at first that this was due to a phenomenon that he termed 'vegetative hybridization', but he later acknowledged it to be an example of tolerance.

Shapiro et al, soon followed by Brent and Gowland, were the first to find that even adult mice could be made specifically unresponsive to skin allografts by the prior multiple inoculation of the recipients with viable cells from the donor strain (in practice, F_1 hybrids to avoid GVHD). Working with a protein antigen, bovine serum albumin (BSA), Mitchison went on to demonstrate that a specific unresponsiveness (tolerance) can be achieved in adult mice at two distinct dosages, high and low. Such mice were subsequently unable to produce anti-BSA antibodies when tested with the antigen with adjuvant.

Although there are numerous animal models of immunological tolerance it has not yet proved possible to apply it to clinical practice. Even so, evidence is accumulating for the development of hyporesponsiveness (tolerance?) to the histocompatibility antigens of donors in long-term renal allograft recipients (see Chapter 8a). The concept of tolerance is important because (i) it has since been shown to be a universal concept applying to all kinds of antigens, (ii) it has shown that the 'insuperable' barrier provided by the immune system can be overcome after all, (iii) it has led to an understanding of self-tolerance and autoimmunity, and (iv) it continues to set the ultimate objective for clinical transplantation.

IMMUNOLOGICALLY PRIVILEGED SITES

Medawar PB (1948) Immunity to homologous grafted skin. III. The fate of skin homografts transplanted to the brain, to subcutaneous tissue and to the anterior chamber of the eye. *British Journal of Experimental Pathology* **29**: 58–69.

Brent L (1990) Immunologically privileged sites. In Johansson BB & Owman C (eds). *Pathophysiology of the Blood – Brain Barrier.* Amsterdam: Elsevier Science Publ. BV (in press).

Tissues grafted to certain sites may not be rejected in the normal way because of an absence of lymphatics and/or vascular supply. Such sites, which include the anterior chamber of the eye, the brain and the cheek pouch of the hamster, are known as 'immunologically privileged sites'. Medawar was by no means the first to describe the survival of foreign tissues transplanted to the brain or the anterior chamber of the eye, and in his 1946 paper references may be found to previous studies by Y. Shirai, J. B. Murphy, K. Tansley (brain); H. S. N. Greene, F. S. Cheever and H. R. Morgan (anterior chamber); and O. Saphir et al and A. Besredka and M. Bardach (testis). To this list we may add the names of W. J. Siebert (1928) and L. Loeb (1930): both found an absence of host responses when foreign tissues were transplanted to the brain. Tansley's experiments may not be entirely relevant for she used not only embryonic donors but 2-day-old rat recipients; though unlikely it is not possible to rule out the induction of tolerance here.

Medawar's 1946 study consisted of a series of controlled experiments in rabbits in which small skin allografts were transplanted to several sites – orthotopically or into a sub-integumentary area, where vascularization would be sure to occur, and into one of the cerebral hemispheres or the anterior chamber of one eye. All recipients had previously been strongly sensitized by the application of eight skin grafts from the donor. The results were complex and somewhat constrained by the protocol, which involved recovery of the grafts after 10 days for histological inspection rather than long-term survival. However, Medawar felt able to conclude that implants in the anterior chamber were exempted from systemic immunization provided that they remained avascular; grafts that had become vascularized (3/9) were rejected promptly, and grafts that had become adherent though without conspicuous blood vessels (2/9) showed partial survival at the end of the observation period. In the brain, 4/6 grafts were destroyed promptly but in the other two epithelial destruction had not been fully accomplished by day 10.

Medawar concluded that vascularization provided the key to the rejection of allografts, though ischaemia following the rupture of blood vessels was not to blame; that the anterior chamber and to some extent the brain provided conditions for tissue survival in the absence of a vascular supply; and that 'lymphatic drainage is required to induce immunity but not to enforce a response to it'. He went on to explain the clinical success of corneal allografts in these terms.

Although Medawar's data have not been wholly corroborated by later studies, they helped to establish the notion that the anterior chamber and the brain are exempted from the rules of allograft rejection, a concept later extended by R. E. Billingham to the cheek pouch of the hamster. It has been questioned more recently in relation to the brain but the transplantation of fetal tissues to the brain, in an attempt to find a new treatment for Parkinsonism, has given it a new impetus (see Chapter 8a).

For an up to date review of this topic see Brent (1990).

KIDNEY PRESERVATION FOR MORE THAN 24 HOURS

Belzer FO, Ashby BS, Huang JS & Dunphy JE (1968) Etiology of rising perfusion pressure in isolated organ perfusion. *Annals of Surgery* **168**: 382–391.

Because organs are often removed as an emergency procedure, and time is required for the identification and preparation of the best tissue-matched recipient, much work has been done to preserve organs for longer periods with prompt function after transplantation. Using a pump perfusion oxygenator circuit, and cryoprecipitated plasma, Belzer and his colleagues in San Francisco showed that preservation of dog kidneys for up to 72 hours was possible. Ten years later R. W. G. Johnson in Manchester had extended the safe storage period to 7 days. A simpler method of cooling the organ by flushing with cold medium has largely replaced the perfusion machine. High osmolar intracellular type fluids such as that developed by G. Collins are just as successful in preserving organs, which can then be transported on ice. Prompt graft function after more than 72 hours preservation is now common for human renal transplants.

MINOR HISTOCOMPATIBILITY AND MHC RESTRICTED RESPONSES

Eichwald EJ & Silmser CR (1955) Untitled communication. *Transplantation Bulletin* **2**: 148–149.

Snell GD (1956) A comment on Eichwald and Silmser's communication. *Transplantation Bulletin* **3**: 29–31.

Counce S, Smith P, Barth R & Snell GD (1956) Strong and weak histocompatibility gene differences in mice and their role in the rejection of homografts of tumors and skin. *Annals of Surgery* **144**: 198–204.

Billingham RE & Silvers WK (1960) Studies on tolerance of the Y chromosome antigen in mice. *Journal of Immunology* **85**: 14–26.

Bailey DW (1963) Histoincompatibility associated with the X chromosome in mice. *Transplantation* **1**: 70–74.

Bailey DW (1971) Recombinant inbred strains. An aid to finding identity, linkage and function of histocompatibility and other genes. *Transplantation* **11**: 325–327.

Zinkernagel RM & Doherty PC (1974) Restriction of in vitro T cell-mediated cytotoxicity in lymphocytic choriomeningitis within a syngeneic or semi-allogeneic system. *Nature* **248**: 701–702.

Bevan MJ (1975) The major histocompatibility complex determines susceptibility to cytotoxic T cells directed against minor histocompatibility antigens. *Journal of Experimental Medicine* **142**: 1349–1364.

Gordon RD, Simpson E & Samelson LE (1975) In vitro cell-mediated immune responses to the male specific (H-Y) antigen in mice. *Journal of Experimental Medicine* **142**: 1108–1120.

Goulmy E (1985) Class I restricted human cytotoxic T lymphocytes directed against minor transplantation antigens and their possible role in organ transplantation. *Progress in Allergy* **36**: 44–72.

Eichwald and Silmser were the first to draw attention to the fact that, within some inbred strains of mice, male skin grafts are rejected by females, a finding for which they had no clear explanation. It was Snell who proposed several hypotheses to account for it, among them the notion that there might be a histocompatibility gene on the Y chromosome that, like the H-3 locus of the mouse, was 'weaker' than H-2 (thus accounting for the relatively slow tempo of rejection). This theme was further developed by Counce et al.

The H-Y antigen, as it become known, proved to be a much studied example of the many minor histocompatibility antigens that were subsequently identified. Billingham and Silvers showed that small numbers of male spleen cells injected into syngeneic female recipients at or some days after birth induced tolerance to subsequently transplanted male skin, and that allogeneic male cells likewise induced tolerance to syngeneic male skin without necessarily inducing tolerance to the skin of the allogeneic donor strain. This may be the only authentic example of tolerance in the absence of cellular chimerism. Bailey was the first to describe histocompatibility genes on the X chromosome of inbred mice and he contributed greatly to the identification of the numerous minor histocompatibility antigens that are now known.

The seminal studies of Zinkernagel and Doherty demonstrated decisively that viral antigens present on the cell surface of infected target cells can be recognized by cytotoxic T lymphocytes only in the context of target cell MHC antigens (in this case the class I antigens of H-2) that are compatible with the MHC antigens of the effector cells. Both Bevan and Gordon et al went on to show that cytotoxic lymphocytes can be generated in vitro to the H-Y antigen and that the cytotoxicity was restricted to male target cells that were at least partially compatible with the strain furnishing the effector cells. Bevan made the same discovery for other minor H antigens and, to explain his data, he examined the dual recognition and interaction (altered self) hypotheses. He concluded that the latter was the more probable, and that his experimental data suggested that the interaction between minor H and H-2 molecules occurred with H-2D, and probably also with H-2K. This proved to be correct.

It has now become accepted that all antigens recognized by T cells, including those of viral and minor histocompatibility origin, are recognized in association with class I and/or class II molecules. This is true for all mammalian species so far examined, including man, mouse and rat. Goulmy has now succeeded in identifying some of the human minor histocompatibility antigens, first H-Y and subsequently several others: they play a role in organ graft rejection and in graft-versus-host disease following bone marrow transplantation.

MIXED LYMPHOCYTE REACTION (MLR) AND THE DISCOVERY OF Ia AND D REGION (CLASS II) HISTOCOMPATIBILITY ANTIGENS

Bach F & Hirschhorn K (1964) Lymphocyte interaction: a potential histocompatibility test *in vitro*. *Science* **143**: 813–814.

Rubin AL, Stenzel KH, Hirschhorn K & Bach F (1964) Histocompatibility and immunologic competence in renal homotransplantation. *Science* **143**: 815–816.

Bain B, Vas MR & Lowenstein I. (1964) Genetic studies on the mixed lymphocyte reaction. *Science* **145**: 1315–1316.

Bain B, Vas MR & Lowenstein L (1964) The development of large immature mononuclear cells in mixed lymphocyte culture. *Blood* **23**: 108–116.

Bach FH & Voynow NK (1966) One-way stimulation in mixed leukocyte cultures. *Science* **153**: 545–548.

Amos DB & Bach FH (1968) Phenotypic expression of the major histocompatibility locus in man (HL-A): leukocyte antigens and mixed leukocyte culture reactivity. *Journal of Experimental Medicine* **128**: 632–637.

Bach FH, Widmer MB, Bach ML & Klein J (1972) Serologically defined and lymphocyte defined components of the major histocompatibility complex in the mouse. *Journal of Experimental Medicine* **136**: 1430–1444.

Sachs DH & Cone JL (1973) A mouse B-cell alloantigen determined by gene(s) linked to the histocompatibility complex. *Journal of Experimental Medicine* **138**: 1289–1304.

van Leeuwen A, Schiut H & van Rood JJ (1973) Typing for MLC (LD). I. The selection of non stimulator cells by MLC inhibition tests using SD-identical stimulator cells (MISIS) and fluorescence antibody studies. *Transplantation Proceedings* **5**: 1539.

McDevitt HO & Tyan ML (1968) Genetic control of the antibody response in inbred mice. Transfer of response by spleen cells and linkage to the major histocompatibility (H-2) locus. *Journal of Experimental Medicine* **128**: 1–11.

McDevitt HO & Benacerraf B (1969) Genetic control of specific immune responses. *Advances in Immunology* **11**: 31–74.

Benacerraf B & McDevitt HO (1972) Histocompatibility linked immune response genes. *Science* **175**: 273–279.

Hauptfeld V, Klein K & Klein J (1973) Serological identification of an Ia-region antigen. *Science* **181**: 167–169.

Bach J-F, Debray-Sachs M, Crosnier J, Kreis H & Dormont J (1970) Correlation between mixed lymphocyte cultures performed before renal transplantation and kidney function. *Clinical and Experimental Immunology* **6**: 821–827.

Sachs JA, Oliver RTD, Paris AMI & Festenstein H (1975) A collaborative scheme for tissue typing and matching in renal transplantation. VII. Relevance of HL-A, donor sex, MLC and other factors on cadaver renal transplants. *Transplantation Proceedings* **7** (supplement 1): 65–69.

Ting A & Morris PJ (1978) Matching for B-cell antigens of the HLA-DR series in cadaver renal transplantation. *Lancet* **i**: 575–577.

Two groups of workers published data in 1964 showing that histocompatibility antigens existed that could not be detected serologically. Bach and Hirschhorn cultured blood lymphocytes from two unrelated individuals and found that after some days this led to the formation of large cells, which had the ability to divide. Further, this form of in vitro reactivity was correlated with the degree of incompatibility as judged by the sharing, or non-sharing, of histocompatibility antigens as determined in a skin graft test following specific sensitization. In their second publication in *Science* that year they concluded that 'This technique of lymphocyte culture offers a new approach to the problem of donor and recipient typing for renal homotransplantation'.

Quite independently, Bain et al demonstrated essentially the same phenomenon using ^{3}H thymidine autoradiography – the generation of large, basophilic cells capable of DNA synthesis and mitosis. Having compared the data from cultures involving unrelated individuals with those obtained from identical and non-identical twins, they suggested that the reaction 'may be related to genetic differences ... and to homograft immunity'.

Bach and Voynow took matters an important step further by converting what had, up to then, been a two-way response (with both sets of cells reacting against each other) into a one-way response. This was achieved by treating the cells from one individual with mitomycin C before culture, thus preventing them from responding without impairing their stimulatory capacity. Further, they measured cell proliferation by estimating the amount of radioactivity incorporated into the cells during culture, in preference to the more cumbersome method of autoradiography. This facilitated the application of the MLR to tissue matching. Amos and Bach explored this possibility further in a study involving 12 families and concluded that a single genetic system, HLA, determines most of the antigens measured by leukocyte antisera and controls reactivity in one-way MLR. They thought that there must be at least 15 MLC antigens, and they described an exceptional case of human siblings who appeared to be serologically identical but responsive to each other in MLC. It must be assumed that these differences have been generated by recombination within the HLA complex.

For once, then, studies with human material led the way and experiments with rodents and other species came later. In 1972 Bach et al, showed that there were two kinds of MHC antigens in the mouse – those defined serologically (SD) and those defined in MLR (the lymphocyte-defined or LD antigens). However, it soon became apparent that even some of the LD antigens could be identified with the help of antisera: for example, Sachs and Cone found that a xenogeneic (rat) antibody raised against murine cells identified an antigen that was preferentially expressed on B lymphocytes; and van Rood's group was the first to identify the DR subregion of HLA, whose genes seemed to be closely associated with the MLC genes and whose products were recognized by antibodies.

A vital parallel development was the first discovery of the immune response (Ir) genes which were originally identified with respect to synthetic polypeptide antigens but shown to cover a wide range of antigens (see the excellent review by McDevitt and Benacerraf). McDevitt and Tyan found that these genes controlled the antibody response in mice and that they were closely linked to the MHC (H-2) region. Hauptfeld et al raised an antibody reacting with a histocompatibility antigen that proved to be controlled by a gene in the Ir region, which they called Ir-1.1, and they went on to show that it was located within the H-2 complex. Although the precise relationship between Ia (I region-associated mouse class II) or D (human class II) antigens and the products of the Ir genes remained uncertain for several years, it was eventually realized as a result of experiments in transgenic mice C that they were, in fact, one and the same. The further subdivisions of the human D region into DP, DQ and DR subregions, most of them serologically identifiable, gave tissue matching a new impetus and a more precise basis. The more recent application of DNA technology in the identification of HLA specificities has provided further refinements.

MLR typing was first used prospectively for living related kidney donors by J-F Bach et al, and for cadaveric donors by Sachs et al; prospective matching for the serologically identifiable DR antigens was introduced by Ting and Morris.

MOUSE MONOCLONAL ANTI-HUMAN CD3 GLOBULIN

Cosimi AB, Colvin RB, Buston RC, Rubin RH, Goldstein G, Kung PC, Hamsen WP, Delmonico FL & Russell PS (1981) Use of monoclonal antibodies to T-Cell subsets for immunological monitoring and treatment in recipients of renal allografts. *New England Journal of Medicine* **305**: 308–314.

A number of monoclonal antibodies have been raised in mice against molecules on human T cells co-expressed with the T cell antigen receptor. One such antibody against CD3, termed OKT3, has been used extensively for the treatment of graft rejection in man. Initially used by Cosimi to monitor the state of immunosuppression by serial measurement of OKT3-positive circulating T cells, this monoclonal was first administered to two patients at the Massachusetts General Hospital for the treatment of steroid-resistant rejection occurring 7 and 16 days after renal transplantation. Both patients recovered near-normal renal function.

A number of clinical trials have since been conducted, with variable results. One problem encountered is the production by the patient of neutralizing antibodies, and attempts are now being made to 'humanize' the mouse monoclonals by replacing the Fc portion with human Fc.

THE THYMUS AND BURSA OF FABRICIUS:
T AND B LYMPHOCYTES

Glick B, Chang TS & Jaap RG (1956) The bursa of Fabricius and antibody production. *Poultry Science* **35**: 224–225.
Mueller AP, Wolfe HR & Meyer RK (1961) Precipitin production in chickens. XXI. Antibody production in bursectomized chickens and in chickens injected with 19-nortestosterone on the 5th day of incubation. *Journal of Immunology* **85**: 172–179.
Miller JFAP (1961) Immunological function of the thymus. *Lancet* **i**: 748–749.

Archer O & Pierce JC (1961) Role of thymus in development of immune response. *Federation Proceedings* **20**(1): 26 (abstract).

Miller JFAP (1962) Effect of neonatal thymectomy on the immunological responsiveness of the mouse. *Proceedings of the Royal Society of London, Series B* **156**: 415–428.

Martinez C, Kersey J, Papermaster BW & Good RA (1962) Skin homograft survival in thymectomized mice. *Proceedings of the Society for Experimental Biology and Medicine* **109**: 193–196.

Archer OK, Pierce JC, Papermaster BW & Good RA (1962) Reduced antibody response in thymectomized rabbits. *Nature* **195**: 191–193.

Dalmasso AP, Martinez C & Good RA (1962) Failure of spleen cells from thymectomized mice to induce graft vs. host reactions. *Proceedings of the Society for Experimental Biology and Medicine* **110**: 205–208.

Arnason BG, Jankovic BD & Waksman BH (1962) Effect of thymectomy on 'delayed' hypersensitivity reactions. *Nature* **194**: 99–100.

Warner NL & Szenberg A (1962) Effect of neonatal thymectomy on the immune response in the chicken. *Nature* **196**: 784–785.

Gowans JL (1959) The recirculation of lymphocytes from blood to lymph in the rat. *Journal of Physiology* **146**: 54–68.

Gowans JL & Knight EJ (1964) The route of recirculation of lymphocytes in the rat. *Proceedings of the Royal Society of London, Series B* **159**: 257–281.

Claman HN, Chaperon EA & Triplett RF (1966) Thymus–marrow combinations. Synergism in antibody production. *Proceedings of the Society for Experimental Biology and Medicine* **122**: 1167–1171.

Roitt IM, Greaves MF, Torrigiano G, Brostroff J & Playfair JHL (1969) The cellular basis of immunological responses. *Lancet* **ii**: 366–371.

The credit for discovering the function of the thymus gland must go largely to Miller, although Archer and Pierce published their abstract in the same year and were clearly working quite independently on parallel lines. Miller, who published his data in full the following year, showed that thymectomy one day after the birth of mice led to severe lymphocyte depletion and the markedly prolonged survival of skin allografts in 70% of animals, compared with rapid rejection when thymectomy was delayed until the 5th day. Syngeneic thymic tissue transplanted later led to the rejection of established skin grafts, a result indicative of the central role played by thymic tissue in this kind of cell-mediated response. Miller put forward two notions in his 1961 paper: first, that the thymus early in life regulates lymphocyte production, possibly by the secretion of a factor, and second, that during embryogenesis the thymus produces the 'originators of immunocompetent cells, many of which would have migrated to other sites at about the time of birth'. He postulated that cells leaving the thymus are especially selected. It is difficult to understand why this vital discovery has not yet been recognized by the award of a Nobel Prize.

Good and his colleagues had previously observed that thymoma can occur in patients suffering from hypogammaglobulinaemia, but their attempts to show that thymectomy in adult animals causes immunodeficiency had proved negative. In 1962 Good and his colleagues published a number of papers describing the effect of early thymectomy in mice on skin allograft survival, antibody formation, graft-versus-host reactivity and other manifestations of the immune response, and Arnason et al demonstrated a reduction in a delayed-type hypersensitivity response (in experimental allergic encephalomyelitis) in rats thymectomized early in life.

Glick et al had demonstrated much earlier that the removal of the bursa of Fabricius from 2-week-old chicks had a highly significant effect on their ability to produce antibodies to *Salmonella typhimurium* antigen. This study was conducted as a result of an experiment in which bursectomized adult chickens had been accidentally used for the production of an antiserum, an enterprise that had failed. Unfortunately Glick et al chose to publish their findings and subsequent papers in a journal unknown to immunologists and it was some years later, when Mueller et al followed a similar approach, before the significance of bursectomy was appreciated by the immunological world.

The scene was thus set for the development of a much closer understanding of the way humoral and cell-mediated responses are controlled, a dichotomy emphasized by Warner and Szenberg, who showed that early thymectomy of chicks (unlike bursectomy) led to skin allograft acceptance; and by the studies of Claman's group, who demonstrated by in vivo experiments that thymus and bone marrow cells co-operate with each other to produce antibodies to sheep red cells. A critically important discovery was made by Gowans in 1959, when he showed that small lymphocytes recirculate from the blood into the lymph on a large scale, thus providing the physiological basis for a closer understanding of the function of lymphocytes. With Knight he went on to demonstrate that the recirculation occurs by entry of lymphocytes into the lymph nodes and their passage through the wall of the post-capillary venules. Later Roitt et al proposed the T and B lymphocyte nomenclature.

6-MERCAPTOPURINE AND AZATHIOPRINE (IMURAN)

Calne RY (1960) The rejection of renal homografts: inhibition in dogs by 6-mercaptopurine. *Lancet* i: 417–418.
Schwartz RS & Damashek W (1959) Drug-induced immunological tolerance. *Nature* **183**: 1682.

Schwartz and Damashek had shown convincingly in 1959 that rabbits given 6-mercaptopurine had a greatly diminished antibody response against heterologous proteins, and that further doses of the same antigen, given after cessation of the drug, evoked no further response. It appeared that a pharmacologically-induced state of tolerance had been created. Calne, working at the Buxton Browne Research Farm, Kent, applied the drug to a canine renal allograft ('homograft') model and revealed a substantial reduction in the severity of graft rejection. He also deduced that 6-mercaptopurine represented a drug with a much better therapeutic index than X-irradiation, and that despite its side-effects it would suppress the immune response without the devastating and irreversible damage inflicted by whole body irradiation.

Shortly thereafter, Wellcome laboratories developed Imuran (azathioprine; the imidazolyl derivative of 6-mercaptopurine), an orally administered immunosuppressant. This drug, combined with steroids, formed the lynch-pin of anti-rejection prophylaxis for two decades, starting with the world's first human recipient to be so treated on 14 April 1960, at the Peter Bent Brigham Hospital.

Index